Exquisite Specificity

EXQUISITE SPECIFICITY

The Monoclonal Antibody Revolution

ALBERTO CAMBROSIO, PH.D.
McGill University

PETER KEATING, PH.D.
Université du Québec à Montréal

New York   Oxford
OXFORD UNIVERSITY PRESS
1995

Oxford University Press

Oxford   New York
Athens   Auckland   Bangok   Bombay
Calcutta   Cape Town   Dar es Salaam   Delhi
Florence   Hong Kong   Instanbul   Karachi
Kuala Lumpur   Madras   Madrid   Melbourne
Mexico City   Nairobi   Paris   Singapore
Taipei   Tokyo   Toronto

and associated companies in
Berlin   Ibadan

Copyright ©1995 by Oxford University Press, Inc.

Published by Oxford University Press, Inc.,
198 Madison Avenue, New York, New York 10016

Oxford is a registered trademark of Oxford University Press

All rights reserved. No part of this publication may be reproduced,
stored in a retrieval system, or transmitted, in any form or by any means,
electronic, mechanical, photocopying, recording, or otherwise
without the prior permission of Oxford University Press.

Library of Congress Cataloging-in-Publication Data
Cambrosio, Alberto, 1950–
Exquisite specificity: the monoclonal antibody revolution/
Alberto Cambrosio, Peter Keating.
p.   cm.
Includes bibliographical references and index.
ISBN 0-19-509741-6
1. Monoclonal antibodies—Research—History.
2. Monoclonal antibodies—Research—Social aspects.
I. Keating, Peter, 1953–
II. Title.
[DNLM: 1. Antibodies, Monoclonal.   QW 575.5.A6 C178e 1995]
QR186.85.C35   1995   616.07'92—dc20
DNLM/DLC for Library of Congress   95-16982

9 8 7 6 5 4 3 2 1
Printed in the United States of America
on acid-free paper

for Fernande Dupuis
AC

for Kemba Kando-Anderson and Yolam Anderson-Golhor
PK

The fact is that he would like not so much to affirm a truth of his own as to ask questions, and he realizes that no one wants to abandon the train of his own discourse to answer questions that, coming from another discourse, would necessitate rethinking the same things with other words, perhaps ending up on strange ground, far from safe paths. Or else he would like others to ask him questions; but he, too, would want only certain questions and not others: the ones to which he would answer by saying the things he feels he can say but could say only if someone asked him to say them. In any event, nobody has the slightest idea of asking him anything.

Calvino (1985:95)

Preface

> Of such techniques are revolutions made.
> Wade (1982:1074)

The technique (and the revolution) alluded to in Wade's quote is associated with two esoteric terms: *hybridoma technology* and *monoclonal antibodies*. Using the former leads to the production of the latter, $573.5 million of which was sold on the U.S. market in 1992 (*Genetic Engineering News* 1993). Monoclonal antibodies also led to the transformation of laboratory and diagnostic practices, the constitution of new biomedical entities, such as new subclasses of white blood cells, and a Nobel Prize for César Milstein and Georges Köhler for having started the revolution. Hybridoma technology and monoclonal antibodies will be the topic of this book, which is also about, or at least indebted to, another revolution that has modified our understanding of scientific and technological activities.

That revolution began about 30 years ago, with the publication of Thomas Kuhn's *The Structure of Scientific Revolutions* (1962). A central part of Kuhn's argument was directed against philosophers, whom he chastised for systematically misrepresenting scientific activity as an exercise in logic. According to Kuhn, the image of science traded in by philosophers was derived mainly from the view of science generated by textbooks. As such, science appeared to function as a series of inductions from clearly defined facts or deductions from logically consistent theories. Not so, argued Kuhn, for if one looked to scientific journals, where the results of scientific research, as opposed to science teaching, were published, then the easily applicable definitions and the idealized logical operations quickly vanished. In the journals, science was a far messier and more dynamic business than had ever been suspected.[1]

Our understanding of the conduct of science has been further transformed by a growing body of studies of scientific practices that have been produced since Kuhn's publication. Going beyond the journal as the primary site of scientific activity, historians, sociologists, and anthropologists have analyzed scientific activity using laboratory notebooks, unpublished correspondence, interviews, and participant observation.[2] More than just a complement to the journal literature, this attempt to follow scientists through the day-to-day work that results in scientific innovation has been undertaken with the understanding that the journal literature misrepresents the untidiness of scientific practices just as surely as the textbook distorts the processes leading to the production of scientific facts and theories.

This emphasis on scientific practices and the networks of people, reagents, and institutions that sustain them may be of little interest to those intrigued by the metaphysical consequences of the results of scientific research as expressed in statements about the organic and inorganic world. For those concerned with the dynamics of scientific development, however, work done in science studies over the last 20 years has called into question, without eliminating, a variety of distinctions that are currently used to describe how science and technology evolve in advanced industrial societies. A brief lexicon would run as follows: scientist/technician, pure/applied, academic/industrial, theory/method, discovery/invention, cooperation/competition, origin/diffusion, public/private, natural/artificial, success/failure. Run together, these dichotomies constitute a cosmology or an account of the origin and structure of the present-day universe of science and technology. In particular, they tell a story about scientists in universities who, through cooperation, make discoveries that are diffused to scientists and engineers in competitive industries. Successful scientists apply methods to solve problems that arise from the articulation of the theory with nature. Innovative companies use this knowledge to invent ways to produce new commodities. It is a story of winners and losers.[3]

The application of these categories to the monoclonal antibody revolution is relatively straightforward. In 1975 academic researchers in Britain working in pure immunology discovered a technique for the bulk production of pure antibodies of unprecedented (and predefined) specificity. Called *monoclonal antibodies*, they had long been known to exist in theory, although impossible to produce in practice. The knowledge diffused to industry, where in the late 1970s industrial scientists invented, among other things, new types of diagnostic kits that, because of their superior quality, replaced the kits then on the market. Those who discovered how to make monoclonal antibodies were awarded the Nobel Prize. Those who first invented the new kits were granted patent monopolies. All these events are, in some sense, real; the story is fiction.

We do not contend that these categories and the dichotomies they generate are false. There probably is no such thing as a true dichotomy. Rather, like all dichotomies it is a question of application and, as everybody knows, dichotomies upon application tend to fade into polarities; some university laboratories are quite industrial, just as it is possible to spot the odd ivory tower in industry. We do not, however, wish to trade in the dichotomies for polarities. Rather, in this book we describe the old ones in use; we show how participants manipulate these categories and how they invent new ones. We look at how science is practiced by looking at how scientists give meaning to their practices, how they decide what counts as science and what counts as technology, what counts as theory and what counts as practice. As we shall see, how they do so often entails redrawing familiar boundaries and reordering symbolic and material constituents of institutions and practices.

We conceived of this study of the monoclonal antibody revolution as an opportunity to investigate the cosmology outlined earlier. As a case of *pure science* and its practical applications, the discovery and diffusion of monoclonal antibodies has given us the chance to follow an *innovation* across the epistemological and institutional boundaries laid out in the many accounts of the origins and development of the revolution. The results of our research can be described as an ethnography in part because it is the investigation of a practical cosmology, local and contingent though it may be, but also because of the method.

Our description of the transformation of a small sector of the biomedical sciences is based mainly on the categories used by the participants. It is therefore the result of mingling with the participants. We have not, however, entirely abandoned the language of academic sociology and history. Our reading of the secondary literature in sciences studies has been constant and clearly informs our narrative. Nonetheless, we try to show, wherever possible, that when the language of academe and the language of native speakers are at odds, the latter is to be preferred as more attuned to the nuances of the "mangle of practice" (Pickering 1991).

In our attempt to make sense of what happened we learned many things. Some of them are in this book. A few deserve mention in the introduction as they illustrate the kinds of problems we came across and how we treated them. It is furthermore possible to arrange these problems in a sequence that corresponds to the development of monoclonal antibodies. This does not imply that we have unearthed the internal logic of the monoclonal antibody revolution. The historical order of this study is not a teleology; it is simply an argument presented in terms of before and after. Similarly, the dynamics of the development of the ever-expanding network through which monoclonal antibodies presently flow is at every point contingent. There were and are no social rules or principles at work.

Like many people in the field, we began with an awareness that science did not produce isolated facts or theories or techniques but that the three were inextricably bound up together in what seemed to be some kind of alchemical brew. Any attempt to speak of either separately seemed doomed to produce fool's gold. However, as readers of Chapter 1 will learn, there is a distinction that is of considerable importance to practitioners, and it is that which separates fact from technique. As regards monoclonal antibodies, this distinction, self-evident after the fact, was one of the products of scientific research and not, as our cosmology would have it, the philosophical basis upon which science is based.

Once one is in possession of a fact or a technique—and if you are a scientist, it is of obvious import to know which one you possess—having it circulate requires more than simply publishing the results. It has long been known in the sociology of science that this is mainly because the methods section of scientific papers simply cannot capture the enormous amount of tacit knowledge that goes into the production of a fact or a technique.[4] This, we learned, is somewhat of a simplification. Mixed cases abound, running from the rare, but not impossible case where nobody *thinks* they can, to the more usual case where some can and most cannot, to the case where most think they can but would not bother. For the practitioner, deciding which tacit knowledge can or should be made explicit entails decisions about what should count as science and what should count as technology, and there are no outside criteria on which to base such a decision.

A technique that practically anybody can or wants to use in a given sector of activity has not simply diffused to other domains. It has undergone a subtle transformation from a technique into a tool. In this respect, an important and partly invisible dimension of the monoclonal antibody revolution lay outside the laboratory. Here a number of variables and not a few expectations had to be standardized. Just as there are no all-purpose tools, however, there is no such thing as universal standardization. Once again, choices had to made about what should and what need not or cannot be standardized. As a collective activity involving a myriad of individual and institutional choices, we term the result *regulation*. Far from being exterior to science, it is an integral part of its functioning.

In the last chapter of this book, we take a closer look at what has possibly attracted the most attention in the monoclonal antibody revolution, and that is the possibility of making money. According to conventional wisdom, the very idea of making money from monoclonal antibodies is contingent upon making them private property. We learned, however, that it was not a simple matter of appropriating a good idea by an individual or corporation; before being appropriated, an idea must be made public. To be made public, the discovery, be it a fact or a technique, has to be redescribed as an invention. Bringing monoclonals under the description of invention entailed the shifting of the boundaries between nature and culture, the production of novel identities, and, hence, the ascription of new intentions (Anscombe 1957). Much of this work took place in a newly established context or, rather, a world of action (Dodier 1993) resulting from the interaction of lawyers and scientists.

As previously stated, we present a case study of scientific innovation and its ramifications. We do not, however, provide a ready-made context (scientific, economic, etc.) for our case. Instead, we have attempted to describe our case from the inside out, showing how contexts themselves are created for the actions and events that, in retrospect, often appear to flow ineluctably from these same contexts. As a case in point, attentive readers will have noticed that while we have used the term *revolution* throughout the introduction, it did not appear in

Preface   xiii

our cosmological vocabulary. Since Kuhn it has become commonplace to oppose normal science to revolutionary science. This distinction does not hold in the case of the monoclonal antibody revolution. It is a different story here, a story of how normal science became a revolution or, in other words, the story of the emergence of a science without a predefined context.

Acknowledgments

First, we were three. We would like to thank Michael Mackenzie, who has in the meantime taken up the career of playwright and theater director, for sharing the initial stages of the project that eventually led to this book. Among our Montreal peers, Camille Limoges deserves special mention, first as a teacher at the Université de Montréal and subsequently for his constant support as a senior colleague, both at the Université du Québec à Montréal and at the Centre Interuniversitaire de Recherche sur les Sciences et les Technologies. AC would like to thank his parents, Athos and Flora Cambrosio, and his brother, Franco Cambrosio. He would also like to extend his gratitude to his colleagues in the Department of Social Studies of Medicine of McGill University, Allan Young, George Weisz, Don Bates, Margaret Lock, and Faith Wallis, for providing him with a most congenial and stimulating academic environment. In addition to his parents, Douglas and Phyllis Keating, PK would like to thank his colleagues at the Département d'histoire at U.Q.A.M. for their warm welcome and open attitude towards the history and sociology of science.

Working in Quebec is often equated to living in a sort of liminal space—or snowdrift—between Europe and North America. During the years it took to produce this book, its content has been shaped by informal interaction with researchers from both sides of the Atlantic. The Centre de Sociologie de l'Innovation of the École des Mines de Paris has been an important reference point; we would like to thank Michel Callon, Bruno Latour, and Jean-Pierre Courtial, as well as several of their students, in particular, Laurent Bibard, for their time and help. Precious insights also resulted from ongoing exchanges with Jean-Pierre Gaudillière, Anne Marie Moulin, and Ilana Löwy, all members of the U158 INSERM team at the Hôpital des Enfants Malades in Paris. Two other Parisians, Laurent Thévenot (Centre d'Études sur l'Emploi) and Nicolas Dodier (CERMES), and a Dijonnais, Daniel Jacobi (Université de Bourgogne), provided more food for thought. On the North-American side, we have been engaged in fruitful discussions with several friends and colleagues, in particular, Joan Fujimura (Stanford University), Susan Leigh Star (University of Illinois, Urbana), Adele Clarke (UCSF), and Michael Lynch (recently moved to Brunel University in London, UK). U.S. historians of immunology have also been exposed to various stages of our work; we thank Arthur Silverstein (Johns Hopkins University) and Alfred Tauber (Boston University).

This book would obviously not have been possible without the collaboration of several scientists and technicians who accepted to be interviewed, sometimes repeatedly, to answer our letters and e-mail messages, and to send us documents. A few chose to remain anonymous; the names of the others can be found in the footnotes. They all deserve our thanks, but we would like to single out Leonard Herzenberg, Melvin Cohn, and Alain Bussard for their particularly helpful and friendly attitude towards our project. Not only did César Milstein share information with us, but also gracefully accepted to write a Foreword that, in its Borgesian inspiration, is in keeping with the spirit of the book.

Research for this book would also not have been possible without the financial support provided by the Social Sciences and Humanities Research Council of Canada and Quebec's Fonds FCAR, to whom we offer our sincere thanks. Finally, we thank Jacques Blanc, who in record time provided us with several suggestions for the cover page illustration.

Previous versions of various parts of this book had been published in article form. We are grateful to the following publishers for giving us permission to use materials from the following:

Cambrosio, Alberto and Peter Keating. 1992. "Between Fact and Technique: The Beginnings of Hybridoma Technology." *Journal of the History of Biology* 25(2):175–230. Copyright © 1992 Kluwer Academic Publishers. Reprinted by permission of Kluwer Academic Publishers.

Cambrosio, Alberto and Peter Keating. 1988. "'Going Monoclonal': Art, Science and Magic in the Day-to-Day Use of Hybridoma Technology." *Social Problems* 35(3):244–260. Copyright © 1988 by the Society for the Study of Social Problems. Reprinted by permission.

Cambrosio, Alberto, Peter Keating, and Michael Mackenzie. 1990. "Scientific Practice in the Courtroom: The Construction of Sociotechnical Identities in a Biotechnology Patent Dispute." *Social Problems* 37(3):301–319. Copyright © 1990 by the Society for the Study of Social Problems. Reprinted by permission.

We are also grateful to the following publishers, associations, and individuals for permission to reproduce the following illustrations:

Figure 1.1: Reprinted with permission from the American Association for Cancer Research, Inc., César Milstein, Georges Köhler, and *Nature* (Köhler, Georges and César Milstein. 1975. "Continuous Cultures of Fused Cells Secreting Antibody of Predefined Specificity." *Nature* 256:495–497. Copyright © 1975 Macmillan Magazines Limited).

Figure 2.1: Reprinted with permission from the *British Medical Journal*. Original source: Llewelyn, Meirion B., Robert E. Hawkins, and Stephen J. Russell. 1992. "Monoclonal Antibodies in Medicine. Discovery of Antibodies." *British Medical Journal* 305:1269–1272.

Figure 2.3 (right side): Original source: Liddell, J. Eryl and A. Cryer. 1991. *A Practical Guide to Monoclonal Antibodies*. Chichester, England: John Wiley & Sons, pp.

14–15. Copyright © 1991 by John Wiley & Sons, Ltd. Reprinted by permission of John Wiley & Sons, Ltd.

Figure 2.4 (right side): Reprinted with permission from César Milstein. Original source: U.S. Congress, Office of Technology Assessment, *Commercial Biotechnology: An International Analysis,* OTA-B-218. Springfield, VA: National Technical Information Service, January 1984, p. 39.

Figure 2.5 Reprinted with permission from Cold Spring Harbor Laboratory and consent from Ed Harlow and David Lane. Original source: Harlow, Ed and David Lane. 1988. *Antibodies. A Laboratory Manual.* Cold Spring Harbor, NY: Cold Spring Harbor Laboratory Press, Figure 6.10 on p. 217.

Figure 2.6: Reprinted with permission from Noyes Publications. Original source: Fazekas De St. Groth, Stephen. 1985. "Monoclonal Antibody Production: Principles and Practice." In *Handbook of Monoclonal Antibodies. Applications in Biology and Medicine,* eds. Soldano Ferrone and Manfred P. Dierich, pp. 1–10, on p. 4. Park Ridge, NJ: Noyes Publications.

Figure 3.6: Redrawn from Gosling, James P. 1990. "A Decade of Development in Immunoassay Methodology." *Clinical Chemistry* 36:1408–1427, Figure 1. Courtesy of the American Association for Clinical Chemistry, Inc.

NOTES

1. A pioneering discussion of the differences between journal, handbook, and textbook science can be found in Fleck (1979), originally published in German in 1935.

2. We shall resist the temptation of introducing here an exhaustive list of books and articles deemed significant in the science studies field. Relevant texts were quoted in the footnotes of the book's chapters, and three anthologies provide a quick overview of work in this field: Knorr-Cetina and Mulkay (1983), Pickering (1992), and Jasanoff et al. (1995).

3. Even Herodotus (1972:43) would have found such stories rather one sided: "I will proceed with my history telling the story as I go along of small cities no less than of great. For most of those which were great once are small today; and those which used to be small were great in my own time. Knowing, therefore, that human prosperity never abides long in one place, I shall pay attention to both alike."

4. This is not, of course, restricted to the sociology of science: "The cookery book is not an independently generated beginning from which cooking can spring; it is nothing more than an abstract of somebody's knowledge of how to cook; it is the stepchild, not the parent of the activity. The book in its turn may help to set a man on to dressing a dinner, but if it were his sole guide, he could never, in fact, begin: the book speaks only to thos who know already the kind of thing to expect from it and consequently how to interpret it" (M. Oakeshot 1951:15, quoted in Cipolla 1965:129).

Contents

Foreword
César Milstein, **xix**

1 Knowing How or Knowing That: Hybridoma Technology's Beginnings, **3**
    Fact or Technique? Discovery Narratives, **8**
    Discontinuity or Continuity? The Koprowski Affair, **11**
    Discontinuity or Continuity (2)? The Schwaber Affair, **18**
    The Cohn Connection, **24**
    Milstein's Founding Tetralogy, **32**
    Conclusions, **37**
    Notes, **38**

2 The Art and Science of (Re)Producing Monoclonal Antibodies, **45**
    Sociological Accounts of Local and Tacit Knowledge, **47**
    The Art of Producing Hybridomas, **50**
    The Objectification of Procedures, **58**
    "Improving" Hybridoma Technology, **62**
    Hybridoma Technology and its Variants, **67**
    The Problem of Codification, **70**
    From Art to Science, **73**
    Conclusions, **76**
    Notes, **77**

3 "From Immunofantasy to Monoclonal Reality": Building a New Tool, **81**
    An Empiricist Account, **85**
    A Contingent Account, **91**
    Building a Tool: Generality Through Standardization, **95**
    Building a Tool: Generality Revisited, **103**

The Domestication of Monoclonal Antibodies, **110**
Providing Exoteric Interpretations, **116**
Conclusions, **123**
Notes, **124**

4 Monoclonals, Herpes, Hepatitis, and Other (not so Dangerous) Things, **131**
RI Goes Monoclonal, **132**
The Herpes Challenge, **137**
The Institution of Hybridoma Technology, **147**
Building an R&D Unit, Tackling Hepatitis, **151**
Hybridoma Technology: A Service Unit, **153**
Notes on Fieldwork at Bio-Bucks, **157**
Notes, **165**

5 Between Nature and Culture: Constructing Novelty, Patenting Inventions, **167**
Milstein Versus Wistar, **172**
Ortho Versus Becton-Dickinson, **174**
Ex Parte Old and *Ex Parte Erlich:* Yes, No, Maybe, **176**
Hybritech Versus Monoclonal Antibodies Inc., **180**
Establishing Identities: Is IRMA a RIA?, **182**
Mere Substitution or Inventive Step?, **189**
Contested Realities: Molecular and Procedural Representations, **193**
Conclusions, **200**
Notes, **202**

Epilogue, **209**
Notes, **212**

References, **213**

Index, **237**

Foreword

CÉSAR MILSTEIN

A book about the meaning of what has come to be called the Monoclonal Antibody Revolution and how it came about should not come as a surprise. Indeed as I read it, I found plenty of good reasons for its publication. The subject is a very suitable example of how technological developments arise from and at the same time reshape or provide answers to basic research into natural phenomena. Furthermore, this story also exemplifies how new techniques and basic developments thereof become the subject of commercial enterprises, with all that this entails (including greed and legal disputes). Yet I find it a strange experience to identify myself with the Milstein of the book, perhaps because I am all too aware that at the time it all seemed to be a mixture of happy coincidences and grabbed opportunities. I am not so sure this is what I would have said today if it were not for the two epigraphs to a partly autobiographical lecture I gave way back in 1981.[1] I do not often use epigraphs but I am glad I did so then. The first was A.J.P. Taylor's remark: "Looking back over my life, everything seems to have happened by accident," followed by an old Spanish proverb: "La oportunidad la pintan calva," meaning, the opportunity is painted bald.[2]

Memories are the essence of interviews. Interviews often tell the interviewer a lot about the other person, but this is not necessarily obvious and in itself is subject to interpretation. Interviews rely mostly on memories that can be not only skewed by personal involvement but also inaccurate in critical details. I remember (!) a young scientist telling me after a lecture about the great impact that the paper by Köhler and I had on him. I asked if he was sure he was referring to the Köhler and Milstein 1975 paper.[3] "Oh yes!" he replied. A hypothetical interviewer might have stopped at this stage, but I was intrigued that someone interested in differentiation had noticed so early the potential of the technology in that area of research. So I persisted by asking in which journal the paper was published. This he did not recall but he remembered bits of the paper. It soon became clear to me and to him that the paper in question was Williams et al. 1977![4]

And then there is the matter of obviousness. Obvious to whom? And at what stage? When I first discussed with Alan Williams the experiments that led to the paper described above, the idea seemed obvious. After all, the hybridomas (the name actually came later) against red blood cells described in Köhler and Milstein must have recognized cell surface antigens. Soon after that discussion, the chairman (Alain Bussard) of a small workshop, part of the European Congress of Immunology, invited me to speculate on further developments to the *Nature* paper. I decided to explain how the method could be used to analyze unknown differentiation antigens. To my surprise no one seemed to have thought about this "obvious" idea, at least that is what the chairman told me. What I did not discuss, though, was that we soon realized that the obvious idea was critically dependent on the outcome of preliminary experiments and that the approach was not as straightforward as it looked in the scheme I had shown on the blackboard. The early essays were based on red cell lysis. Other types of cells were not so easy to use in the same way.[5] Furthermore, differentiation antigens occur in discreet numbers of copies per cell. So the first experiments we performed—and never published—were designed to determine whether binding assays (on which Williams was a recognized expert) were suitable to detect surface antigens present in the expected number of molecules per cell. It was only then that the approach became obvious.

Is the written word more reliable? Written records rarely tell us how science operates as a daily activity. In addition, some scientists like to unfold their inner thoughts while others prefer to do so in conversation with close colleagues or to keep them to themselves. How to know if certain texts are cautious because the author is uncertain, or does not like to sound dogmatic, or thinks the style is likely to be more palatable to the reviewers, or simply because a change of the text was demanded by a reviewer?

Many of these issues repeatedly arise in this book and I must confess that I have been most impressed by the way in which the authors have been able to sieve through a vast amount of material and come to interesting and meaningful conclusions. I only read the typescript when it was finished. I therefore remain free to keep my own views on details to myself, and for this I am immensely grateful to the authors.

By 1984 my thoughts had shifted towards some of the issues discussed above. At least this is what my choice of epigraph for my Nobel lecture suggests. It was written by Jorge Luis Borges (italics in the original): *"Cuando se acerca el fin,* escribió Cartaphilus, *ya no quedan imágenes del recuerdo; sólo quedan palabras.* Palabras, palabras desplazadas y mutiladas, palabras de otros, fué la pobre limosna que le dejaron las horas y los siglos. (*"As the end draws near,* wrote Cartaphilus, *there remain no longer images of memories; there remain only words.* Words, displaced and mutilated words, others' words, these were the pitiful gifts left to him by the hours and the centuries". With apologies to J.L.B.).

NOTES

1. César Milstein. 1982. "The Thirteenth Lynen Lecture: Messing About with Isotopes and Enzymes and Antibodies." In *From Gene to Protein: Translation Into Biotechnology*, Miami Winter Symposia, vol. 19, eds. Fazal Ahmad, Julius Schultz, Eric E. Smith, and William J. Whelan, pp. 3–24. New York: Academic Press.

2. The correct proverb is "La ocasión la pintan calva". It is inspired by the roman goddess Occasion depicted with plenty of hair in front but totally bald behind, to symbolize that you grab it by the hair, but if you let it pass, it is too late (J. M. Iribarren. 1944. *El porqué de los dichos*, p. 110. 7th ed. Pamplona: Departamento de Educación y Cultura, Gobierno de Navarra).

3. Georges Köhler and César Milstein. 1975. "Continuous Cultures of Fused Cells Secreting Antibody of Predefined Specificity." *Nature* 256:495–497.

4. Alan F. Williams, Giovanni Galfré and César Milstein. 1977. "Analysis of Cell Surfaces by Xenogeneic Myeloma-Hybrid Antibodies: Differentiation Antigens of Rat Lymphocytes." *Cell* 12:663–673.

5. Indeed the difficulties emerged in parallel work and gave rise to the concept of synergistic lysis by monoclonal antibody pairs (J.C. Howard, G. W. Butcher, G. Galfrè, C. Milstein, and C.P. Milstein. 1979. "Monoclonal Antibodies as Tools to Analyze the Serological and Genetic Complexities of Major Transplantation Antigens." *Immunological Reviews* 47:139–174).

Exquisite Specificity

1
Knowing How or Knowing That: Hybridoma Technology's Beginnings

> La question, refoulée par notre appareillage logique, ne cesse pourtant de nous revenir: comment penser le dynamisme *au travers même* de la disposition? Ou encore: comment toute situation peut-elle être perçue *en même temps* comme cours des choses?
> Jullien (1992:11)

In 1984, Georges Köhler and César Milstein won the Nobel Prize in Medicine for the development of hybridoma technology, which is used to produce monoclonal antibodies (Fig. 1.1). Hans Winzgell, of the Karolinska Institute, noted in his presentation speech that hybridoma technology had "revolutionized the use of antibodies in health care and research" because "rare antibodies with a tailor-made fit for a given structure" could now be made and because "the hybridoma cells [could] be stored in tissue banks and the very same monoclonal antibody [could] be used all over the world with a guarantee for eternal supply" (quoted in Wasson 1987). He could have added that substantial sales based on the industrial exploitation of hybridoma technology had begun by the early 1980s, thus turning monoclonal antibodies into one of the success stories of modern biomedical research *and* of commercial biotechnology (Wasson 1987; Rothman and Parkinson 1988; Mackenzie, Cambrosio, and Keating 1988). Succinctly put, Köhler and Milstein's hybridoma technology "revolutionized serology, provided tools for the examination of basic immunological mechanisms, and created an industry" (Goldsby, Srikumaran, and Albert 1984).

From the point of view of science studies, hybridoma technology has a number of attractions as an object of inquiry. It spans basic research, clinical investi-

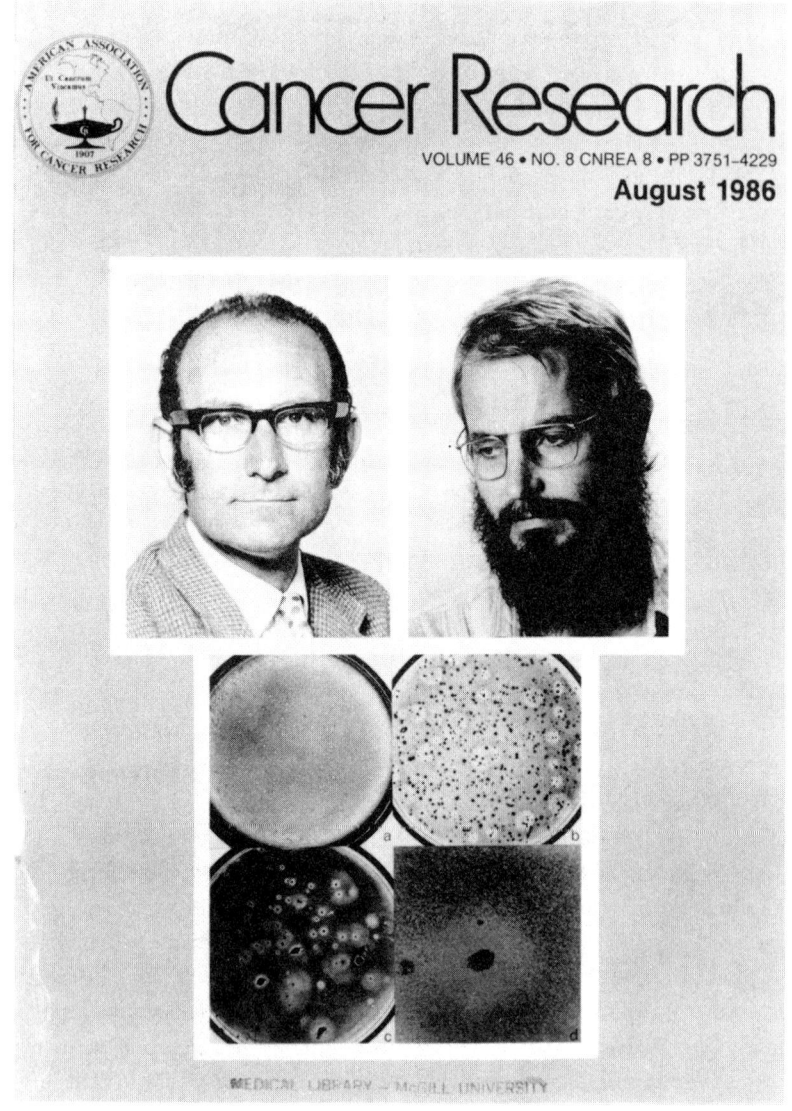

Figure 1.1. Cover page of the August 1986 issue of *Cancer Research* commemorating the award of the 1984 Nobel Prize in medicine to Milstein and Köhler. Part of the cover legend reads as follows: "Pictured are Cesar Milstein (*left*) and Georges Köhler (*right*). The figure, from the *Nature* article of 1975, is on the isolation of one anti-sheep red blood cell-secreting clone."

gations, industrial research and development (R&D), and commercialization. The technology thus provides fascinating possibilities for a variety of traditional inquiries about such issues as patterns of discovery, the reception of innovations by the scientific community, their transfer from university to industry, and the development of clinical and commercial innovations. The effort to produce a comprehensive account of hybridoma technology however—an account that would examine and integrate all these aspects—is hampered by the fact that different disciplines, such as R&D economics, cognitive psychology, history of science, and sociology of science, construct their object differently.[1] Faced with this situation, our strategy will be to adopt an anthropological stance, following the technology around as it is translated into a tool of widespread application and a commercial innovation. We begin in this chapter by asking: How did hybridoma technology come to be viewed as a discovery and a technology?

Our endeavor is not entirely new, of course. Brannigan's (1981) attributional model of discovery comes readily to mind. According to this model, mentalistic and social-historical accounts of discovery, although apparently opposed, can both be described as naturalistic, insofar as they treat discovery as a natural phenomenon to be explained by a set of psychological, sociological, or historical causes. Brannigan (1981:11) contrasts these accounts with an attributional model that "focuses on how persons confer the status of 'discovery' on social events and how they determine and sanction the appropriateness of this category both for their own achievements and for those of others." Stripped of their naturalistic aura, discoveries become problematic events: The task is to account for their constitution as discoveries.

Along somewhat similar lines, Jan Sapp (1990), in his analysis of an alleged fraud concerning the German biologist Franz Moewus, points out that the problem is not to decide whether a fraud has been committed but to delineate the social and technical processes that led to the categorization of Moewus's work as fraudulent. After all, Mendel's results—to take a widely cited example—have long been known to be too good to be true, but they are not regarded as fraudulent. In other words, fraud is the mirror image of discovery: Both are attributions, even if of an opposite sign. The historian's task, then, is to "follow the scientists as they negotiate the validity of [a scientist's] work" (Sapp 1990:306).

One aspect of Sapp's reconstruction of the Moewus saga is of particular interest here. Had Moewus's work not been discarded as fraudulent, then a plausible argument could be made that it anticipated the work of two American biochemical geneticists, Beadle and Tatum, the 1958 Nobel Prize winners. Moewus could then be viewed as an alternative candidate for the title of founding father of biochemical genetics. This, in turn, would imply a conflict over scientific priority and discovery. But of which "discovery" are we speaking? As Sapp points out, in the case of Beadle and Tatum it is not at all clear why they received the Nobel Prize. Was it for their one gene–one enzyme theory? Several other geneticists had advanced a similar hypothesis; moreover, at the time of the award, the meaning and status of that hypothesis had not been settled. Perhaps it was for their methodological developments that focused on the use of microorganisms. As Sapp (1990:55) puts it: "The discovery was not a theoretical achievement of *solving* the problem of gene action; it was a technical achievement of showing how to use microorganisms for biochemical genetics and for *creating* and investigating various problems." But if this is so, one could also argue that Moewus's work with microorganisms, independently of the status (fact or fraud) of his results, was a remarkable technical achievement. Indeed, one of the few American geneticists who continued to support Moewus long after accusations of fraud began to shower upon him espoused precisely this point of view, as he came to see the issue "as a debate between two principles of hierarchization in scientific practice: the debate between the principle of giving primacy to observation and data, with all that it entails, on the one hand, and the principle that privileges the establishment of techniques and theory and its correlative interest, on the other" (Sapp 1990:284).

In this example we clearly see not only that scientists' accounts are central to the establishment of knowledge claims, but also that the description and classification of research findings as fact or as technique is part of the process of establishing their status as a discovery (or as a fraud). We would go so far as to claim that the division of knowledge into fact and technique precedes discovery and is actually constitutive of the latter. This is what we will attempt to show by providing a series of closely related narratives of the "discovery" of hybridoma technology. We have chosen this expository strategy because it corresponds to the methodological stance of following the scientists. The reader will not be provided with authoritative statements of how things really happened and what hybridoma technology is really about. Rather, he or she will be confronted with participant-centered accounts; these accounts focus on the novelty status of hybridoma technology, and they do so by constituting, in different ways, a distinction between fact and technique.

Let us begin with an article published in *Science* on the 1984 Nobel Prize in Medicine, which Köhler and Milstein shared with Niels Jerne. Here one reads: "The choices reflect an interesting blend: recognition to Milstein and Köhler for a methodological breakthrough that has profound practical significance, and in the case of Jerne for theoretical advances that have shaped our concepts of the immune system" (Uhr 1984). By that time, the status of hybridoma technology as a technology had apparently been settled, and, correlatively, *hybridoma technology* had been constituted as a discrete entity with a distinct set of attributes.

In order to follow scientists in their construction of the fact/technique distinction, established classifications must be put aside and no *a priori* distinctions, or even entities to which such distinctions would apply, should be taken for granted. Our methodological stance thus entails the impossibility of classifying *a priori* the production of monoclonal antibodies into established categories such as the confirmation of a theory, the establishment of a fact, the development of a technique, etc. In other words, while it is now possible to take for granted the present status of a scientific technique such as hybridoma technology, it is also important to understand how this relatively stable status as a new technology was acquired. This involves understanding the imputation of novelty status. In turn, the definition of *novelty* hinges on the identity (factual? technical? "merely" technical?) of the entity that is claimed to be new.

The distinction between fact and technique is not without precedent in the historical or sociological literature on science. Referring to previous work by Gaston Bachelard, who coined the term *phénoménotechnique,* Latour and Woolgar (1986:63–69) question the division between material and conceptual components of scientific work. They point to Bachelard's insight that pieces of apparatus should be considered as "reified theory," insofar as they embody the results of debates from other areas. Correlatively, they argue that no *a priori* distinction should be made between *facts* and *(mere) technique.* This distinction is the result of at least two different processes: black-boxing and routinization. In the first case, while the establishment of a fact constitutes the *raison d'être* of a given research group, this same fact, once its status as fact has been secured, can be transferred to other groups, where it can function as a tool or technique. In the second case, Latour and Woolgar point out that what are now purely technical matters handled by technicians, previously mobilized Ph.D.'s, who devoted much time to their development, fine-tuning, and the like. The purely technical, in other words, is the result of scientific work whose traces disappear once the problems they inspired are deemed settled.

Our endeavor is slightly different from that of Latour and Woolgar. We do not intend to show that some fact was transformed into a (routinized) technique or that establishing a technique involved scientific, as opposed to merely technical, work for we were confronted with research results that, from the very beginning, were construed as both technique *and* fact. Monoclonal antibodies thus appeared simultaneously as a fact and as a technique used to establish such a fact. Our purpose is to focus on the negotiations surrounding the early characterization of the research that only a few years later would become reified under the term *hybridoma technology.*

The significance of our inquiry is not limited to the case of monoclonal antibodies. Indeed, one of the central problems scientists (and industrialists) have when confronted with a novelty is deciding exactly what is new about it, for nothing can be completely new if it is to achieve the minimal status of a thing, and the part of the thing that is new is not the same for everybody. In other words (for instance, Lakoff 1987), novelty is a prototypical category. The work of separating the new from the old is an essential part of the constitution of new and old technoscientific objects. This implies that it is necessary at some point to establish limits for what is to count as old and thus to reinterpret the context in which the new emerged. This has both practical ramifications, for instance, when lawyers debate the patentability of an alleged innovation (see Chapter 5), and epistemological consequences, such as when philosophers claim that techniques and instruments account for the stability of laboratory sciences (Hacking 1992). On the basis of the argument developed in this chapter, it will be seen that attributions such as *technique* and *instrument* are both the source and the result of scientific work. In particular, we shall see that such attributions are useful resources in the constitution and management of continuities and discontinuities between and across different lines of work.

To sum up, what follows is not the history of a discovery. It is not even the history of how research results came to be seen as a discovery. Rather, it is the history of how the distinction between fact and technique was constituted in relation to what became known as hybridoma technology and of how, through this work, hybridoma technology was itself constituted as an object. To put the matter slightly differently, we are not dealing here with the now classical problem of the (social) construction of a fact; rather, we are dealing with the (epistemological) constitution of an object.

Fact or Technique? Discovery Narratives

There is a striking similarity between the conclusion of Watson and Crick's 1953 *Nature* paper, which announced the elucidation of the double-helical structure of DNA and the final sentences of Köhler and Milstein's 1975 paper, also published in *Nature*, which reported the successful performance of what became hybridoma technology. Watson and Crick's conclusion reads as follows: "It has not escaped our notice that the specific pairing we have postulated immediately suggests a possible copying mechanism for the genetic material." Köhler and Milstein conclude: "Such [hybrid antibody-producing] cells can be grown *in vitro* in massive cultures to provide specific antibody. Such cultures could be valuable for medical and industrial use." In both cases, by evoking the potential consequences of their findings, these papers seem to suspend their own closure, thereby creating the possibility that future achievements will be retrospectively read as naturally flowing from their contribution.

Some (fictional) reader will quickly point out that the similarities end here. In fact, he or she will argue, whereas the elucidation of the double-helical structure of DNA was immediately perceived as an important discovery, as shown by the participants' self-consciousness of its potential Nobel Prize value and the circumstances surrounding the publication of the findings,[2] the editor of *Nature* noticed nothing revolutionary in Köhler and Milstein's paper.[3] In fact, hybridoma technology had to wait at least three years, until 1978, before achieving the status of a revolutionary discovery, and even then, only in restricted circles. The reader could further argue that the difference between the two cases is hardly surprising, because in the case of the double helix we are dealing with a scientific fact, while in the case of monoclonal antibodies we are dealing with a technique. According to this line of reasoning, the importance of a fact is bound to be immediately appreciated (the fact that sometimes it was not appreciated only confirms the general rule), whereas in the case of a technique it takes time to establish its operational status and wide applicability. Facts belong to the logical world of theory and lie outside time and space, while techniques evolve in the contingent realm of material reality.[4] Is it really so?

At this point we could discuss the difference (or lack thereof) between science and technology (e.g., Latour 1987). In both Watson and Crick's, and in Köhler and Milstein's cases, however, our starting point was a paper: We were not confronted by science or technology but by a few pages of text. So, let us begin by analyzing a particular sort of evidence, texts, which will eventually lead us to other kinds of evidence, such as tumor cells, actors' oral statements, attributed skills, and priority claims.

A canonical genealogy of hybridoma technology, established through the inspection of the bibliographies of papers published in the area,[5] links Köhler and Milstein's 1975 paper—the foundational paper—to two subsequent contributions. Together they form a trilogy of founding papers. They are as follows:

Köhler and Milstein (1975); henceforth MILSTEIN 75
Köhler and Milstein (1976); henceforth MILSTEIN 76
Galfré et al. (1977); henceforth MILSTEIN 77a

For reasons that will become clear, a fourth paper can be added:

Williams, Galfré, and Milstein (1977); henceforth MILSTEIN 77b.

A quick look at the authors' address shows that these papers were produced in one institution: César Milstein's MRC Laboratory of Molecular Biology (Cambridge, England).[6] So the papers have led us to a particular laboratory, and some readers may find this reassuring; the flimsy paper has been given a solid institutional foundation. There are, however, complications. For instance, during the 1975–1977 period, the output of César Milstein's MRC Laboratory of Molecular Biology was not limited to these four papers.

Even if we restrict ourselves to the collaborative work involving both Köhler and Milstein, other papers were published, such as, for instance, a 1977 paper, "Fusion of T and B Cells" (Köhler, Pearson, and Milstein, 1977) or a 1976 paper, "Fusion Between Immunoglobulin-Secreting and Nonsecreting Myeloma Cell Lines" (Köhler, Howe, and Milstein 1976). To a newcomer to the field, these titles sound intriguingly similar to those singled out as the founding papers of hybridoma technology: Cell fusion (sometimes implied by the use of the term *hybrid*) seems a common feature, as well as the presence of such entities as myelomas, antigens, and antibodies.

So, even if the analysis of these papers shows that they do not deal with hybridoma technology, narrowly (and retrospectively!) defined, we should not just brush them aside on the basis of some *a priori* distinction. In addition, other papers published during the same period, even if they do not focus on hybridoma technology as such, clearly mention aspects that will be later perceived as constitutive of it.[7] The following question can thus be raised: How was the canonical tetralogy of papers constituted? Could it be that it is based on hindsight?

These questions have interesting consequences. For example, it has been convincingly argued by both scientists (e.g., Medawar 1993) and sociologists (e.g., Knorr-Cetina 1981) that scientific papers misrepresent the order and direction of laboratory activities: The development of a paper's argument rarely corresponds to the order of the hands-on laboratory work. The same argument applies, even more forcefully, to the literary production of an entire laboratory. Here the links between the different texts are inevitably *a posteriori* constructions.

Another, and slightly more radical, way of putting the same argument is to claim that the constitution of an object (for instance, hybridoma technology) is not to be differentiated from the construction of accounts concerning that object, and that therefore no *a priori*, intrinsic links exist among the different contributions that are later summed up under the term *hybridoma technology*. While papers do refer to each other through the use of citations, different links could have been established between the papers constituting the 1975–1977 output of Milstein's laboratory or, for that matter, any other paper that has been categorized under the rubric *hybridoma technology*. Indeed, different genealogies could have been established, different narratives told. For instance, some authors denied a foundational status to MILSTEIN 75 and simply listed it as one contribution among others, thus replacing discontinuity with continuity. In turn, the issue of (dis)continuity raises the question of what should count as a fact and what should count as a (mere) technique. Let us open a new section to explore this question.

Discontinuity or Continuity? The Koprowski Affair

Let us start by briefly following a central character of MILSTEIN 75, namely, the P3-X63Ag8 myeloma cell line.[8] Although we shall have a closer look at MILSTEIN 75 later in this chapter, let us for the moment focus on MILSTEIN 75's central claim that by fusing antibody-producing cells from the spleen of a particular strain of inbred mice (so-called BALB/c mice) immunized with sheep red blood cells[9] with a specific myeloma cell line (a tumor of plasma, or antibody-producing, cells)[10] called P3-X63Ag8, one obtains hybrid cells (later to be dubbed *hybridomas*) that have retained properties of both parental cells, that is, the capacity of secreting antibody against sheep red blood cells and the capacity of reproducing indefinitely in cell culture (antibody-producing spleen cells are unable to survive in cell culture). It will be noticed that in reproducing MILSTEIN 75's claims we are not indulging in any generalization based on hindsight.

In MILSTEIN 75, no particular attention is paid to the first fusion partner, antibody-secreting spleen cells, which can be easily produced in the laboratory by immunizing BALB/c mice, obtained from commercial companies specializing in laboratory animals.[11] MILSTEIN 75, however, treats P3-X63Ag8 as a central character, insofar as it is a) an important element of a specific line of research (more later), referred to both in the text and in footnotes; b) a decisive factor in the success of the particular experiment reported in MILSTEIN 75; and c) a rare object that initially could only be obtained from Milstein's laboratory.[12] By following P3-X63Ag8 we can thus identify the first laboratories that attempted to perform experiments based on MILSTEIN 75 claims.

The first three places to which P3-X63Ag8 leads us are the laboratories of Alain Bussard (Institut Pasteur, Paris), Klaus Rajewsky (Institute of Genetics, University of Köln), and Hilary Koprowski, head of the Philadelphia-based Wistar Institute (Milstein, personal communication; Rajewsky, letter to the authors, January 3, 1991). Papers originating in these laboratories could be said to be the first reporting the successful adoption and use of the technique described by MILSTEIN 75 and MILSTEIN 76. Could be? Were they or were they not? The answer is not straightforward, and to understand why let us turn to the original papers, namely,

Bussard and Pages (1978); henceforth BUSSARD 78

Hämmerling et al. (1978); henceforth RAJEWSKY 78a

Rajewsky et al. (1978); henceforth RAJEWSKY 78b

Lemke et al. (1978); henceforth RAJEWSKY 78c

Koprowski, Gerhard, and Croce (1977a); henceforth KOPROWSKI 77.

Bussard's case is somewhat idiosyncratic. For several years he had been involved in experiments designed to show that peritoneal cells, which are not normally considered part of the immune system, are immunologically competent, that is, that they secrete antibodies (Bussard 1966).[13] The idea had been met with skepticism. Upon reading Köhler and Milstein's paper, Bussard saw a way of vindicating his thesis. Bussard invited Milstein to Paris in December of 1976 and, under Milstein's guidance, he and his wife, a virologist already familiar with cell culture techniques, were able to immortalize antibody-producing peritoneal cells.[14]

Thus Bussard replaced the antibody-producing lymphocytes with a cell whose antibody-producing capacity had until then been in doubt, therefore claiming to have "adapted to the mouse peritoneal cell, the immunocyte we have used most frequently as our experimental model, the original technique of Köhler and Milstein" (BUSSARD 78:167). The point here is that Köhler and Milstein are represented as a new beginning, having succeeded where others had failed: "Since 1965 several attempts have been made to fuse immunocytes with myeloma cells, but little success was realized until 1975 when Köhler and Milstein succeeded in fusing a plasmocytoma cell with an antibody-producing cell, namely an anti-sheep red blood cell (SRBC) lymphocyte" (Ibid.).[15]

RAJEWSKY 78a–c explicitly represent their contribution as flowing from MILSTEIN 75 and MILSTEIN 76, which are therefore singled out as the founding papers. Whereas Bussard speaks of adaptation, Rajewsky goes further and presents his case as one of adoption. For instance, the Introduction of RAJEWSKY 78a reads:

> Recently Köhler and Milstein [wrong ref.: MILSTEIN 75[16]] reported that hybridization of myeloma cells with sheep red blood cell (SRBC) sensitized lymphocytes resulted in hybrid cells secreting anti-SRBC antibody. This cell fusion technique which opens new ways for the mass production of monoclonal antibodies of predefined specificity has been established in our laboratory and it has also been extended to construction of permanent T-cell tissue culture lines by fusion of T-cell tumors with selected T lymphocyte subpopulations.

This introduction, while acknowledging the paper's own contribution (i.e., the extension of the technique to T-cell lines) explicitly claims that the underlying technique is the same as that developed by MILSTEIN 75: It had been borrowed and established in the German laboratory. At the same time, this opening paragraph attaches a definite meaning and purpose to, and therefore an identity for, the technique by claiming that it "opens new ways for the mass production of monoclonal antibodies of predefined specificity." In other words, the technique is defined in relation to a particular use and is actually constituted, *qua* technique, by this translation. There are various levels of generality, however, at which such a translation can be implemented; for instance, RAJEWSKY 78a clearly defines hybridoma technology as a general technique, a technique potentially leading to the production of antibodies against all sorts of antigens (as opposed to the antigens used in the experiments described in the paper).

Similarly, RAJEWSKY 78b opens with the following sentences: "A detailed analysis of the antibody repertoire requires the isolation of individual antibody species out of the complex mixture of antibodies produced in most immune responses. Such an approach has been dramatically facilitated by the cell fusion technique as recently introduced by Köhler and Milstein [wrong ref.: MILSTEIN 75[17] and MILSTEIN 76]." Here again we see the double process of grounding the genealogy of the paper in Köhler and Milstein, and of attaching a particular meaning, purpose, and identity to the technique; the only difference this time is that the meaning of the technique becomes more specific. From a tool for mass production (a general technique), hybridoma technology becomes, in application, a tool for the analysis of the antibody repertoire (a technique for a specific goal). Apart from *Nature*'s more telegraphic style, the opening sentence of RAJEWSKY 78c plays a similar role: "Hybridisation of a myeloma cell line with hyperimmunised spleen cells can provide cell lines secreting monoclonal antibodies of predefined specificity [MILSTEIN 75 and MILSTEIN 76 are cited]."

Things are very different in KOPROWSKI 77. The opening paragraphs read:

> Monoclonal antibodies specific for antigenic determinants of viruses such as influenza [ref. to a 1976 paper by co-author Gerhard] or parainfluenza I [ref. to a 1977 paper by co-authors Gerhard and Koprowski] have been produced *in vitro* in the splenic fragment system. Until now, however, the production of antibody by spleen foci in culture has been declining after 30–40 days and ceasing altogether after 90 days. In our observation, any attempts to transform cells of the splenic fragments by either simian virus 40 or Abelson murine leukemia virus ended in failure. The selection *in vitro* of continuous cell lines that produce antibodies of given specificities would greatly facilitate antigenic analysis of viral determinants. The availability of such antibody might also be useful in immunotherapy. In the present study we have succeeded in the selection of somatic cell hybrids between influenza virus–primed mouse spleen cells and mouse myeloma cells. These hybrids can be maintained indefinitely in culture and continue to produce anti-influenza antibodies.

Two things should be noted. In the first place, the opening sentence refers to a technique, splenic fragments,[18] that had been developed to produce monoclonal antibodies before hybridoma technology existed. Therefore, the production of monoclonal antibodies is not a novelty, as it has already been carried out by, among others, the authors of KOPROWSKI 77.[19] In the second place, the focus of the opening paragraph, as compared with the corresponding lines in RAJEWSKY 78a–c, is narrower: The text speaks of viruses and, even more specifically, of anti-influenza antibodies. This is somewhat surprising, because, as sociologists of science have pointed out (e.g., Law 1983), the opening lines of a scientific paper often function as a "funnel of interest," that is, the reader is guided, through successive steps or translations, from some very general initial statement (e.g., in RAJEWSKY 78b, the study of antibody repertoires) to the specific topic of the paper (e.g., in RAJEWSKY 78b, the study of antibodies specific for group A streptococcal carbohydrate).

At stake, however, in KOPROWSKI 77 is the establishment of both originality *and* continuity: continuity with previous cell hybridization experiments, so that MILSTEIN 75 no longer can be said to represent a novelty, as well as continuity with the production of anti-influenza monoclonal antibodies, which did not have to wait for Köhler and Milstein's technique. Originality is involved insofar as hybridoma technology had not yet been shown to be operational in the production of anti-viral antibodies: Köhler and Milstein had only produced antibodies against sheep red blood cells, whereas here one is confronted with a technique to produce antibodies against viral antigens, "a matter which was not addressed in any of the prior Milstein publications" (Koprowski and Croce 1980).

The sentences that follow in the paper freely admit the limits of the splenic fragment technique (the production of antibodies ceases after 3 months) and also point to the failure of methods tried in order to overcome this problem. Summoning these limits and failures serves as a backdrop against which the successful alternative is presented, that is, the new technology based on the production of "somatic cell hybrids between influenza virus-primed mouse spleen cells and mouse myeloma cells." Unlike RAJEWSKY 78a–c, however, no reference is made to Köhler and Milstein; they are not presented as the originators of the new technique.

The next section of the paper, Materials and Methods is, from this point of view, revealing. MILSTEIN 75 and MILSTEIN 76 are quoted only in relation to the P3-X63Ag8 myeloma cells, which, the paper acknowledges, "were obtained through the kindness of Cesar Milstein." The production of hybrids, however, is described as based on "established fusion procedures,"[20] and a 1964 paper by Littlefield[21] is quoted. In other words, Milstein's contribution is limited to the supply of raw materials (i.e., the myeloma cell line used as one of the fusion partners), and the actual production of hybrids through a fusion procedure is presented not as the discrete achievement of Milstein's lab but as a result of more diffused and continuous technical developments, of which MILSTEIN 75 and MILSTEIN 76 are only one step.

A gloss of KOPROWSKI 77 would thus read as follows. At the time of Köhler and Milstein's publication, monoclonal antibodies were not a theoretical or conceptual novelty. In theory all antibodies were monoclonal antibodies because, according to the clonal selection theory of antibody formation—the paradigm of modern immunology—a single plasma (spleen) cell secretes one and only one kind of antibody. Monoclonal antibodies were also already available in practice; for instance, through Klinman's (1969) splenic fragment system[22] researchers were able to isolate single B lymphocytes that secreted a single type of antibody.[23]

The novelty of hybridoma technology is thus not that it created a new theoretical entity or made that entity available for the first time. In retrospect, what hybridoma technology did do was to make monoclonal antibodies easily available. Moreover, while this might be called a breakthrough, it is a breakthrough that hinges not on the development of specific methods, because, for instance, cell hybridization was well known, but on the use of a specific fusion partner, the P3-X63Ag8 cell line, which happened to be available in Milstein's laboratory.

This gloss of KOPROWSKI 77 is not the result of the overinterpretation of a few, isolated passages. It summarizes interviews with researchers of the Wistar Institute, including Hilary Koprowski, Zenon Steplewski, Carlo Croce, and Walter Gerhard. Let us begin with Gerhard, who had been a postdoctoral student of Norman Klinman, the originator of the splenic fragments culture technique. In this technique, mice are irradiated to destroy antibody-producing cells in the spleen. They are subsequently injected with immunocompetent B and T cells, some of which lodge in the spleen. The latter is then removed and cut into small cubes. Each cube is put into an individual culture well, to which antigen is added. If an immunocompetent cell is present in a given cube, it will be stimulated to expand clonally and to start producing (monoclonal) antibodies, which can be harvested in the culture medium.

Working with the influenza antigens with which he was familiar, Gerhard had succeeded in keeping fragments producing antibodies for up to three months. Therefore, with this technique "you could make a sufficient amount of monoclonal antibodies that you could actually start analyzing them, that you could do something with the monoclonals" (interview, September 29, 1987). This is consonant with Koprowski's claim that researchers at Wistar, prior to MILSTEIN 75, were already familiar with monoclonals as a technique. Thus, as Gerhard put it (interview, September 29, 1987), when MILSTEIN 75 was published "many people may have said, it's nice but so what, what can we do with it? I didn't have to say that."

If the product (monoclonals) was known, what about the cell hybridization procedure? Both Koprowski (interview, September 28, 1987) and Steplewski (interview, September 28, 1987) referred to their (and their collaborator Barbara Knowles') "pioneering work" in the field of somatic cell hybridization in the 1960s. Since then, cell fusion had become "almost a standard technique" at Wistar.[24] Of course, the line of work pursued at Wistar was not Milstein's immunogenetics. Wistar's researchers used cell fusion as a tool in cancer research and, more precisely, in research related to the viral (SV40) transformation of normal cells into malignant cells.[25] Moreover, most of the time the cells used were not cells from the immune system but, rather, fibroblasts (connective tissue cells) or fibroblastlike cells.

The techniques involved in producing cell hybrids were, however, for all practical purposes, identical. Furthermore, lymphocytes were also used; Knowles, for instance, had co-authored a 1971 paper with researchers at the Albert Einstein College of Medicine in New York in which a mouse fibroblast was fused with a myeloma and whereby the resulting hybrid ceased to produce immunoglobulin (Coffino et al. 1971).[26] This and related work on immunoglobulin synthesis was reviewed in a 1974 paper by Koprowski and Knowles. The somatic cell genetic line of work was expanded with the arrival at the institute of Carlo Croce in 1970.

The idea behind the use of cell fusion in somatic cell genetic experiments was that the resulting hybrid soon starts segregating chromosomes; by determining the functions that are lost, one can hope to locate a function on a particular chromosome. This, in turn, could lead to mapping the genes responsible. From a practical point of view, immunoglobulin-producing cells were a good system to work with because the presence and characteristics of immunoglobulins could be easily detected by immunological techniques. Steplewski claims to have discussed with Knowles the possibility of fusing mouse lymphocytes with human fibroblasts. Preferential segregation of the human chromosomes would have led to a hybrid cell that still produced antibody.

So if Wistar's researchers claim to have undertaken experiments similar to Milstein's, how do they account for the fact that these experiments did not lead to hybridoma technology?[27] One could, of course, point out—as Steplewski openly admitted—that Wistar's researchers were not looking for monoclonal antibodies; they were mapping (immunoglobulin) genes. But so, as we shall see, was Milstein! Thus, according once again to both Koprowski and Steplewski, the reason they did not produce monoclonal antibodies was that they did not have "the right partner," that is, the myeloma cell line P3-X63Ag8: "After the [MILSTEIN 75] paper appeared on the right partner, we got the cells from Milstein and we made the first monoclonal antibody against influenza virus" (Koprowski, interview, September 28, 1987).

It was not, however, sufficient merely to have access to a cell line available only in selected places. As we shall see, although myelomas had already been produced, they had not been adapted for cell fusion. Myeloma cell lines later became available, but, in the meantime, researchers at Wistar had become convinced that antibody production after cell fusion was a biologically unattainable goal: "The problem, ours and everybody else's, was that as a partner of fusion we were using fibroblasts which shut off the genes of antibody production. So we never got anything. This was in 1966. . . . So that idea was around probably every lab. Everyone was looking for the right partner. We couldn't succeed so we decided that probably the genes that are responsible for antibodies need to be in vivo and in vitro you can't get them out and we gave up." (Steplewski, interview, September 28, 1987).[28]

The evidence gathered by comparing RAJEWSKY 78a–c with KOPROWSKI 77 shows that genealogical links between papers are the result of operations performed by later papers on earlier ones, such as a) the simultaneous construction of a discontinuity and of a point of origin through the attribution of a foundational role to earlier papers, and b) the derivation of a linear sequence of papers from this point of origin through, among other things, the stabilization of their meaning(s), leading to the establishment of not only a chronological, but also a substantive, continuity.[29] The (fictional) reader might object that the above example is rather unusual, and extremely vicious. Don't you know, the reader will continue, that Koprowski and co-workers were planning to appropriate Köhler and Milstein's technique by filing (in 1978) two patent claims—on a method for producing monoclonal antibodies against viral and tumor antigens—which were eventually granted in 1979 and in 1980 in the United States (but not in the United Kingdom; see Chapter 5)? Haven't you realized that this explains their behavior? No other scientist behaved the way they did, and anyway Köhler and Milstein's Nobel Prize has settled this matter. In order to understand this you should abandon your obsession with discourse and representations and look at real world interests![30]

To this we would reply, Koprowski and co-workers might well have been moved by an interest in securing a patent, but that does not automatically disqualify their arguments as mere opportunism. Furthermore, our reader's reasoning could be turned around: It could be argued that Koprowski and co-workers did not stress continuity in order to appropriate Köhler and Milstein's technology but, rather, that it is precisely because they perceived continuity in the way they did that they felt legitimized in securing patent protection for their work. Finally, and more importantly, perhaps KOPROWSKI 77 is an extreme example, but what is important is that it is not unthinkable in the literal sense of the word; one can impute hidden agendas to its protagonists, treat it as a biased account but not discard it as nonsense. Maybe it is close to the borders of what could be plausibly argued, but it is still within the domain of the arguable. In any event, our argument does not depend solely on KOPROWSKI 77. We have another example that does not involve patents or other purported obvious interests: Let's call it the Schwaber affair.

Discontinuity or Continuity (2)? The Schwaber Affair

In May 1982, *Science* published a reply to a February News and Comments item that used the by then widespread revolution metaphor to describe the development of hybridoma technology. It is worth reproducing this short letter (Schwaber 1982) in its entirety:

> Nicholas Wade, in his article "Hybridomas: The Making of a Revolution" (News and Comments, 26 Feb., p. 1703), discusses Köhler and Milstein's use of lymphocytes as fusion partners of mouse myeloma cells as though it were a radical departure from the science of the time. In fact, fusion of human lymphocytes with mouse myeloma cells to give rise to hybrid cells which secreted myeloma and lymphocyte-derived immunoglobulins was described in 1973 [ref.: Schwaber and Cohen 1973], concurrent with the first myeloma-myeloma fusions [ref.: Cotton and Milstein 1973], and again in 1974 [ref.: Schwaber and Cohen 1974]. Köhler and Milstein acknowledged this work in their 1975 description of mouse splenocyte-mouse myeloma hybrid cells. The mouse immunoglobulin secreted by these mouse-human hybrid cells was an antibody (*Pneumococcus C* polysaccharide). The germinal contribution of Köhler and Milstein to this process was the use of immunized spleen cells that secreted antibodies which would be determined by prior immunization and which could then be selected from the general population.

This is an interesting letter because of its denial of the revolutionary status ("radical departure from the science of the time") of some of the key elements of MILSTEIN 75. Notice that this denial is not made with respect to the consequences (scientific, commercial, and other) of hybridoma technology that were the main topic of Wade's article, but with respect to "the science of the time." From this point of view, it is similar to KOPROWSKI 77. There is, however, a difference. While KOPROWSKI 77 claimed that monoclonal antibodies of predetermined specificity were not a novelty, whereas the immortalization of the cell lines (hybridomas) producing them was, Schwaber's claim is that MILSTEIN 75's novel contribution lies not in the development of hybridomas but in the production of monoclonal antibodies of predetermined specificity. In other words, the continuity claims advanced by KOPROWSKI 77 and by Schwaber's letter are based on different components of the hybridoma technique.[31]

In addition to MILSTEIN 75, the three papers mentioned in Schwaber's letter are the following:

> Schwaber and Cohen (1973); henceforth SCHWABER 73
> Schwaber and Cohen (1974); henceforth SCHWABER 74
> Cotton and Milstein (1973); henceforth MILSTEIN 73

Despite Wade's purported oversight, these papers did not go un-noticed. For instance, according to the *Science Citation Index*, SCHWABER 73 was cited 40 times between its publication and 1984. What was it cited for? Here are two excerpts from citing papers:

> The first successful hybridization of neoplastic cells with normal lymphocytes was performed between mouse myeloma cells and human normal lymphocytes and it led to permanent hybrid cell lines secreting both mouse and human immunoglobulins (Schwaber & Cohen 1973). But the specificities of the human immunoglobulins secreted by these hybridomas remained unknown. Two years later, in 1975, Köhler & Milstein succeeded in the hybridization of mouse myeloma cells with immunized mouse spleen cells. The resulting hybridomas secreted monoclonal antibodies with specificity towards sheep red blood cell antigens which had been used for immunization. (Lemke, Hämmerling, and Hämmerling 1979:176).

> In 1973, Schwaber & Cohen fused mouse lymphoma cells with human peripheral blood cells and obtained hybrid lines that secreted both mouse and human immunoglobulin. This showed that fusion of a malignant and a normal lymphoid cell could result in a continuous cell line producing the products of the normal cell. However, [this study did not lead] directly to the hybridoma technology.
> (Yelton and Scharff 1981:660–661).[32]

What these quotes seem to say is as follows: Well, SCHWABER 73 almost did it, but not quite. The actual breakthrough came with MILSTEIN 75. Although this interpretation seems compatible with Schwaber's letter to *Science*, let us look at another quote:

> Cotton and Milstein (1973) demonstrated that fusion of two antibody-producing mouse myeloma cell lines resulted in hybrids expressing the products of both parental lines. In the same year Schwaber and Cohen (1973) demonstrated that fusion of human lymphocytes with mouse myeloma cells resulted in hybrids that secreted myeloma- and lymphocyte-derived immunoglobulins. Thus, the stage was set for the now classic observation by Köhler and Milstein (1975) in which they demonstrated that fusion of immunized spleen cells to mouse myeloma cells resulted in hybrids that secreted antibodies determined by prior immunization.
> (Shay 1985:7–8).

Well, there is a subtle difference: SCHWABER 73, rather than "not leading directly" to hybridoma technology, "sets the stage" for it; it is only a shift in emphasis, but one that introduces continuity in place of a discrete break. Let us continue:

> In vitro production of human immunoglobulins by somatic cell hybridization was first reported by Schwaber and Cohen [ref.: SCHWABER 73]. Kohler [sic] and Milstein [ref.: MILSTEIN 75] subsequently produced murine monoclonal antibodies. (Schwaber et al. 1984).

Here there is a stronger sense of continuity: SCHWABER 73 first did it with human material, then MILSTEIN 75 came along with mouse material. Wait a second!, says the (fictional) reader. This is a quote from a paper co-authored by Schwaber. I understand that you don't believe in authors, but you should come up with a less openly biased example. OK, what about the next two quotes:

> Continuous production of a human immunoglobulin by a human lymphocyte immortalized by fusion to a mouse myeloma line was first reported by Schwaber and Cohen [ref.: SCHWABER 73], 2 years prior to Köhler and Milstein's work describing murine hybridomas producing antibodies of predefined specificity [ref.: MILSTEIN 75] (Abrams et al. 1986:110).

> Human-mouse hybrids secreting nonspecific Ig of both parental types were first described in 1973 [ref.: SCHWABER 73]. The field of murine antigen-specific monoclonal antibody production of pre-defined specificity was established in 1975 by the work of Köhler and Milstein [ref.: MILSTEIN 75] who showed that a mouse could be immunized to an antigen, and that the spleen cells from that mouse could be fused with an aminopterin-sensitive myeloma line to develop hybrid cell lines producing high titers of monoclonal antibody directed towards the immunizing antigen [ref.: MILSTEIN 75]. Finally, in the 1980s human monoclonal antibodies derived from hybridization were developed, initially using patients' lymphocytes and most recently normal human peripheral blood lymphocytes as the fusion partners with aminopterin-sensitive human or mouse myeloma lines. . . .
> (Fauci, Lane, and Volkman 1983).

Here MILSTEIN 75 is one step, admittedly an important one, but still one step, in a series of contributions leading from SCHWABER 73 to the production in the 1980s of human monoclonal antibodies. MILSTEIN 75 stands out less dramatically than in the revolutionary version of the story.

This is easily accounted for, our (fictional) reader will point out. Just notice that these two papers, as well as the one from which the previous quote was taken, deal with human monoclonals. As you surely know, the production of human monoclonals is more difficult than the production of murine monoclonals, for reasons ranging from ethical concerns (you cannot inject human beings with multiple antigens, take their spleens out, etc.) to the natural properties of human cells (poor performance of HAT-sensitive human cells, inefficient growth, inefficient fusions, etc.) (Thompson et al. 1986). On the other hand, the production of human monoclonals, while certainly not a practical source of day-to-day reagents in a research laboratory, is potentially very important for in vivo diagnostics and for therapeutic use, because of possible allergic reactions to murine material. So, no wonder the production of human monoclonals has developed into a discrete subspecialty and that within that specialty SCHWABER 73, which used human lymphocytes as a fusion partner, is given prominence.

To this, we would reply: There is some point to what you say. Consider, for instance, two books devoted to hybridoma technology, both featuring, in their introduction, a chronological list of "landmark discoveries" leading to the production of monoclonal antibodies (Shay 1985; Goding 1983). Both lists contain MILSTEIN 73 and, of course, MILSTEIN 75, but only the list appearing in the book devoted to human monoclonals mentions SCHWABER 73.

This being said, your remark is not an objection. First, what you have done is to stress the socially and technically contingent nature of discovery narratives. Second, you must understand that human hybridomas could be described as "human hybridomas" only after the establishment of the narrative web that came to be centered around MILSTEIN 75. In other words, the claim, brought forward in one of the earlier quotes, that first SCHWABER 73 produced human immunoglobulin-secreting hybridomas, and subsequently MILSTEIN 75 developed murine immunoglobulin-secreting hybridomas, has to be inverted: Human immunoglobulin-secreting hybridomas were a logico-semantic consequence, despite their status as a historical precursor of murine immunoglobulin-secreting hybridomas, because there were no "hybridomas," as we now understand the term, before MILSTEIN 75 or, it could be argued (see below), before MILSTEIN 77a.

So, let us return again to the original papers written by Schwaber and Cohen, and by Cotton and Milstein. We quote the opening lines from each of these three papers, which summarize their content:

> Hybrids between two distinct differentiated cell types usually do not express the differentiated characteristics of either parental cell. The synthesis of enzymes necessary for the metabolism of the cell continues, while the synthesis of specialized products of differentiation often is suppressed [ref.: Ephrussi 1972]. Mouse myeloma cells, after fusion with mouse fibroblasts, follow this pattern; that is, the hybrid cells cease synthesis of immunoglobulin [ref.: Coffino et al. 1971, Periman 1970]. A myeloma × lymphoma hybrid, however, continues secretion of immunoglobulin [ref.: Mohit and Fan 1971, Mohit 1971]. We report here the isolation of a hybrid clone, resulting from fusion of mouse myeloma cells secreting immunoglobulin of known specificity and human peripheral blood lymphocytes not secreting detectable immunoglobulin. The hybrid cells continue secretion of mouse immunoglobulin and initiate synthesis and secretion of human immunoglobulin. (SCHWABER 73:444–445).

> Fusion of human peripheral blood lymphocytes, not forming detectable immunoglobulins, with mouse myeloma cells (TEPC-15), secreting mouse immunoglobulin A with known antibody activity, yielded a somatic cell hybrid clone that secreted both human and mouse immunoglobulins. (SCHWABER 74:2203).

> Each immunoglobulin chain is the integrated expression of one of several V and C genes, coding, respectively, for their variable and constant sections [ref.: Milstein

and Munro 1970]. The restricted expression of these genes leads to molecules of a single class and type with identical combining sites at both halves of the antibody molecule [ref.: Bernier and Cebra 1964, Mellors and Korngold 1963, Pernis 1967]. This symmetry is essential for the formation of the antigen-antibody lattice. Its importance is emphasized by allelic exclusion, whereby each cell expresses only one of two possible alleles [ref.: Pernis 1967]. To understand this problem further we have studied the expression of these genes in hybrid cells obtained by fusion of two cell lines producing different immunoglobulins. Successful fusion of this type has not yet been demonstrated but fusion between immunoglobulin-producing cells and non-immunoglobulin-producing cells has been reported. Thus myeloma cells have been fused to fibroblasts [ref.: Periman 1970, Coffino et al. 1971, Bevan et al. 1972] and also to a non-immunoglobulin-producing lymphoma line [ref.: Mohit 1971]. Substantial immunoglobulin production in the hybrids was observed only in the latter case. Here, we demonstrate that fusion between two immunoglobulin-secreting cell lines produces hybrid cells which secrete immunoglobulin of both parental types. (MILSTEIN 73:42).

One possible way of making sense of these passages is to look at a passage in MILSTEIN 75 that cites them jointly[33]:

When two antibodies-producing cells are fused, the products of both parental lines are expressed [ref.: MILSTEIN 73, SCHWABER 74], and although the light and heavy chains of both parental lines are randomly joined, no evidence of scrambling of V and C sections is observed [ref.: MILSTEIN 73]. . . . We conclude that, as previously shown with interspecies hybrids [ref.: MILSTEIN 73, SCHWABER 74], new Ig molecules are produced as a result of mixed association between heavy and light chains from the two parents. (MILSTEIN 75:495).

Notice, first of all, that SCHWABER 74 is not cited for its technical achievement, that is, the fusion of a myeloma and a lymphocyte, which, as Schwaber would later argue in its letter to *Science,* could be seen as corresponding to part of the procedure reported in MILSTEIN 75. Rather, it is cited for the production of two "facts," namely, that "when two antibodies-producing cells are fused, the products of both parental lines are expressed" and that "Ig molecules [of interspecies hybrids] are produced as a result of mixed association between heavy and light chains from the two parents." By referring to what Schwaber and Cohen have done as a fact, Köhler and Milstein (intentionally or not is not the question) are fencing them off, preventing them from having technical continuity with their own work. The credibility of Köhler and Milstein's work as an autonomous technical achievement is thereby increased.

The equivalence between MILSTEIN 73 and SCHWABER 74 is further enhanced by the fact that MILSTEIN 75 speaks in both cases of the fusion of "two antibody-producing cells." Although, technically speaking, this definition is correct, it obscures the fact that in the case of MILSTEIN 73 one is dealing with the fusion of two (a mouse and a rat) myelomas, and in the case of SCHWABER 74 with the fusion of a (mouse) myeloma and a (human) lymphocyte.[34] The preceding remarks should not be read as an indictment of MILSTEIN 75 for (un)consciously misrepresenting SCHWABER 74. Rather, our point is that the way in which MILSTEIN 75 treats similar or related papers, such as SCHWABER 74, is an indication of MILSTEIN 75's still unsettled status, of its oscillation between the report of a technical procedure and the report of a fact. In the latter case, distinctions concerning the identity of fusion partners are less relevant than in the former.

Notice, secondly, that MILSTEIN 75 clearly equates MILSTEIN 73 with SCHWABER 74; by extrapolation, SCHWABER 73 could be easily added to this equation. And indeed, through simple inspection of the co-citation pattern of the introductory lines of SCHWABER 73 and MILSTEIN 73, as quoted earlier, a similar case could be easily made. Both extracts are located in the field of somatic cell hybridization by co-citing previous work by Coffino et al., Periman, and Mohit. A closer analysis of the papers shows that MILSTEIN 73 insists more on the molecular-genetic aspect (citing previous work by Milstein and Munro,[35] Mellors and Korngold, and Pernis).

It also shows that this can be seen from the difference between the tools and entities mobilized by the two papers. MILSTEIN 73, for instance, speaks of genes and immunoglobulins' heavy and light chains, and uses tools such as autoradiographs and isoelectric focusing; SCHWABER 73 invokes more "traditional" entities, such as chromosomes, and uses tools such as chromosome analysis (metaphase chromosome spreads) and fluorescent antibody experiments. Correlatively, and using Pinch's (1985) notion of externality,[36] one could further argue that SCHWABER 73 has a lower degree of externality than MILSTEIN 73 insofar as the first paper looks only at the immunoglobulin secretion pattern, while the second paper draws inferences from that pattern concerning the underlying genetic determinants.

What interests us, however, is that both papers claim to have established some facts concerning the successful production of immunoglobulins of both parental types, a result that MILSTEIN 73 relates to the phenomenon called *allelic exclusion*. There is an oscillation here between what could be called a *practical* breakthrough, as expressed by an emphasis on the *operational* side ("we succeeded in producing hybrid cells secreting. . . "), and a *factual* breakthrough ("experiments show that hybrid cells secrete . . . and this tells us something about allelic exclusion"). In both cases, however, no particular emphasis is laid on the fusion technique as such.

Where does all this leave us? We started this section with a letter by Schwaber, who argued that, when put in context, MILSTEIN 75 did not constitute a radical departure from the science of the time and pointed, as evidence of this, to a 1973 paper he co-authored with Cohen. We then saw that SCHWABER 73 had not been ignored by subsequent papers in the field, some of which explicitly looked for an appropriate way of fitting his work into a narrative on hybridoma technology. In some cases, it was used as a backdrop against which one could reaffirm the fundamental discontinuity introduced by Köhler and Milstein's contribution. In other cases, namely, when the production of human monoclonal antibodies was at issue, papers stressed the more or less continuous nature of the different contributions to the constitution of hybridoma technology.

Rather then attempting to set things straight, we took Schwaber's injunction to look at the science of the time seriously by examining the ambiguous way MILSTEIN 75 referred to the 1973–1974 contributions from both Schwaber's and Milstein's laboratories. To further develop this point, we shall devote the next section to the science of the time. For reasons that will soon become clear, the section is entitled "The Cohn Connection."

The Cohn Connection

During interviews concerning the origins of hybridoma technology, we came across a number of allusions to the fact that other researchers had tried to fuse normal lymphocytes and myeloma cells before Köhler and Milstein, and that they had failed. As Walter Gerhard (interview, September 29, 1987) put it, "I still remember, in one of the meetings, I asked people who did somatic cell fusions: 'Can you fuse plasmacytomas with B cells?' And they would say, 'No, people have tried. [The hybrid cells] always stop secreting antibodies.'"[37]

Indeed, as the story goes, when Köhler suggested to Milstein the by now famous fusion experiment, Milstein warned him about previous failures. As one commentator put it, "lymphocytes were known to be bad fusers" (Wade 1982).[38] We decided to find out more about these alleged "previous and failed attempts," the quotation marks referring to the fact that we are aware of the problematic status of such a description. It is only in retrospect that such attempts can be described as previous and teleologically assigned a place in the path leading to hybridoma technology; correlatively, what can be counted as a failure often depends on the meaning and purpose projected back onto those experiments.

Several indications led us to Melvin Cohn, a well-known immunologist at the Salk Institute and, as we were soon to find out, the head of the laboratory from which Milstein received the P3 myeloma cell line out of which the P3-X63Ag8 cell line, used in the 1975 fusion experiment, was developed. Basically, Melvin

Cohn confirmed what we had heard from other researchers, namely, that he had tried fusion experiments similar to Köhler and Milstein's, but that those experiments had not worked because the cells did not fuse. This story is worth being told in more detail because of what it tells us about experimental practice. It is a story in which cryptically labeled cell lines play a central role. We shall try, as far as possible, to avoid confusion by dropping any pretense of comprehensiveness and retaining only those details relevant to our present purpose. Accordingly, in what follows, we focus on three issues: a) cell fusion and the production of cell hybrids, b) the so-called HAT selective medium, and c) the origin and circulation of myeloma cell lines. Points a and b are discussed only because they are of importance in understanding point c, which is the item of interest.

The use of the term *hybridoma* to designate the result of the fusion between a myeloma cell and a normal lymphocyte is fairly recent. It postdates the development of what became known as *hybridoma technology*. Hybrid cells, however, have a longer history. Standard accounts state that the formation of somatic cell hybrids through cell fusion was first noticed in cultured mouse cells by French researchers working in Paris under Georges Barski in 1960 (Barski, Sorieul, and Cornefert 1960). Conflicting histories of the origins of this specialty are provided in books by two of its pioneers: Boris Ephrussi (1970:ch.2) and Henry Harris (1970:1–9).[39]

For our present purpose, suffice it to say that, as noted by Buttin and Cazenave (1980), in the five years following Barski et al.'s observation several techniques were developed to induce fusions and to select the results of such fusions. The original procedure was rather tedious, depending, as it did, on the spontaneous fusion of the cells that required up to three months of co-culturing of the cells to be fused. A Japanese researcher had demonstrated the possibility of inducing cell fusion with viruses in 1958 (Okada 1958),[40] and the technique was introduced into somatic cell genetics in 1965, the Sendai virus being used as a fusogen (Harris and Watkins 1965). The same fusogen, inactivated Sendai virus, was used in the initial Köhler and Milstein experiments. Two other key elements were used in those experiments: myeloma cells and the use of a selective medium, called HAT, to separate fused from unfused cells.

As far as the selective medium is concerned, its introduction into research is recorded in a paper published in 1964 by Littlefield (1964a).[41] In order to survive and grow in cell culture, cells need a series of enzymes that allow the cell to use the substances supplied in the culture medium. Two of these enzymes are known as TK (thymidine kinase) and HGPRT (hypoxanthine guanine phosphoribosyl transferase). Littlefield's trick was to choose as one fusion partner a cell that had lost HGPRT activity and as the other fusion partner a cell that had lost TK activity.

These fusion partners were isolated by adding genetic markers to the cells.

Markers such as 8-azaguanine or 6-thioguanine allow for the selection of cells having lost HGPRT activity. 5-Bromodeoxyuridine allows for the selection of cells that have lost TK activity. In normal conditions cells can work around the absence of TK and HGPRT by using other metabolic pathways; however, the activity of both TK and HGPRT is necessary for survival in a special medium called HAT (hypoxanthine aminopterin thymidine), in which the cells are grown after treatment with a fusing agent such as Sendai virus. Only fused hybrid cells have both enzymes; thus, unfused cells or cells that fused with the same kind of cell would die because of the absence of one of the two enzymes. This very system was used by Köhler and Milstein with only one difference. Because in their case one of the fusion partners, normal lymphocytes, do not survive in cell culture (Nabholz, Miggiano, and Bodmer 1969), only the other fusion partner, myeloma cells, needed to have lost either TK or HGPRT activity; hybrid cells (hybridomas) would be supplied with the missing enzyme by the normal lymphocyte, which is both TK and HGPRT positive.

The third element, and the one to which we devote more attention, is myeloma cell lines (also known as plasmacytomas). *Plasmacytoma* is the name given to a plasma-cell tumor[42] found in mice in the early 1950s and shown to be analogous to the human plasma-cell cancer known as multiple myeloma. Both multiple myeloma and plasmacytomas have played a central role in modern immunological research, for instance, in the study of the structure of antibodies (multiple myeloma) and in the study of antibody synthesis in vitro and the structure of immunoglobulin genes (murine plasmacytoma).[43] By the end of the 1950s, plasmacytomas had become easily producible following the serendipitous discovery in Michael Potter's laboratory at the NIH that they could be induced in mice—more precisely, in a particularly susceptible strain of laboratory mice known as BALB/c—through the injection of mineral oil (Potter 1986). While plasmacytomas could now be easily induced, the establishment of in vitro continuous lines of plasmacytoma was more difficult. It was only in the mid-1960s that work in Melvin Cohn's laboratory at the Salk Institute succeeded in showing the feasibility of in vitro culture of plasmacytomas, thus substantially increasing the degree of experimental manipulability of this system (Melchers, Potter, and Warner 1978:ix–xxiii).

Michael Potter's plasmacytoma induction program, instituted in the early 1960s, resulted in the establishment of a so-called myeloma library, that is, a collection of myeloma cell lines that were made available to other researchers. One of these lines was named MOPC 21 (the acronym MOPC stands for Mineral Oil PlasmaCytoma). At the Salk Institute, Melvin Cohn, who, as a student in Paris had learned cell hybridization from Boris Ephrussi, decided around 1967 to launch a similar induction program. While waiting for the first results of his local induction program, he asked Potter to send him some of his cell lines. Potter's cell lines were renamed by order of arrival, P1, P2, P3, ..., with P standing, of course, for Potter.[44] MOPC 21 became P3 and was adapted to growth in culture.

After initial experiments the cell line was not recovered from the freezer and was therefore lost. A continuous line of P3 was, however, soon reestablished, modified with genetic markers, and named P3K, the K standing for the first name, Kengo, of Horibata, Cohn's Japanese student who handled that project (Melchers, Potter, and Warner 1978:ix–xxiii; Horibata and Harris 1970). P3K was later sent, on request, to Milstein, who introduced additional genetic markers and cloned it. The P3-X63Ag8 used in MILSTEIN 75 was thus clone 63 of the P3K cell line, containing the marker 8-azaguanine.[45]

Let us step back. What were these researchers doing with these various and variously (re)named myeloma cells? First of all, as we pointed out, myelomas played a key role in immunological research. According to Yelton et al. (1980), Potter's and Cohn's induction programs had an enormous impact, "[n]ot only were the tumors themselves important, but their distribution promoted an interchange of ideas and reagents that has played a crucial role in the progress of modern immunology." Melvin Cohn (1967) agrees: "[Michael Potter] established a collection of cell lines which are to this field what the T-phages were to molecular biology."

Why were the tumors themselves important? Myelomas were deployed at the crossroads between immunology and somatic cell genetics. On the one hand, once the identity between the homogeneous proteins produced by myelomas and normal antibodies was established in the early 1970s,[46] myelomas became a very practical tool for the study of the normal immune response, as exemplified by the analysis of the biochemistry of immunoglobulin production. Unlike the normal cells of the immune systems, they could be maintained in continuous culture. On the other hand, myelomas often produced variant immunoglobulin molecules, and the mutant gene product could be easily obtained by injecting myelomas back into mice, thus providing a very useful experimental system for somatic cell genetics. Furthermore, as we have seen in the previous sections, by fusing myeloma cell lines one could hope to gain insights into the regulation and expression of immunoglobulin genes.

As previously stated, Milstein requested and obtained from Cohn the P3 (MOPC 21) cell line. What for? In a series of papers published in the early 1970s (Milstein and Svasti 1971; Svasti and Milstein 1972a; Svasti and Milstein 1972b), Milstein and collaborators first analyzed the biochemical structure of an immunoglobulin (IgG1) of the MOPC 21 myeloma and established the amino acid sequence of the immunoglobulin's light chain. They then shifted their attention to the messenger RNA, which directs the synthesis of this protein and sequenced it (Brownlee et al. 1972; Milstein et al. 1972; Brownlee et al. 1973; Milstein et al. 1974). Judging from the Materials and Methods sections of these papers, Milstein and collaborators used both the MOPC 21 line obtained from Potter and maintained by transplantation in BALB/c mice and the P3K line obtained from Horibata. The evidential context of these papers was the analysis of the mechanisms of immunoglobulin secretion and of the molecules involved in the synthesis of the constant and variable regions of the immunoglobulin molecule. Milstein and co-workers presented their contribution as a necessary, albeit preliminary, step in the study of immunogenetics based on hybridization techniques, as exemplified in MILSTEIN 73.

The use of myelomas also had its drawbacks. It was next to impossible to know the specificity of the myeloma immunoglobulins. While thousands of myelomas were generated, it was possible to identify the corresponding antigens in only a few cases. This was done by brute force screening against a battery of potential antigens (Yelton et al. 1980:5).[47] Interestingly, in the fall of 1974 Milstein had suggested to Köhler that as a start for further immunogenetic studies he should try to discover the specificity of P3-X63Ag8's immunoglobulin by brute force screening. Köhler demurred. Instead, on the basis of a recent successful experiment in which he had fused P3-X63Ag8 with a derivative of another of Cohn' cell lines, P1, Köhler decided to attempt the fusion of P3-X63Ag8 with normal lymphocytes and performed the experiment reported in MILSTEIN 75 (Wade 1982).

The difficulty of determining the specificity of the myeloma immunoglobulins had two distinct consequences that should not be confused. On the one hand, it drastically reduced the utility of myelomas as possible sources of reagents that could be used as tools in other research projects. Klinman's splenic fragments technique, which, as we have seen in the section on the Koprowski affair, did succeed in producing monoclonal antibodies, provided one solution to this problem. On the other hand, the utility of myelomas in immunogenetic studies such as those pursued by Milstein and Cohn was also hampered, insofar as the absence of information on the myeloma immunoglobulin made testing for genetic transformations following cell hybridization very difficult. Attempted solutions to this problem[48] included the induction of myelomas in animals that had been previously hyperimmunized with a given antigen, in the (unrealized) hope that one of the myelomas would secrete immunoglobulin against that antigen (Bazin 1986; Yelton and Scharff 1981), and the viral transformation of antibody-producing cells, in the hope of "immortalizing" them.[49]

As we saw in the section on the Koprowski affair, researchers at the Wistar Institute claimed that although they had done extensive work with cell fusion, they did not develop hybridoma technology because they lacked the right fusion partner (i.e., the P3 myeloma cell line). When myeloma cell lines became available, they had given up the idea that hybrid cells could be made to produce antibodies in vitro. The situation is different in Cohn's case. His team developed P3 in cell culture and supplied it to Milstein.[50] Because he had the right partner and because the idea of producing hybrid cells was in the air, did he actually try to fuse myelomas and lymphocytes, and, if so, what happened to those fusions? The answer to the first question is that Cohn's group tried both myeloma/myeloma and myeloma/lymphocyte fusion experiments.

The aim, as in Milstein's case, was not to produce monoclonal antibodies as reagents: "It never crossed my mind as a way of making reagents" (Cohn, interview, March 15, 1990). The point was, as with Milstein, to study the pathway of immunoglobulin synthesis by looking at different stages of B cell differentiation. So what happened to those experiments? As the following two quotes make clear, the experiments failed: The cells did not fuse. In the first excerpt, having first explained that they had established several myeloma and two lymphoma cell lines, the authors continue:

> Analysis of the genetic control of Ig synthesis could be carried much further if we had a method for the deliberate induction of and/or selection for new mutations [of myeloma cells] and a technique for somatic cell hybridization applicable to myeloma cells. The Sendai virus induced fusion technique which has been successfully employed by other workers with other cell types has not been effective with our Ig secreting myeloma cells, because they are not agglutinable by that virus.
> (Harris and Cohn 1970:275–276).

Similarly, in a second excerpt, we read that

> An alternative method of genetic analysis involves the formation and isolation of hybrids between myelomas and other cell types. Unfortunately, the use of Sendai virus to form artificial hybrids . . . has not been successful since we have found that none of the Ig secreting myeloma cell lines (nor S49) are agglutinable by the virus, although the Ig negative mutant cells and the S1A lymphoma cells are agglutinable (unpublished results). Application of the drug resistant mutant cell hybrid selection system [ref.: Littlefield 1964] is also difficult with the myeloma cell lines due to their near-tetraploid state and the consequent gene dosage of the thymidine kinase and the guanine-hypoxanthine phosphoribosyl transferase (PRTase) loci.
> (Horibata and Harris 1970:74–75).

An explanation for this failure has been offered by Yelton et al. (1980:5):

> Most of the early attempts to fuse myeloma cells employed inactivated Sendai virus to increase the very low spontaneous frequency of myeloma myeloma hybrids. This was not successful presumably because most, if not all, mouse myeloma cells do not contain receptors for Sendai (P. Mauces and M. Cohn, personal communication). However, Cotton and Milstein (1973) were able to obtain hybrids between mouse and rat myeloma cells.

More recently, Cohn (interview, March 15, 1990) suggested another explanation:

> So we studied a little bit, why didn't these cells fuse? We discovered that they carried a virus which excluded the Sendai. We needed something else if we were going to do fusion. In the meantime, Milstein using that same line in his first paper got fusion with Sendai and that I will never understand. I think what has happened is, he put more markers into it or he treated it in some way and by chance got a line that did not carry this excluding virus.[51] Therefore it fused with Sendai.

An additional sense of the capricious and unpredictable nature of work with cell lines[52] can be gathered from a 1978 letter that Renato Dulbecco, another Salk researcher, wrote to Milstein, requesting a seed culture of a derivative of the P3 cell line: "We have already made a determined effort using other myeloma lines obtained locally but so far we have had no success. We would like, therefore, to try your line" (Dulbecco to Milstein, April 27, 1978). Milstein had meanwhile already sent cell lines to the Salk Institute (where they originated!), specifically, to Cohn. So Dulbecco added: "I know that sublines of your line are available locally, but I would very much prefer to obtain them from you in order to avoid the possibility that there has been any confusion or special selection."

What did Cohn do upon reading MILSTEIN 75? Not much. He did not try the fusion: "We didn't even attempt to reproduce the first Milstein P3/Sendai experiment. We knew that it wouldn't work with our line" (interview, March 15, 1990). Moreover, Cohn seems to have been unimpressed with Köhler and Milstein's results: "In his first *Nature* paper with Köhler, . . . that fusion is very low frequency. If we had gotten it, we would have published it the way he did, but we would have considered it marginal" (interview, March 15, 1990). This might explain why he waited until January 1977 before writing to Milstein to request a sample of the P3-X63-Ag8 myeloma cell line: "Having heard five speakers talk about your derivative of P3, X63 Ag8, that is used in fusions, I am hoping that the line is available to the scientific community. I did not dare write to you previously and I have been too lazy to put the thioguanine marker into P3" (Cohn to Milstein, January 17, 1977).

Another factor played an important role in Cohn's decision to adopt hybridoma technology. In 1977 Milstein and collaborators published a paper (MILSTEIN 77a) in which, instead of Sendai virus, they used a chemical fusogen known as polyethylene glycol (PEG). PEG had been introduced to somatic cell hybridization by Pontecorvo (1975) in a paper that, after having been rejected by the first journal to which it was submitted, has now attained the status of a citation classic.[53] Upon reading MILSTEIN 77a, Cohn, already aware of Pontecorvo's paper, tried the fusion with his own standard line and it worked "beautifully."[54] As Cohn (interview, March 15, 1990) put it: "So they [Milstein et al.] made it work. The polyethylene glycol technique was what made the difference here."[55]

By now the (fictional) reader might have noticed a curious pattern. Scientists who "almost did it" argue as follows: First, they point out that everything was already in place when Köhler and Milstein performed their famous experiment; then, they transfer responsibility for the near miss to nonhuman actors. For Wistar's researchers the culprit was the missing "right partner"; for Cohn it was an insidious virus that had infected his myeloma cell lines. Theirs was not an intellectual failure, it was merely technical:

> The principle is very old. Cell hybrids of various kinds have been done between everything. It is a standard genetic technique. But even before, Harris did all this work on fusing cells and so on. So the introduction of it into the immune system was in the wind. The one who makes it work is the one who makes the advance. Intellectually, though, it was nothing. . . . Techniques are very often stumbled upon, a general principle is stumbled upon and then somebody improves it and improves it and so on and so forth. A thousand people can make hybridomas, it's opened up all sorts of industry and clinical diagnosis and all the rest of it. . . . If it works you're famous and if it doesn't work you've done nothing. It's not something that excites me, you see. . . . I think techniques are second order. You can't have science without the techniques, that's true. But it is the framework in which you do the experiment that's important. (Cohn, interview, March 15, 1990).

That this is not a resentful position, dictated by the bitterness of having missed it, can be seen by recalling a short-lived debate concerning the obviously forthcoming Nobel Prize for hybridoma technology. Should it be attributed to both Köhler and Milstein or to Milstein alone? In a paper in *Science*, Wade (1982) strongly argued for the former alternative.[56] In his reconstruction of the events leading to the "discovery," the idea and the decision to perform the experiment are attributed almost solely to Köhler, the postdoctoral student. Milstein, the head of the laboratory, is described as a somewhat reluctant partner, whose insight consisted in not opposing the conduct of the experiment, despite his knowledge of earlier failures by other researchers.

Opponents of Wade's argument quickly pointed out that, while this may indeed be true, Köhler's experiment could not have been performed elsewhere. Both the material and conceptual infrastructure of that experiment was provided by Milstein. What Köhler did was an additional, "merely technical" step, which rested on Milstein's previous work. In recalling this debate, our point is not to investigate, even less to settle, the matter of who did it.[57] Rather, we wish to point to the striking similarity between the argument of Wade's opponents and the argument of researchers such as Cohn. The main difference is that in one case it applies to workers within the same laboratory, whereas in the other case it applies to different laboratories involved in related lines of work.

This does not mean that Köhler and Milstein's contribution was inconsequential. As Malcolm Gefter, an MIT immunologist, put it (interview, November 8,

1985): "The major impact of Milstein' discovery was to show that it could be done.... An idea without an experiment is neither right nor wrong, it's just an idea." However, several interviewees also pointed out that the potential importance of monoclonal antibodies from the practical and scientific point of view was not immediately realized. Again, according to Cohn (interview, March 15, 1990): "Even after the Milstein paper appeared, most people wanted to use it for somatic cell genetics. We used [hybridoma technology] mostly for that. We did not use it to make reagents. I don't think we really appreciated how important that part would be technically."[58]

Gefter (interview, November 8, 1985) attributes this lack of appreciation to the fact that the initial experiments were performed in a scientific environment in a precommercialization era. It was only two or three years later, with the excitement generated by the patenting of recombinant DNA techniques, that people began to realize that monoclonal antibodies were an important milestone. According to Gefter, they became exciting molecules "in the midst of the whole hysteria for biotechnology." This explanation, however, while emphasizing the importance of socioeconomic contingencies, takes hybridoma technology for granted, as an entity that passively waited for the world to discover it. Against this possibility we shall show how a close analysis of the hybridoma technology foundational papers sheds light on its translation from a mere technique for a limited group of insiders into a powerful new tool for biology and medicine.

Milstein's Founding Tetralogy

Is it now time to return to our starting point and take a closer look at MILSTEIN 75? Well, not quite yet. We shall first look at MILSTEIN 77a and MILSTEIN 77b, because of the strategic place they occupy between the initial announcement of the successful development of what would become known as hybridoma technology and the description of this achievement as an event. It is indeed claimed that these papers correspond to a decisive turn in the career of hybridoma technology. Following their publication, requests for myeloma cell lines began to inundate Milstein's laboratory as well as other laboratories known to have received the cell line (Milstein, personal communication; Cohn to Milstein, June 9, 1977). In order to understand how this came about, let us start by looking at the opening paragraph of MILSTEIN 77a:

> Fusion between myeloma cells and spleen cells from immunised donors have been shown to be a successful method of deriving homogeneous anti-SRBC (anti-sheep red blood cell) and anti-TNP antibodies [ref.: MILSTEIN 75, MILSTEIN 76]. One of the most powerful features of this approach is that, by cloning, one may easily

derive cell lines synthesising monoclonal antibodies despite using non-purified immunogens. The multiple components of a heterogeneous population of hybrid cells are resolved by cloning techniques. This feature makes the system a very powerful tool in the study of complex antigenic structures. The established cell lines offer the further advantage of unlimited permanent supply of material, and the possibility of worldwide standardisation.

The first sentence of this opening paragraph refers to the fact that hybridoma technology, as devised in 1975, works, that is, it is a "successful method" to produce antibodies of predefined specificities. The two preceding papers, MILSTEIN 75 and MILSTEIN 76, however, applied this "successful method" to the production of anti-SRBC and anti-TNP antibodies, that is, of antibodies of no intrinsic scientific (or commercial) interest. SRBC and TNP were chosen because they were good immunogens and because the anti-SRBC system is part of a routine immunological technique (the Jerne plaque assay) for antibody activity detection; they were, in other words, a "convenient experimental device" (Milstein 1984). Moreover, they were easily and widely available, as opposed, for instance, to antigens of clinical interest that are sometimes very difficult to obtain, both because of the necessity of belonging to the "invisible college" where those antigens are available[59] and because of the need to develop an expertise in handling them.

As pointed out by MILSTEIN 75, "it remains to be seen whether similar results can be obtained using other antigens."[60] This is the question that MILSTEIN 77a had been designed to answer in the affirmative, establishing at the same time a strong genealogical link between MILSTEIN 75, MILSTEIN 76, and MILSTEIN 77a and redefining our understanding of the previous contributions. While in the original experiment the production of anti-SRBC antibodies could have been seen as an end in itself (an experimental system for immunogenetic studies), it became a necessary, preliminary step toward the constitution of hybridoma technology as a general technique.

MILSTEIN 77a presents itself as a demonstration of the usefulness of hybridoma technology, that is, of its applicability to scientifically, clinically, and commercially relevant antigens. Such a demonstration is carried out not only by reporting the production of monoclonal antibodies against some "interesting" antigen, but also by showing the advantages of hybridoma technology over preceding methods. The second sentence explains that you can actually use nonpurified immunogens (unavoidable when dealing with complex antigenic structures, such as the major histocompatibility antigens mentioned in the paper's title) and still get antibodies against the antigenic determinant you are interested in. This powerful feature is likely to appeal to a wide audience insofar as the purification of antigens was regarded as the most tedious and difficult part of anti-sera production. It is made possible by hybridoma technology's use of cloning techniques (third sentence), which thus becomes one of its distinctive features. As a result of this powerful feature, one is provided with a powerful tool for the potentially rewarding, and previously difficult and cumbersome, study of complex antigenic structures (fourth sentence).

The choice of major histocompatibility antigens as a target is particularly apt. Histocompatibility antigens, which establish the unique identity of a given organism's tissues, are of practical value for organ transplantation and of theoretical value. The distinction between self and non-self remains one of modern immunology's foundational metaphors (e.g., Moulin 1990; Tauber 1994). The final sentence of the opening paragraph completes the enrollment (Law 1983) of the reader by referring to two other overwhelming "advantages" of the technique: "unlimited permanent supply of material" and "worldwide standardization."

The latter claims were less descriptive than prospective, as permanent supplies were not immediately forthcoming. For example, a year later one reads in the Preface to the proceedings of the first major meeting on hybridomas (Melchers, Potter, and Warner 1978:xiii–xiv):

> Probably *the* major technical problem in this field is the difficulty to maintain a functional stable hybridoma. Although numerous examples were presented of functionally active and specific hybridomas that have been maintained for many months, the predominant pattern seems to be of loss of activity from the hybrid after a few months of culture. . . . Clearly the resolution of the problem of stability has not yet been found, and all efforts should be made to preserve lines at an early stage, during their functionally active state by freezing.

The claim of an unlimited permanent supply of material, in other words, played on the in principle/in practice distinction: "*In principle,* an unlimited supply of a monogeneous antibody specific for almost any antigen can now be obtained. *In practice,* a number of technical problems persist that can be understood by examining the hybridoma experiments in a little more detail." (Yelton and Scharff 1980, our emphasis).

Following the major histocompatibility antigens, MILSTEIN 77b tackled differentiation antigens. The paper's introduction summarizes the importance of this target. As defined in 1969 by Boyse and Old, differentiation antigens refer to cell surface molecules that are "not generally distributed on all tissues" and have therefore a double relevance: They "can be very useful in marking functional subpopulations of cells, and may also be the molecules which are involved in tissue-specific cell surface phenomena."[61] Antibodies are, in principle, powerful tools in the study of differentiation antigens. Major problems were encountered, however, in raising antibodies against specific differentiation antigens.

MILSTEIN 77b discusses the various attempts,[62] including Klinman's splenic fragments technique, to solve these problems. Finding them wanting,[63] the paper proposes MILSTEIN 75 and 76 as a solution. MILSTEIN 77b then performs a retrospective operation. Recall that sheep red blood cells were used as an antigen in the original MILSTEIN 75 experiment and that this choice was based on purely "technical" reasons (it is a good immunogen) rather than on its scientific interest. Now MILSTEIN 77b points out that the experiment actually resulted in the definition of three erythrocyte cell-surface molecules, thus retrospectively linking the study to the field of differentiation antigens. In fact, MILSTEIN 77b goes well beyond sheep red blood cells: "subpopulations of lymphoid cells in bone marrow and thoracic duct lymph," that is, cells of interest for clinical and basic research, are its main target.

Are we overinterpreting the case? In his Nobel Lecture, Milstein (1986) provided a gloss of papers such as MILSTEIN 77a and MILSTEIN 77b by noting that some time after his (and Köhler's) initial experiments, "it dawned on me that it was up to us to demonstrate that the exploitation of our newly acquired ability to produce monoclonal antibodies *à la carte* was of more importance than our original purpose. . . . For several years I shelved the antibody diversity problem to demonstrate the practical importance of monoclonal antibodies in other areas of basic research and in clinical diagnosis." The "practical importance of monoclonal antibodies" did not flow naturally from some alleged intrinsic properties of these entities: It was carefully constructed.[64]

As a contrast to MILSTEIN 77a and MILSTEIN 77b, and to finish our argument, let us return to MILSTEIN 75, a paper that, given the importance later attributed to it, is surprisingly short, three pages, half of which are taken up by figures.[65] We focus on two mutually constitutive tensions underlying the paper.

The introductory paragraph claims that while "the manufacture of predefined specific antibodies by means of permanent tissue culture cell lines is of general interest," available cultures (myeloma cells) are "not a satisfactory source of monoclonal antibodies of predefined specificity."[66] One might expect the paper to go on to explain that a general technique for establishing cultures secreting monoclonal antibodies of predefined specificity has been found. However, the paper is modest; it promises only to describe "the derivation of a number of tissue culture cell lines which secrete anti-sheep red blood cells (SRBC) antibodies." An initial, general statement captures the readers' interest only to draw them into the restricted topic of the paper (Law 1983).

The final section of the paper, however, reverses this procedure by leaving the narrow topic (anti-SRBC antibodies) and suggesting that: "Such [hybrid antibody-producing] cells can be grown *in vitro* in massive cultures to provide specific antibody. Such cultures could be valuable for medical and industrial use." This statement, in turn, is preceded by a more cautious one: "it remains to be seen whether similar results can be obtained using other [than SRBC] antigens." The rhetorical strategy of the paper is sustained by a continuous tension between well-documented specific claims and more or less cautious and open-ended claims concerning the possible transformation of those results into more general results. These claims, as we have seen, were taken up in later publications, starting in 1977, and were retrospectively used as evidence of a strong continuity between the initial experiments and what, after multiple translations, had by then become *hybridoma technology*.

This underlying tension is correlative with a second. As we pointed out during our discussion of the Schwaber affair, the oscillation between the reporting of facts and the description of a technique was clearly displayed in MILSTEIN 75. The introductory section of the paper announced a technique. The next three paragraphs dealt with the genetic basis of the cellular production of immunoglobulin (antibody) molecules, as reconstructed from experiments involving the fusion of two myelomas cell lines (as opposed to the fusion of a myeloma cell line with immunized spleen cells, which characterizes what will become known as hybridoma technology).

This section summarized previous work by recalling established "facts." Its explicit conclusion is a good indicator of its content: "we conclude that, as previously shown with interspecies hybrids, new [immunoglobulin] molecules are produced as a result of mixed association between heavy and light chains from the two parents," and "we conclude that in syngeneic cell hybrids (as well as in interspecies cell hybrids) V-C integration [i.e., integration of the genes coding, respectively, for the variable and constant sections of immunoglobulin molecules] is not the result of cytoplasmic events." This section can be read in at least two different ways: a) as a sort of a factual background that acts as a condition of possibility for the innovative, procedural work reported in the paper; and b) as a framework that gives meaning to the work reported in the paper. From this point of view, the legitimation of the technique lies not in the fact that it works, but, rather, in the existence of biological principles that account for it. In other words, we are confronted simultaneously with a biological fact and a technique. As we saw in the section on the Schwaber affair, this ambiguity is entertained by explicit reference to factual elements of previous work by Schwaber and Cohen, and by Cotton and Milstein.

An additional confirmation of the ambiguity of MILSTEIN 75 can be found in one of the earliest papers to cite it. In a 1976 article, Scharff and colleagues noted that even though the fusion of mouse myeloma cells to mouse fibroblasts or lymphoid cells [ref.: Periman 1970, Mohit 1971, Coffino et al. 1971] or to fibroblast and lymphoid cells from other species [ref.: MILSTEIN 73, SCHWABER 74] had been previously reported, the fusion of mouse myelomas had been extremely difficult to achieve. Describing a method for "routinely obtaining" such hybrids, they added: "While this manuscript was in preparation, Köhler and Milstein (1975) also reported the successful fusion of *mouse myeloma to mouse myeloma*" (Margulies, Kuehl, and Scharff 1976, our emphasis).

With hindsight such a characterization of MILSTEIN 75 might appear as a blunder ("Hey, they missed the 'real' meaning of that experiment"). Indeed, the same blunder can be found in MILSTEIN 75, which, as we saw in the Schwaber affair section, equated the fusion between two myelomas described in MILSTEIN 73 with the fusion between a myeloma and a lymphocyte described in SCHWABER 74. Last but not least, in the months following the publication of MILSTEIN 75, in papers given at conferences such as the Cold Spring Harbor Symposium, "Origins of Lymphocyte Diversity," held in the summer of 1976 (Milstein et al. 1977), or the Lake Placid conference, "Gene Expression and Regulation in Cultured Cells," held in the fall of 1976 (Milstein et al. 1978), Köhler and Milstein presented the experiments described in the 1975 *Nature* paper as little more than a way to study the genetics of antibody diversity.[67] Clearly, in 1975 and 1976 the hybridoma technique had not yet achieved the status of technology. The fate of the results presented in MILSTEIN 75 was not contained in that paper. It was in other people's (and other papers') hands. This will be the topic of Chapter 3.

Conclusions

More than once we have used a well-known rhetorical device: An argument was made, a fictional reader voiced objections, and we answered those objections, thus closing, at least temporarily, our argument. The use of this device raises a question: How is the presence of the fictional reader to be understood? Is it a mere rhetorical tool, or does this character designate somebody? Depending on the context, it could be seen as aimed at a number of straw men: traditional sociologists, whiggish historians, well-intentioned philosophers of science. Actually, none of these characters is the fictional reader. In fact, the latter refers to any of the scientific actors (Milstein, Schwaber, Koprowski, Cohn, and so on) who inhabit our narratives. In other words, the fictional reader is an icon for the "native" reader/writer who simultaneously produces and questions the products of that literary activity known as scientific texts by explicitly and implicitly raising the issue of the distinction between fact and technique.

By following the dispute over the novelty of Köhler and Milstein's contribution, we saw that it is not exactly clear which of the different elements of hybridoma technology should be regarded as novel. Was it the use of the P3 myeloma line? Was it the theoretical framework related to the notion of allelic exclusion? Was it. . . ? In each and every case, arguments for or against continuity or discontinuity with previous work can be made. And in each case the determination of novelty, as presented in the continuity/discontinuity issue, appeared to hang on the previous attribution of an epistemological status to the object that had allegedly been discovered: Was it a fact or a technique?

If one focuses on the relatively narrow network of immunogenetics, one could argue that a series of "facts" had been established that, when transferred to other fields, such as the virological research pursued in Koprowski's Institute, were translated into a technique. As we have seen, however, even from an immunogenetic point of view, the production of monoclonal antibodies can be seen as being simultaneously a fact and a technique to establish that fact. Not only was Milstein not seeking to develop a technique for the production of monoclonal antibodies when the original experiments were carried out, as he himself noted (Milstein 1980), but the significance later imputed to those experiments was not the same as their initial meaning. The paper was seen as one of a number of papers that used cell fusion techniques to dissect the genetic control of antibody diversity.

Distinctions that now appear crucial (e.g., were the fusion partners two myelomas or a myeloma and a spleen cell?) were easily overlooked. At some point, around 1977, the production of monoclonal antibodies became a goal in itself, independent of the initial immunogenetic network. The transformation of MILSTEIN 75 into the foundational event of hybridoma technology was thus achieved. This transformation did not flow naturally from the original experiments. Rather, as we shall see in Chapter 3, it involved specific investments that mobilized the activity of a large number of other scientific and industrial actors.

A tentative generalization can be deduced from our argument so far. The dichotomy between fact and technique that underlies much of contemporary science studies seems to be fundamentally misconceived insofar as the determination of what counts as a fact and what counts as a technique is not possible on *a priori* grounds. Historians and sociologists of science are confronted with a field of heterogeneous interventions in which parcels of work are constituted as discrete entities and simultaneously attributed a technical or a factual identity. Novelty and innovation are the result of such polymorphic attributional processes.

NOTES

1. For a critique of the assumption of epistemological unity see Hacking (1986).
2. See, for instance, the classical account by one of the co-discoverers: Watson (1968).
3. Fjermedal (1984:6–7) provides a journalistic account of this alleged blunder:

When the break finally came, it arrived well hidden within the August 7, 1975, issue of the prestigious British scientific magazine *Nature*. The editors of *Nature* will probably go to their graves trying to explain why they didn't see the full significance of the report, which was to cause immediate waves of excitement and communications throughout the world of medical research.

The cover of the August 7 issue of *Nature* was dedicated to desert locusts. The featured articles were "The Origin of Nucleic and of Eukaryotic Cells," "Paleolithic Remains at the Hadar in the Afar region," and "Integration of Viral Genomes."

Drs. César Milstein and Georges Köhler, of great Britain's Medical Research Council Laboratory of Molecular Biology in Cambridge, had offered their findings to *Nature* as an article, but instead it was relegated to the Letters to *Nature* section where it was preceded by letters on "Defensive Stoning by Baboons," "Three Remains in Southern Penine Peats," "Evidence for Visual Functions Mediated by Anomalous Projection in Goldfish," and 12 other similarly esoteric, though I would think interesting, subjects. Upon reaching the 16th letter, the perhaps bleary-eyed reader would have come across the title "Continuous Cultures of Fused Cells Secreting Antibody of Predefined Specificity."

See also Teitelman (1989:20): "Milstein and Köhler...submitted a short paper to *Nature,* the British scientific journal, but the editors buried it among the letters describing baboon behavior and goldfish physiology." These narratives are, of course, topical stories of unrecognized geniuses. As we shall see, it is, to say the least, not at all evident that Köhler and Milstein's paper "was to cause immediate waves of excitement and communications throughout the world of medical research." Moreover, the title of Köhler and Milstein's paper is, to a nonscientific reader, hardly less esoteric than the other titles quoted by Fjermedal, which, in any event, are not addressed to nonscientific readers.

4. From this point of view, the "right" comparison would be between Köhler and Milstein paper and the 1973 discovery of rDNA techniques by Herbert Boyer and Stanley Cohen.

5. This has also been done through scientometrics. See Rothman and Parkinson (1984).

6. MILSTEIN 77a is also linked to the ARC Institute of Animal Physiology and MILSTEIN 77b to the MRC Immunochemistry Unit, Department of Biochemistry, University of Oxford.

7. For instance, the following three papers (published in the Proceedings of three conferences): Milstein et al. (1978); Köhler, Hengartner, and Milstein (1978); Milstein et al. (1977).

8. This can be done in two ways. One is to follow the myeloma line by looking at the correspondence between Milstein and the laboratories that requested the myeloma line. We would like to thank Dr. Milstein for allowing us to make copies of this correspondence. It should, however, be pointed out that in the case of both Dr. Rajewsky and Dr. Koprowski, Dr. Milstein was unable to provide a written record of their request. Another way of following myelomas, is to consult the Materials and Methods and the Acknowledgments sections of the scientific articles in question.

9. We shall comment later on the choice of sheep red blood cells as the antigen.

10. Myelomas are also known as plasmacytomas. They can be "easily" produced by injecting mineral oil into the intraperitoneal cavity of BALB/c mice. See the later discussion.

11. See, however, the discussion in Chapter 3 of the complex infrastructure that makes such an "easy" task possible.

12. See later in this chapter and Chapter 3 for a more detailed account of the origins and circulation of myelomas.

13. For a discussion of Bussard's work on peritoneal cells, see Gaudilliére (1991).

14. Bussard, interview, August 20, 1989; Bussard, letters to the authors, August 8, 1991 and August 28, 1991; see also BUSSARD 78.

15. It is interesting to note that for BUSSARD 78:167–168 the reasons for this success remain somewhat obscure: "The success was probably due to their [Köhler and Milstein] careful choice of different parameters: the type of plasmocytoma used (called X63 Ag8), the mode of fusion, the screening procedures used to detect the antibody-producing cells, the subcloning procedure, etc."

16. The publication year of MILSTEIN 75 is erroneously cited as 1976.

17. Once again, the publication year of MILSTEIN 75 is erroneously cited as 1976.

18. See the later discussion for more details on Klinman's splenic fragments technique.

19. In a letter to *Science,* Hilary Koprowski and Carlo Croce (1980) reported that they had written

to Milstein in August 1976, "informing him that techniques for production of monoclonal antibodies against viruses were already developed at The Wistar Institute and requesting that Dr. Milstein furnish the myeloma cells in order to study further production of such antibodies;" one might easily surmise that the techniques "already developed at The Wistar Institute" involved the splenic fragments technique.

20. See later discussion for more details on cell fusion.

21. See later discussion for more details on Littlefield's selective medium technique.

22. The opening sentence of Klinman (1969) establishes a causal link between the clonal selection theory and the splenic fragments technique:

The currently accepted hypothesis concerning the mechanism of the immune response was stated by Burnet and others . . . and postulates that an antigen stimulates specific cells which possess the genetic information for the production of the appropriate antibody. Two assumptions implicit in this hypothesis are (a) that reactive cells have a limited genetic capacity to make antibody, and (b) that upon stimulation with antigen, such cells will proliferate and their clonal progeny will make identical antibody molecules. Thus the antibody produced by a cell and its clonal progeny should be homogeneous in its specific interaction with antigen.

The paper then goes on to explain how such clonal progeny could be isolated from spleens to obtain homogeneous antibodies.

23. Actually, Klinman's technique remained in competition with the hybridoma technique for a number of years following Köhler and Milstein's work. See note 63.

24. For a review of early work on cell fusion, see Steplewski and Koprowski (1970). For a popularized account of this work, see Koprowski (1969). For a review of later work (up to November 1973), see Koprowski and Knowles (1974).

25. This is true even after 1975. The first monoclonal antibodies produced at Wistar were directed against influenza virus and tumor antigens; in other words, monoclonal antibodies were used as a technique for molecular virology and tumor biology, as opposed to immunological research.

26. Matthew D. Scharff, head of the Albert Einstein College of Medicine's team, is a key figure in immunogenetics. He did extensive work with mouse myeloma cells, adapting them for cell culture, developing methods for detecting variants, and analyzing their synthesis, assembly, and secretion of immunoglobulins. His line of work was closely linked to Milstein's. See Chapter 3 for more details on Dr. Scharff.

27. From the point of view of the historian, this is a whiggish question; from the point of view of the actors, it follows from their previous argument.

28. A somatic cell geneticist from the Pasteur Institute in Paris, Gérard Buttin (interview, September 18, 1989), pointed out to us that in order to avoid the segregation of the immunoglobulin-producing genes, fusions must be performed between cells belonging to the same differentiation path (for instance, plasma cells and myelomas). Fusion of cells from different differentiation paths (for instance, myelomas and fibroblasts) results in segregation of characters that are not common to both cells. According to Buttin, cell biologists and somatic cell geneticists had long been familiar with this phenomenon; therefore, the failure of immunologists to act accordingly is a good example of disciplinary compartmentalization. The problem with this kind of account is that it is based on hindsight and assumes that immunologists were trying to produce monoclonal antibodies.

29. This operation can be performed not only retrospectively but also prospectively by, for instance, so-called essay reviews. While generally presented as a passive assessment of "the state of the art," they most often play a performative role, constituting the object and its meaning through the mapping of its future use(s). See chapter 3 for a detailed discussion of this issue.

30. It could be wondered why we have introduced the "interest" problem, because the fictional reader could have raised many other issues. The reason is quite simple: The interest problem figured prominently in all the interviews and discussions with scientists that broached the Koprowski case.

31. Compare this with the following anecdote, reported by in Wade (1982): When a member of the Horowitz Prize Committee of Columbia University was asked why the 1980 prize had been given to Milstein alone and not jointly to both Köhler and Milstein, he replied that "Milstein had previously

done work on rat-mouse hybridomas, from which this [hybridoma technology] was a logical consequence." Wade comments that "however, the rat-mouse hybrid cells studied by Milstein and Cotton were not hybridomas: they were hybrids between two myelomas, whereas a hybridoma is the fusion of a myeloma with a lymphocyte."

32. In the first part of the same paragraph, Yelton and Scharff evoke the contribution of another alleged precursor:

> It is a historical curiosity that a monoclonal antibody may have been generated by cell fusion as early as 1966. Sinkovics et al. . . . report injecting a diploid virus producing lymphoma into the peritoneal cavity of a mouse and recovering a tetraploid line that secreted a putative virus-neutralizing activity and two types of immunoglobulin. It was suggested that the immunoglobulins were the neutralizing factors and that the cell line arose by an in vivo fusion of a lymphoma cell to an antivirus-producing lymphocyte(s). The experiment was never successfully repeated, nor was it conclusive that cell fusion occurred.

Sinkovics (1981) had himself claimed priority in a letter to *Cancer Research:*

> The purpose of this correspondence is to direct attention to tetraploid murine lymphoma cell lines developed by us at the M.D. Anderson Hospital in the mid-1960's. . . . These cell lines resulted from the fusion of diploid, leukemia virus producer lymphoma cells (lymphoma 620), and immune spleen cells producing neutralizing antibodies to the leukemia virus. . . . The process of fusion was proposed and illustrated by us first in 1969. . . .
>
> The fused cells retained malignancy, grew in continuous cultures in spinner bottles or as ascites tumors in mice . . . , and produced leukemia viral antigens and particles, as well as immunoglobulins . . . that specifically neutralized a virulent mouse passage strain of the leukemia virus in mice. . . . These cell lines (in particular, cell line 818) were carried in continuous suspension cultures for a decade; now they are stored deep frozen.
>
> We did not propose in print that the fused cells may serve practical purposes as sources of antibodies; we did not call the fused cells "hybridomas." Instead, we suggested that fusion of this type should occur in the natural process of lymphoproliferative diseases.

On the priority of Sinkovics, see also Wainwright (1992:378), in which the following quote is attributed to Dr. Sinkovics:

> We made many mistakes, it was a "marketing error." In the late sixties medical research was practised in "noble purity." In the last ten years everybody has begun to patent all discoveries and promote them using the services of a marketing agent. We made a discovery but did not market it. We should have called it what it was, we should have called a press conference on it. We should have made lots of noise about, and of course patented it. It never occurred to us to patent it, or to call a press conference about it. At the time we were absolutely devastated that no one at meetings made adversarial or even complimentary comments about our work.

33. It actually cites only MILSTEIN 73 and SCHWABER 74, but SCHWABER 73 and SCHWABER 74 can be considered to contain similar material. One could question MILSTEIN 75's choice of citing the later article, rather than the earlier one, which, chronologically speaking, would have been contemporaneous with MILSTEIN 73.

34. This seems to correspond to a larger (mis)perception. In a table summarizing different fusion experiments, Buttin and Cazenave (1980) list SCHWABER 73 along with MILSTEIN 73 as reporting a fusion between two myelomas.

35. Milstein and Munro (1973) is a comprehensive review of previous work on immunogenetics.

36. The degree of externality increases with the number of inferential steps that one is ready to take from the rough data to the imputation of their meaning. Pinch also relates different degrees of externality to different evidential contexts.

37. See also another immunologist's recollection: "It was not the first time that people thought about trying to do cell-cell fusions, but this [Köhler and Milstein's experiment] was the first time it was successful." (Ita Askonas quoted in Tansey and Catterall 1994:325).

38. In a letter to the authors (September 10, 1991), César Milstein points out that his recollections of the events are "quite different" from those of Georges Köhler reported by Wade. On the occasion of the joint award by the Lasker Foundation, Milstein and Köhler issued a statement that was never published, in which they pointed out that "both conception and execution of the work was [sic] the result of close collaboration," and that "the combined effect which resulted from such collaboration was of a synergistic nature." Milstein claims not to have replied to Wade's account because of "a previous [bad] experience with him regarding the Koprowski patent." On the other hand, Georges Köhler (letter to the authors, January 20, 1992) states that "[m]ost information about hybridomas has been well summarized by Wade in *Science 215:* 1073, as you are probably aware of."

39. See also Littlefield (1987), who notes that Ephrussi's and Harris's views "are personal, sometimes contrasting."

40. See also Okada (1962). Okada's fusogen, a strain of the parainfluenza I group of myxoviruses known as the HVJ virus, is now called Sendai virus.

41. See also Littlefield (1964b). Littlefield's work, as he himself pointed out (Littlefield 1973), built on previous work by Szybalski. See, for example, Szybalski, Szybalska, and Ragni (1962).

42. Plasma cells were later shown to be the antibody-producing cells.

43. Chapter 6 ("A Crucial Experiment of Nature: Multiple Myeloma and the Structure of Antibodies") in Swazey and Reeds (1978) provides a historical overview of immunological research related to multiple myeloma. For the mouse side of the story, see Potter (1986).

44. Locally produced cell lines were similarly named after the name of the technician who produced them: S1, S2, S3 . . . for Stanley; J1, J2, J3 . . . for Jones; and so on (Cohn, interview, March 15, 1990).

45. MILSTEIN 73 uses a derivative of another cell line obtained from Horibata, P1, which is fused with a rat tumor cell line developed by a Belgian researcher, Hervé Bazin.

46. See the references in Yelton et al. (1980).

47. For a short history of the screening of myeloma proteins, see Potter (1986).

48. It should also be mentioned that in an attempt to produce antibodies with molecular uniformity for studies of the chemical structure of the immunoglobulins, some researchers attempted immunization with simple antigens with small, repeating structural subunits; see Krause (1970).

49. Both Koprowski and Cohn tried this technique and failed (Gerhard, interveiw, September 29, 1987; Cohn, interview, March 15, 1990).

50. Cohn (interview, March 15, 1990) claims to have supplied genetically marked P3 cells to Milstein, whereas the latter (letter to the authors, September 10, 1991) claims that he received "a wild type clone, which was not genetically marked in any way." Milstein claims further that the introduction of the markers was indeed a major problem, whose solution was decisive: "For the [two years prior to Köhler's arrival], we tried to make a mouse azoguanine-resistant line, including several attempts at P3. We (me and my assistant, Shirley Howe) failed to do so. However, out of a very long-term culture of a subclone of P3 (almost a year in continuous culture, and used for the isolation of spontaneous mutants), Georges Köhler tried once again, and obtained the azoguanine-resistant line, which became the parental line which is widely used for hybridoma technology." (Ibid.).

51. See note 50. Milstein (letter to the authors, September 10, 1991) points out that he and his co-workers "only put the markers which were suitable for the Littlefield procedure. The line we received did not contain any such biochemical markers." He, however, adds that "it is also true that the long-term culture from which the azoguanine resistant line was selected may have been a reason why our cell line was better than others, tried at a later stage."

52. See also, on this topic, the very entertaining book by Michael Gold (1986).

53. The circumstances surrounding this work are described in Pontecorvo (1990). In addition to Milstein's laboratory, researchers from both the Wistar Institute (Steplewski, Koprowski, and Leibovitz 1976) and the Albert Einstein College of Medicine (Gefter, Margulies, and Scharff 1977) quickly adopted PEG as a fusogen in mammalian somatic cell hybridization.

54. Actually the PEG technique did not work right away. PEG is available in various sizes. The PEG of the size used by Milstein did not work in Cohn's laboratory, and it was only when he used

another size that Cohn, who by now knew that it could be done, was able to produce a successful fusion (Cohn, interview, March 15, 1990). As noted by Buttin et al. (1978): "PEG concentration is difficult to control locally in most reported fusion procedures which rely on 'gentle pipetting' for the removal of the culture medium and timer-controlled resuspension of the cell pellets in a PEG solution." For more details on this issue, see Chapter 2.

55. Cohn's opinion is shared by Yelton et al. (1978) when they note that "*[w]ith improvements in the techniques of fusing myeloma cells. . .* , the basic approaches described by Köhler [sic] and Milstein. . .have gained wide acceptance" (our emphasis). Reference to a paper on PEG fusion makes clear that the introduction of this chemical fusogen ranks among the decisive "improvements." Similarly, Buttin et al. (1978), note: "The high efficiency of polyethylene-glycol (PEG) as a fusing agent for fibroblasts and its ability to yield hybrids *in cell combinations recalcitrant to Sendai virus. . .* has led most groups to substitute this simple chemical for the agglutinating virus" (our emphasis).

56. The awarding of the Nobel Prize is routinely preceded by the attribution of other prizes, including, for instance, the Lasker Prize. Some of these prizes were awarded to Milstein alone, and this was denounced by Wade.

57. On Milstein's assessment of Wade's reconstruction of the events leading to the discovery of hybridoma technology, see note 38.

58. See also Springer (1985:xi): "Soon after the publication of the hybridoma technique in 1975, it was not widely appreciated what a dramatic impact it would have. Widespread use of monoclonal antibodies came first in the field where they were developed, immunology."

59. For instance, it is not surprising that one of the leaders in the production of monoclonal antibodies directed against cell surface antigens of human leucocytes, Stuart F. Schlossman, could count on an extensive leucocyte cancer cell bank accumulated over the years in connection with Harvard Medical School and the Dana Farber Cancer Institute; see Keating and Cambrosio (1994).

60. As we have seen, this point was indeed raised by Hilary Koprowski to counter accusations that he had patented the basic Köhler and Milstein technique. Moreover, in the months following the publication of MILSTEIN 75, the operational status of the technique was still uncertain. In a paper presented in the fall of 1976 at Lake Placid in New York, Köhler and Milstein commented on their *Nature* paper as follows: "These experiments suggest that it *may* be possible to fuse myeloma cells and normal antibody-producing cells so that the resulting hybrid line could carry the antibody-producing capacity of one parent and the ability to grow in vitro or as tumors of the other parent" (our emphasis); see Milstein et al. (1978).

61. A contemporary example, unfortunately familiar to most readers, of the clinical relevance of differentiation antigens is the identification of a depletion of T4 cells in AIDS; T4 cells are a subpopulation of T cells (lymphocytes), as defined by the presence of differentiation antigens. The classification of lymphocytes on the basis of differentiation antigens is said to have been revolutionized by hybridoma technology. On this issue see Cambrosio and Keating (1992). Another much vaunted possible clinical application of differentiation antigens is the presence of tumor-specific antigens that could differentiate cancer cells from normal cells, thus making them the possible target of diagnostic and (immune) therapeutic measures.

62. One approach is allogeneic immunization (raising antisera within a species), which detects polymorphic molecules (i.e., no antibodies are raised against molecules that are common to the tissues of that particular species). Major problems are that sera raised in this way are weak and many cell surface molecules go undetected. The other approach is xenogeneic immunization (one species immunized with material from another species). Here the problem is that the resulting immune response is very complex.

63. In 1978 some researchers still presented Klinman's technique as an alternative to Köhler and Milstein's. See, for example, Levy, Dilley, and Lampson (1978): "If the intent is to examine the mouse repertoire of evokable antibody responses to human cell surface antigens, and to quickly define as many antigens as possible, then we prefer the technique of fragment culture [Klinman' technique]. However, if large quantities or stable sources of standard reagents are to be produced, then somatic cell hybridization [Köhler and Milstein's technique] is preferred."

64. For further elaboration of this point, see Chapter 3.

65. Historians of molecular biology will, however, not be so surprised. The 1953 Watson and Crick paper on the double helix was even shorter, two pages.

66. See the earlier discussion in the Cohn connection section. Köhler and Milstein's claim that myeloma cells are not a "satisfactory" source of monoclonal antibodies can be glossed in the following way: a) Their usefulness as a research *model* is limited by the fact that it is very difficult to find out which antigen is the target of such an immunoglobulin, and b) the specificity of the immunoglobulin secreted by a myeloma cell line cannot be predetermined by the researcher, and this eliminates its usefulness as a *general research tool*.

67. An interesting twist, in this respect, is provided by the question of secreting versus nonsecreting myelomas. When using as a fusion partner a myeloma that secretes it own immunoglobulin, the resulting hybrid will secrete a mixture of immunoglobulins, from which the immunoglobulin of *predefined specificity* must then be isolated. By using nonsecreting myelomas, only the immunoglobulin produced by the parent spleen cell will be secreted by the hybrid. It is therefore often maintained that the production of nonsecreting myelomas constituted a major advance in the technique. It is, however, important to note that Köhler himself continued to study hybridomas using myelomas, which secreted immunoglobulins for some time after the isolation of nonsecreting myelomas. In the initial experiments, hybridomas obtained from the fusion of spleen cells with secreting myelomas were considered interesting in their own right. The way antibodies were assembled out of elements of both parent cells offered important insights into the genetic constitution of antibody proteins; see Köhler, Hengartner, and Shulman (1978).

2
The Art and Science of (Re)Producing Monoclonal Antibodies

> *Dire ce qui reste non-dit* quand tout semble dit n'est pas l'opération ultime d'une synthèse confinant au délire, car le discours de ce non-dit ne peut en aucun cas être ajouté, pour le compléter, à celui qui semblait pouvoir tout dire.
> Descombes (1977:178)

In January of 1976, less than a year after the publication of MILSTEIN 75, Dr. Allan Jones, a researcher in the Department of Clinical Microbiology at a major London hospital sent the following letter to César Milstein (Jones to Milstein, January 20, 1976): "I understand from Professor Scharff of Albert Einstein College of Medicine, N.Y., that your group is working with a clonable myeloma (P3) which behaves rather similarly to the MPC 11 which has been cloned by him. I am interested in attempting some work with such a system. Would it be possible to supply me with such a culture?"[1]

Milstein complied and by March Jones had the culture well established in his lab (Jones to Milstein, March 14, 1976). However, nine months later, in December of 1976, he was still unable to repeat Köhler and Milstein's work "on the production of cell lines secreting monoclonal antibodies" (Jones to Milstein, December 24, 1976).[2] Believing that the cell line Milstein had sent him was different from the one used in the production of hybridomas, Jones wrote again to Milstein, asking whether the explanation for the difficulties he was experiencing "might not lie in some special property of the P3-X67Ag8 clone used by you" and requesting a culture of the latter (ibid.).

In his reply, Milstein noted that while there had been some confusion over the nomenclature of P3 derivatives, the cell line Jones had received was the same as the one he was now requesting (Milstein to Jones, January 12, 1977).[3] As for the problems Jones had encountered, Milstein acknowledged the existence of various "bugs" that were liable to creep into the system, mentioning problems related to the use of horse serum, Sendai virus, and toxic HAT concentrates; a shift from horse to fetal calf serum and the replacement of Sendai virus with polyethylene glycol fusion had apparently taken care of the most acute problems (ibid.). Nonetheless, even with this information, by March of 1977 Jones was still experiencing difficulty and, following the suggestion of several colleagues, arranged a visit to Milstein's lab in order to master the technique (Jones to Milstein, March 28, 1977; Milstein to Jones, May 4, 1977).

This is an episode in the transmission of knowledge. It illustrates the relation between written instructions and "hands on," experiential learning, between the well-ordered world of experimental protocols and the unpredictability of recalcitrant materials and reagents. It has been reported, as the letter exchange mentioned earlier confirms, that following the initial success both Milstein and Köhler (who had in the meantime returned to Basel) were unable to reproduce the experiment for about six months.[4]

The problem of replication resurfaced with a vengeance when other researchers attempted to implement the procedure developed in Milstein's lab. Some researchers told us that they had been able to implement hybridoma technology almost immediately, while others acknowledged that it had taken them several months to reproduce the technique, and still more time before producing "useful" monoclonals on a routine basis. Because replication is a precondition of diffusion, it seems appropriate to discuss the problems in using hybridoma technology before moving on, in Chapter 3, to an analysis of how it was transformed into a success story of modern biomedical technology.

The problem of replication and the various levels of knowledge involved in daily laboratory practice concern not only scientists; they have also become a standard topic in the sociology of scientific knowledge.[5] This is not surprising, because the latter is often characterized by an ethnographic approach. Issues of relevance to the "natives" ought to loom large in this kind of sociology. There are, however, different ways of understanding the relationship between actors' accounts and sociological accounts. It is often held, for example, that the categories used by sociologists are ignored or unrecognized by the actors they study, both because of some alleged epistemic privilege of the observer over the observed and because, as a condition of their efficacy, the forces and interests that supposedly account for the actors' behavior ought to remain inaccessible to them.[6] In contrast, we shall argue that categories such as tacit or local knowledge are not only accessible to the actors, often in the form of categories such as art and magic, but that they are consciously manipulated by them as part of their effort to determine the status of a procedure such as hybridoma technology, that is, in order to *make* procedures reproducible by regulating, among other things, the circulation of people, protocols, and biological materials.

In what follows we first provide a brief overview of how sociologists have translated the question of replication into the examination of the different kinds of knowledge—local, tacit, etc.—at work in scientific practices. We then move to a participant-centered account of how scientists view and manage the implementation of hybridoma technology in their laboratories and how they categorize the components of the technology according to the kind of knowledge they embody.

Sociological Accounts of Local and Tacit Knowledge

As we pointed out in the introduction, the sociology of science has moved from the study of scientific communities to the problem of the construction of scientific knowledge (Knorr-Cetina and Mulkay 1983). This change of interest has resulted in a shift in the scope and object of sociological inquiry, as evidenced by the many laboratory studies and analyses of scientific controversies, both of which have tended to highlight the contingent elements of scientific knowledge. Laboratory studies, for example, have described the local dimensions of scientific knowledge and the processes whereby the latter are integrated into the sanctioned corpus of science (Latour and Woolgar 1986; Knorr-Cetina 1981; Lynch 1985; Star 1983). Similarly, research bearing on the conduct of scientific controversies has stressed the negotiable elements in these episodes and the role played by tacit understanding in the replication of disputed experience (Collins 1985; Pinch 1986). In this context, the categories of *local knowledge* and *tacit knowledge* have gained central importance. However, the meaning given to these notions is hardly uniform, and there is indeed some confusion surrounding their use.

While the terms *local knowledge* and *tacit knowledge* have often been used as either synonymous or overlapping, some authors have taken great pains to distinguish them. Knorr-Cetina (1981:37–40 and 127–130), for example, has proposed an analysis of scientific knowledge that distinguishes public knowledge, tacit knowledge, and local knowledge (know-how). The first two categories are separated from the third on the basis of *availability*. According to Knorr-Cetina, public knowledge and tacit knowledge refer to scientific knowledge that is "generally available" to the scientific community, while local knowledge is composed of the largely inaccessible idiosyncrasies of the individual researcher or laboratory. Knorr-Cetina's classification of knowledge corresponds, on the one hand, to the categories of scientific institutions used by sociologists and historians (i.e., field, discipline, institute) and, on the other, to the classification of knowledge used by scientists in their daily practice (i.e., science, art, magic).[7]

Michael Lynch's notion of tacit knowledge is similar to Knorr-Cetina's notion of local knowledge. Lynch (1982, 1985), however, has gone further in removing all reference to individuals as possible repositories of knowledge. For Lynch, tacit knowledge, unlike Knorr-Cetina's local knowledge, is "not anybody's knowledge." In fact, Lynch's ethnomethodological approach is an attempt to go beyond the description of the unwritten knowledge that circulates within a given scientific discipline in order to describe a more fundamental form of knowledge, incorporated in the practices themselves. This knowledge is taken for granted by the researchers and, although un-noticed, plays a central role in the conscious evaluation of experiments and experimental results, giving rise to what Lynch terms *endogenous critical inquiry* (as opposed to professional sociological inquiry).

Harry Collins's work on scientific controversies also relies to a great extent on the notion of tacit knowledge. In contrast to Knorr-Cetina and Lynch, however, Collins (1987) is less interested in the actors' practices than in using the notion of tacit knowledge as the key to constructing his emerging "science of knowledge." In particular, Collins has proposed a division of the domain of cognition into four components: facts and rules, heuristics, manual and perceptual skills, and cultural skills. The last two elements of Collins's analysis are members of the category of tacit knowledge, which is the knowledge required to use formal and informal rules but which cannot, without being fundamentally transformed, be verbalized or formalized.

Applied to the analysis of scientific controversies, Collins's approach shows that at the heart of a dispute lies the *experimenter's regress*, which is described as the following situation. Because of the artisanal nature of scientific experiments, a researcher's competence and the reliability of his or her experiment can only be assessed on the basis of the results obtained. Because, however, the results can be considered valid only if they are obtained from reliable experiments, any assessment is necessarily flawed by circular reasoning. Collins argues that scientists are able to break this circle of reason and hence close controversy by negotiation, the consensual resolution of which depends upon the prior existence of a network of social relations and therefore an institutionalized "form of life" for the researchers (Collins 1985).

This model of scientific practice, referred to as *enculturational*, allots tacit knowledge the key role in the production of new knowledge and is thus at variance with what Collins terms the *algorithmic model* defended by researchers when they are asked to account for their activity. According to this latter model, scientific practice is described by scientists themselves as the application of rules (scientific knowledge being composed solely of formal and informal rules). Insofar as Collins's model is opposed to the scientist's model of scientific practice, it is reducible to the distinction between what can be said and what cannot: "the crucial division in knowledge is not the separation between information and heuristics . . . but between the articulateable and the tacit" (Collins, Green, and Draper 1985:329).[8]

In more recent contributions, Collins has specified his position by resorting to two mutually constitutive sets of distinctions (Collins 1990; Collins, de Vries, and Bijker 1990).[9] The first distinction is between *embodied capabilities*, that is, those human capabilities that can only be transferred through socialization, and *repertoires*, that is, those capabilities that can be transferred through inscriptions, in a context-free, material form. The second distinction is between *regular action*, characterized by a flexible instantiation of behavior, and *behavior-specific* or *machinelike action*, which corresponds to the instantiation of a repertoire. For our present purpose, the relevant point is how these distinctions apply to the transmission of knowledge.

According to Collins, embodied capabilities can be learned only through apprenticeship or socialization. Machinelike behavior can similarly be learned through apprenticeship or socialization, but it can be also learned by following instructions or rote repetition (in the case of simple machinelike behavior) or simulation (in the case of complex machinelike behavior). The essential thing here is that "regular action cannot be learned except through socialization or apprenticeship" (Collins, de Vries, and Bijker 1990).

Whether one agrees with it or not, Collins's argument is certainly relevant to philosophical discussions about the possibility of artificial intelligence, in relation to which it has indeed been developed. The extent to which his argument has any utility for an ethnographic account of scientific practice, however, is far less clear. From the latter point of view, the question is not whether or not a certain kind of action—regular or machinelike—or a certain form of knowledge—skills, explicit knowledge, etc.—can *in principle* be learned in a given way but to understand how actors classify actions and how they regulate the transmission of knowledge. In addition, because Collins's scheme is scarcely predictive of the category in which a given particular action should be classified or, in other words, of which domains will eventually be transformed into machinelike domains, his approach does not offer any advantage over postfactum narratives.

The various conceptions of local or tacit knowledge supplied by sociologists[10] suggest that tacit knowledge is impossible to articulate, and yet it is not clear why this should be so. If tacit knowledge is that which one knows without knowing how to say it, then there are certainly things that are known and cannot be said that can nonetheless be shown and formally transmitted in this manner. In this respect, Ferguson's (1985) work is quite instructive. According to this author, there is, in the area of machine production, "an enormous quantity of nonverbal knowledge which has accrued and which has been diffused through published diagrams."[11] Surely the transmission of nonverbal knowledge may in some way count as an instance of the articulation of the tacit.

Indeed, it is rarely specified why certain kinds of knowledge cannot, by their nature, be enunciated. One could easily imagine, on the contrary, that some things are left unsaid not because of the impossibility of their being said but for a variety of other reasons. For example, an individual's silence may be the result not of an inability to verbalize, but of the perception of the trivial nature of what might have been said. Surely, some things are generally accepted as being known to all within a given discipline and hence trivial. One could, moreover, conceive of knowledge unspoken for fear of sanctions or knowledge unspeakable within a certain conceptual framework (or paradigm, or disciplinary matrix). In other words, the restriction of the tacit to the unsaid does not necessarily entail that the tacit is by nature nonverbal; much that is unsaid clearly has the possibility of being verbalized but remains, for many reasons, unsayable, unthinkable, trivial, secret, or censored (Descombes 1977:41).[12] In other words, what we need is not a science but an ethnography of (tacit) knowledge.

One of the effects of ascribing a nonverbal, inaccessible, nontransmissible nature to tacit knowledge has been to reinforce the assumption that we are here dealing with a form of knowledge largely beyond the control and manipulation of scientists, that we have entered the unconscious or, at least, nonconscious realm of science. As previously indicated, we shall argue to the contrary, that the unsaid is indeed a part of conscious scientific practice and hence subject to negotiation, discussion, and (re)construction. Questions of local knowledge, tacit knowledge, and magic, far from being ignored by scientific researchers, are explicitly a part of their daily practice.[13] These questions give rise to a series of social *and* technical distinctions that are constitutive of scientific work. It follows then that the establishment of a typology of knowledge is not only the preoccupation of the sociologist but is also a recognized issue for scientists.

The Art of Producing Hybridomas

Several observers have noted that, since its inception in 1975, the procedure used to manufacture monoclonal antibodies has remained for the most part unchanged (French et al. 1986; Westerwoudt 1985).[14] That is to say, according once again to scientists, that it has remained a largely *artisanal* technique. Before looking into the possible meaning of the characterization of hybridoma technology as artisanal, let us recap very briefly the various steps involved in the procedure (some of these steps have been discussed in Chapter 1; see also Figure 2.1).

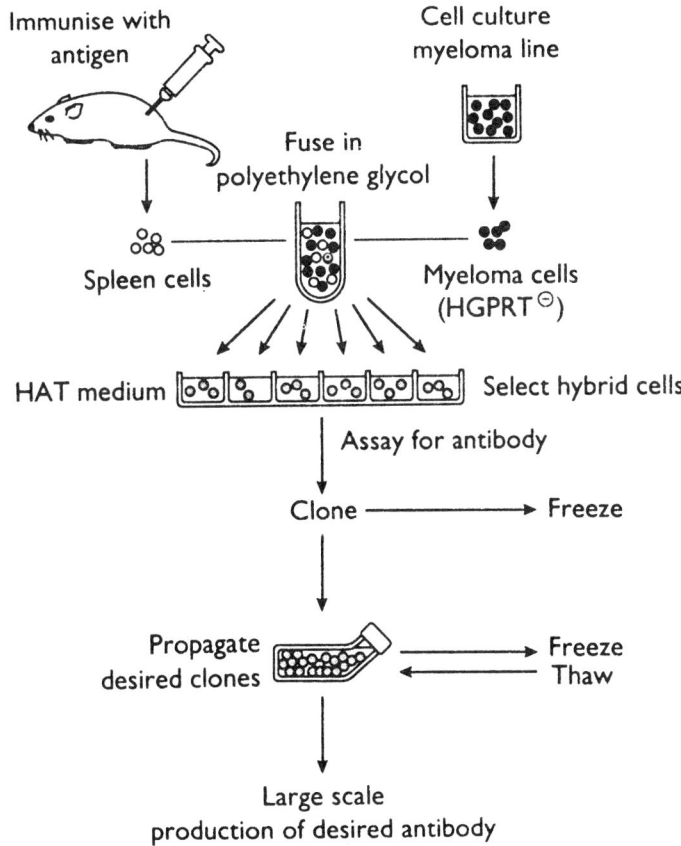

Figure 2.1. A schematic representation of the procedure for producing hybridomas, (Source: Llewelyn, Hawkins, and Russell 1992.) See Figure 2.6 for a different schematic representation of hybridoma technology.

The animals (mice and, more recently, rats) must first be injected with the chosen antigen in order to be immunized. After a delay of several weeks, the spleen of the immunized animal is extracted, the antibody-producing cells of the spleen are suspended in a medium, and they are mixed with myelomas in the presence of an agent that promotes cell fusion (as discussed in Chapter 1, Sendaï virus, used in the initial experiments, was replaced in 1976 by a chemical substance, polyethylene glycol [PEG]). Following fusion, successfully fused cells or *hybridomas* are separated from the unfused cells; this is accomplished by placing the mixture in a solution (so-called HAT medium) in which only the hybrids will survive.

After a period of growth in culture, hybridomas producing the required antibodies are selected using a variety of techniques (for example, immunoassays).

The selected hybridomas are then cloned, cultivated, and frozen for conservation. Subsequently, the hybridomas may be either cultivated in vitro in order to harvest antibodies secreted in the medium or injected into animals, where they generate ascitic tumors, which in turn secrete antibodies into the animal's internal cavity. Depending upon the reason for which the antibodies were produced, the latter may be submitted to a series of additional manipulations, including purification, immunochemical characterization, and conjugation with radioactive or enzymatic labels.

Hybridoma technology is thus composed of a series of steps that call upon different domains of expertise loosely identified with different disciplines. The initial immunization, for example, is most closely related to immunology, the fusion procedure falls within the realm of cell biology or cell genetics, and the immunoassays used for the selection of the hybridomas as well as the various procedures used to characterize the antibodies are more closely identified with immunochemistry or biochemistry. Hybridoma technology invariably draws upon expertise in cell culture, the sterile manipulation of biological material, as well as the disciplines related to the antigen of interest (virology in the case of viral antigens, bacteriology in the case of bacterial antigens, etc.). This breakdown of the procedure into a series of domains of technical expertise is not an analytical artifact but is to be found in both written and oral reports of success in implementing hybridoma technology, when, for instance, scientists account for their proficiency by mentioning their previous disciplinary training in some of the techniques involved in hybridoma technology.

What makes hybridoma technology artisanal, and what does it mean to be so? In order to answer these questions, we shall consider both written sources, such as technical manuals, and informal statements gathered through interviews and laboratory discussions. We shall thus be able to assess what counts as artisanal and to show that this category is indeed a component of scientists' discourse.

It is well known that knowledge and know-how in hybridoma-related fields have long circulated informally. According to Goding (1983:3), "[i]mmunochemistry has an oral tradition, and a surprising number of key elements are not easily accessible from the literature." The artisanal nature of hybridoma technology is evident in the fact that the training necessary for its manipulation takes the form of an apprenticeship. As an academic researcher remarked (interview, winter 1986), "it's difficult to learn a technique which is art from a paper." Even manuals offering instruction in the technique maintain a similar opinion:

> The newcomer to hybridization is well advised to learn the technique in a laboratory which is already practicing fusion. It has been a frequent observation that newcomers to the technique are relatively unsuccessful initially and obtain many hybrids after some practice, although an experienced observer cannot see any

> difference between the technique used on the first day and in subsequent, successful experiments. The best approach is therefore to learn from an experienced laboratory and practice until hybrids are obtained. (Zola and Brocks 1982:4–5).

Art, in other words, inevitably has a local dimension, both in terms of a particular lab and of the particular kind of biological material one is working with.

> Every lab developed their own tricks. They are very simple things but if it works and you know why you keep it that way. So some people fused them in a Petri dish on a flat surface. We always used centrifuge tubes. And the product is always the same.... The conditions, almost for each lab, have to be developed.... Because different cell lines behave differently and so on.
> (Interview with an academic researcher, fall 1987).

The artisanal features of the technique are further reinforced by the often unpredictable nature of the results obtained.

> The waywardness of the original method, repeatedly commented upon by its originators, is best demonstrated by comparing tests set up and run under identical conditions. The wide scatter of results is typical: the odds of obtaining hybrid clones in all culture cups or in none is about the same.
> (Fazekas De St. Groth and Scheidegger 1980:5).

> It is quite common for a laboratory to have success for several months and then failure for as long a period. So the immediate record of a laboratory is more important than the long-term one. Even within a research group one individual may fail where others succeed and this is a reason for encouraging separate reagents and cell lines. (Campbell 1984:156).

> The fusion does not invariably work. Often a repeat of the fusion process without obvious changes results in successful hybridization.
> (*Hybridoma Techniques* 1980:4).

While the rate of successful fusion does indeed increase with time, expertise is not identified with the possibility of succeeding every time. Rather, expertise is equated with the ability to operate confidently in an experimental situation characterized by a high degree of uncertainty (Star 1983). This persisting state of uncertainty is said to follow from the interaction of "nature" and a given researcher's professional trajectory: "the diversity of published approaches [to hybridoma technology] reflects both individual biological problems and previous experience" (Goding 1983:56).

To be experienced in an art, to have expertise, implies the mastery of specific ways of seeing and doing. The nature of these skills and the difficulty of their transmission can best be seen in the following example. After a certain growth period, it is necessary to transfer the hybridomas from a 96-well microplate to another in order to ensure their continued survival (Figures 2.2 and 2.3). If they are transferred too soon, there is a possibility they will not survive the transfer; if too much time elapses, there is a possibility they will die in the original microplate wells. It is furthermore necessary that the hybridomas be left in the original wells long enough to have secreted sufficient antibody to make possible their screening as producers of the desired antibody. The moment of transfer is thus a crucial step in the procedure, and its determination requires scrutiny of the color of the culture liquid (which contains a pH indicator), the form of the cells, and their size. These parameters, however, cannot be analyzed in isolation. The decision to transfer depends upon the perception of a synthetic variable referred to as the *viability of the culture*. The perception of culture viability allows the experienced researcher to decide when the fused cells should be transferred and requires learning how to look at cells (Figure 2.4):

> As the cells become very dense, *they start to look unhealthy*, and viability drops.
> (Goding 1983:67, emphasis added).

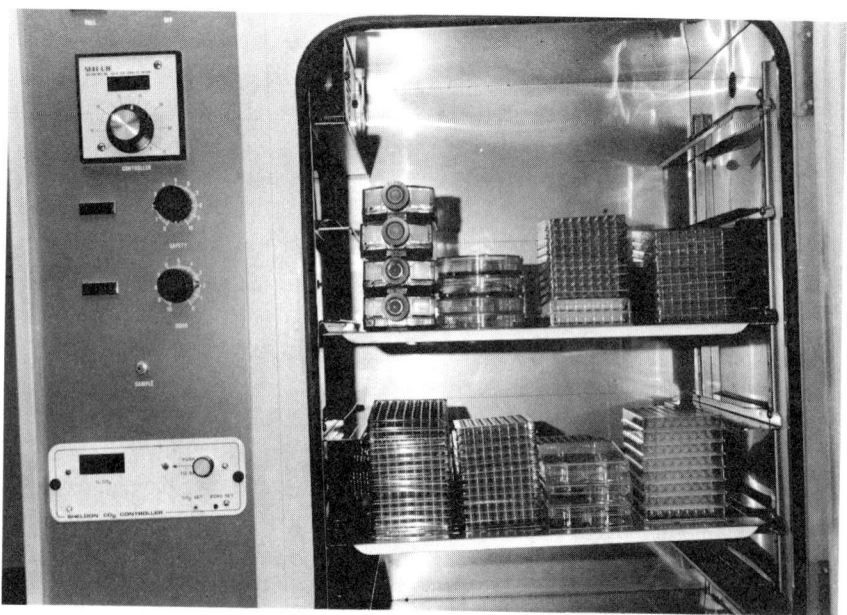

Figure 2.2. Cell-culture plates in a CO_2 incubator (photo: Jack Goldsmith). Compare with Photograph 2 in Latour and Woolgar (1986:93).

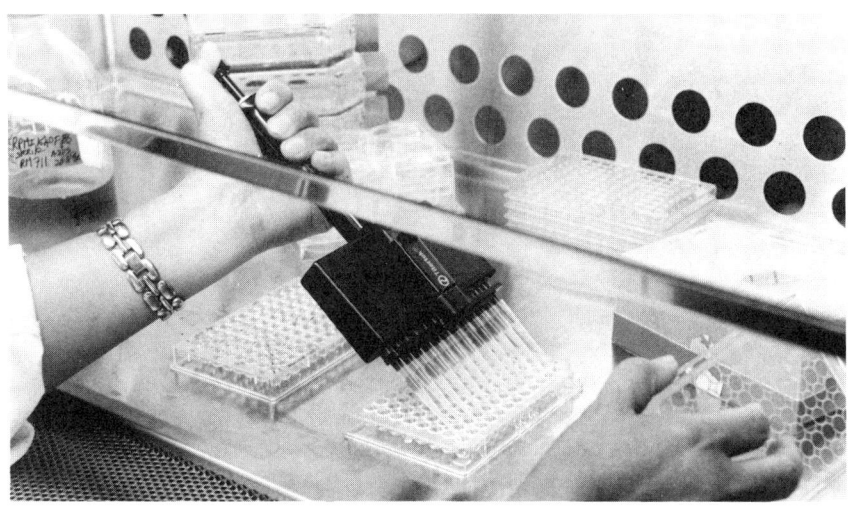

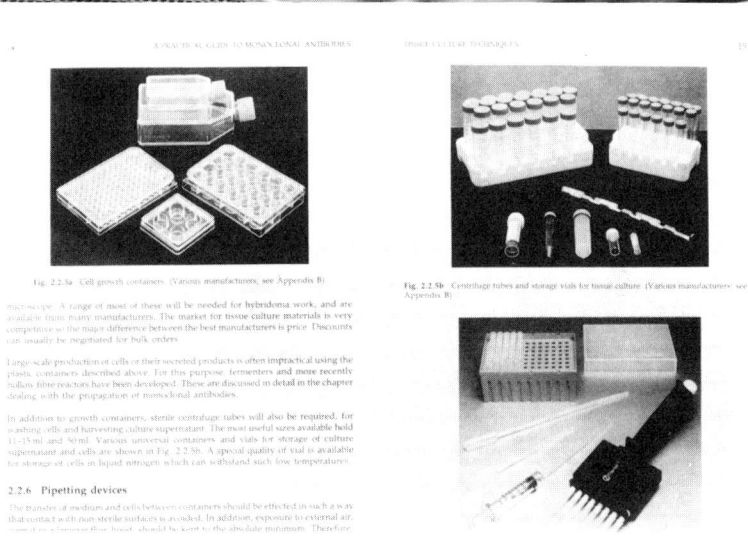

Figure 2.3. Transferring cells with a multipipettor. *Top:* A technician at work (photo: Jack Goldsmith). *Bottom:* Cell-culture equipment as represented in a laboratory manual. (Source: Liddell and Cryer 1991.)

> Sometimes the hybridomas *do not look "happy"* after the replacement of hybridoma technology with normal growth medium.
> (Eshhar 1985:22 emphasis added).

> When inspecting cells by phase microscopy, you get a feeling for just what the cells are doing, and how healthy they are by looking at them. A good hybrid should look like a little beach ball. (Interview with an industrial researcher, winter 1986).

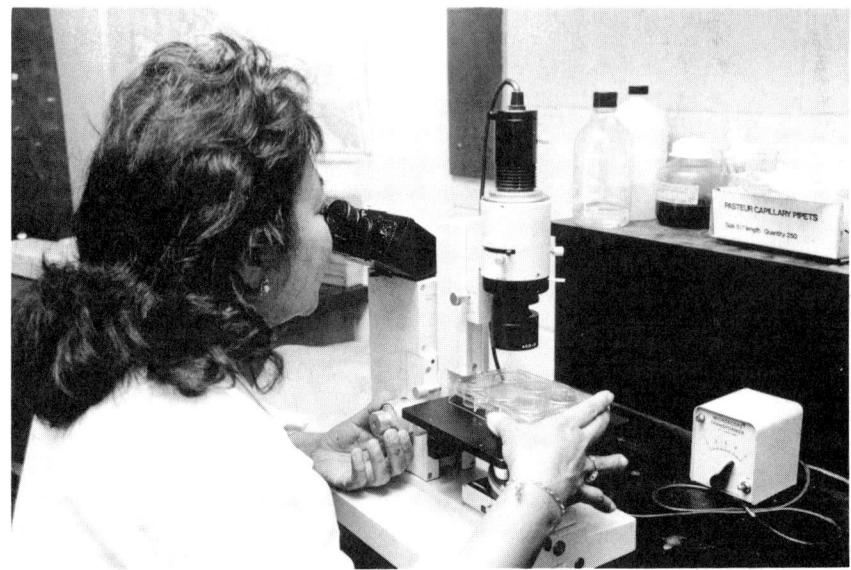

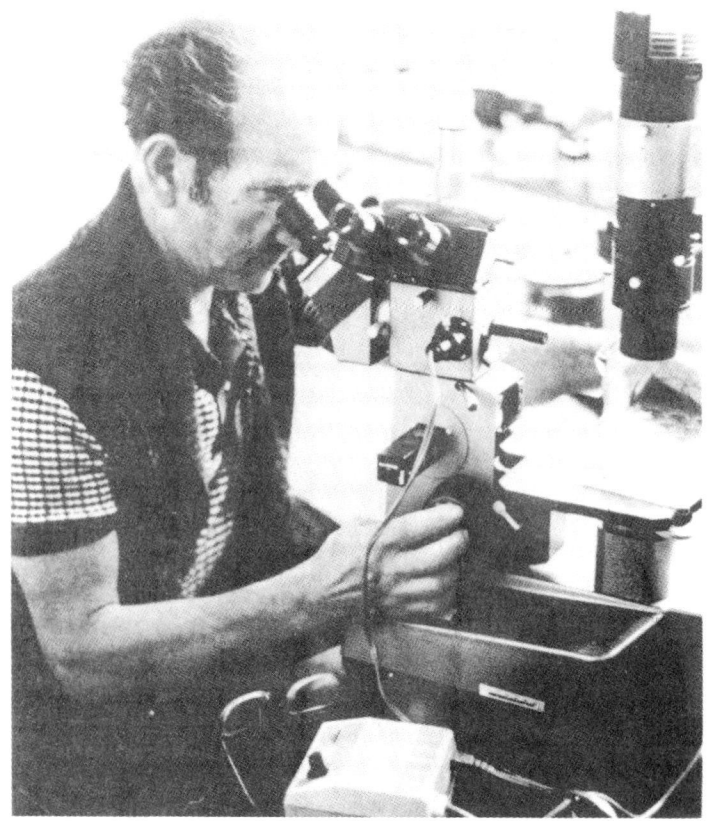

Figure 2.4. Observing "the viability of cells" with an inverted microscope. *Top:* A technician at work (photo: Jack Goldsmith). *Bottom:* César Milstein at work. (Source: OTA 1984.)

> You look in the microscope at cells growing: Are they healthy or are they not healthy? You learn that by association. The professor says, these are healthy, those are not. You learn by association, without knowing what you are looking at; you learn to know when it looks good.
> (Interview with an academic researcher, fall 1985).

Apprenticeship in hybridoma technology requires not only learning to interpret visual clues, it also necessitates the development of motor skills related to the handling of cells. Asked why some researchers were unable to reproduce hybridoma technology from published papers and had to visit his lab in order to learn it, a cell biologist who had been among the very first scientists to adopt hybridoma technology answered:

> They couldn't reproduce it? Well, because there were small tricks. For example, when you add polyethylene glycol to the cells they become very fragile. People who work for years with the cells, they are used to vigorous mixing, shaking. So if you pipet those cells strongly, you disrupt them and you would lose your experiment. Things like that. (Interview with an academic researcher, fall 1987).

Another example of this taming of the performer can be found in the fact that apprentices have to be taught to control and coordinate their gestures in order to preserve sterility. The interesting thing, in this respect, is that a lack of sterility, unlike, for instance, a lack of precaution in handling hot material, does not provide immediate feedback to the performer. Once contamination of cell cultures is noticed, it is difficult to ascertain which undisciplined gesture provoked it. The solution to this problem lies in the replacement of minute feedback adjustments with the repetitive performance of a set of ritual gestures.

To sum up, when apprentices are taught the procedure, the instructor (technician, graduate student, or professor) usually stresses the importance of the variables that have not been written down. The latter, as we have seen, refer more often than not to visual and motor aspects of the procedure that contribute to the learning of a gestalt. The learning of particular ways of seeing and acting is not restricted to experimental practice per se but is also essential to the understanding of formal written instructions. To illustrate this we draw upon our experience.

At the beginning of this study, one of us undertook a comparison of several different experimental protocols for the production of hybridomas. He had not yet been able to attend a fusion experiment but relied, to a great extent, on his previous biological training. While one might expect that it would be relatively easy to detect differences between the protocols, this was only true in a mechanical or literal sense; to the untrained eye, the protocols appeared to be arbitrary lists of instructions lacking any overall sense. The situation changed fundamentally once he was able to attend a training session in the technique. Once these instructions were embodied in a series of gestures, they became confounded with other factors, such as the manual skills of a given person or that person's degree of familiarity with a given piece of equipment. The comparison between protocols now became possible, each line of instruction evoking shapes, colors, time spans, and gestures that could be compared.

Ethnomethodology has developed the theme of the passage from written instructions to actual experimental practice. On this view, much of what is important to the understanding of an experimental protocol is not contained in the instructions but is incorporated in the various visual and corporal movements that make up the actual practice. It is further maintained that the experimental gestures themselves constitute an important part of the reasoning peculiar to specific disciplines (Lynch 1985). This fact has not escaped scientists.

Scientific researchers perceive the circulation of fellow scientists (most notably postdocs) between laboratories as the circulation of incorporated knowledge. In one of the academic laboratories we visited, for example, a postdoc had introduced a particular way of shaking test tubes containing recently fused cells that, following centrifugation, had a tendency to stick to the walls of the tube. This gesture, at first sight somewhat innocuous, was quickly adopted by the other researchers in the laboratory, who pointed out that it often made the difference between the success or failure of a fusion. Bioindustrial laboratories are also well aware of the importance and source of this dimension of scientific practice and, hence, frequently offer postdoctoral fellowships in addition to maintaining consultantships with university researchers.

The Objectification of Procedures

The fact that the hybridoma technique has features that are widely recognized as artisanal has not stifled attempts to objectify the know-how. Not only do written protocols exist, as previously noted, but it has indeed been possible for researchers to learn the technique through such protocols.

This does not imply that hybridoma know-how was transmitted in this way alone. Insofar as hybridoma technology links together a set of previously existing techniques, it is simply the case that the learning by doing happened at an earlier point. This was clearly the case for the early users of the technique (Drs. Bussard, Koprowski, and Rajewsky) discussed in Chapter 1. As noted by Collins (1987), the problem here is the distribution of know-how within a given field. Widely distributed know-how is taken for granted and not perceived as know-how.[15] In what follows, we shall examine the ways the tacit is articulated through the objectification and formal transmission of the technique.

There are essentially four kinds of written documents describing the hybridoma technique. The first is the Materials and Methods section of scientific papers. The brevity of these descriptions may be taken as a sign that the information contained therein is destined for members of the same discipline or the same technical area. They are of little use to researchers unfamiliar with the procedure.

A second form in which the technique is described is the experimental protocols produced in manuscript form by university laboratories for internal use. The protocols are also sent to researchers who request them. Industrial laboratories tend to produce more formal versions of this type of document (standard operating procedures). The informal nature of some university laboratory protocols, however, does not prohibit their transfer to industry. This is carried out either through transfer of a researcher or as part of a commercial package. Taggart Hybridoma Technology, for example, developed by an academic scientist and sold under license by the HyClone Company, provided buyers with a specific myeloma cell line, an experimental protocol, and direct technical assistance through an 800 telephone number. Research protocols offer a condensation of a particular laboratory's experience with a technique. They contain a combination of scientific, artisanal, and idiosyncratic rationales and hence require strict adherence. As Eshhar (1985:10, emphasis added) has remarked: "Fusion protocols are simple and easy to follow and usually successful, *if one sticks to them.*"

Books dedicated solely to hybridoma technology offer a third kind of description and are generally justified by the importance of this technology for disciplines other than that in which it emerged. For although the production of monoclonal antibodies draws upon a variety of skills from different disciplines, it is not uniformly accessible to members of all disciplines. Thus an individual with experience in cell culture (e.g., a virologist) would have a certain advantage in learning the technique over, for example, a biochemist. As a technical manual notes, however:

> It is not necessary to have extensive cell culture experience or to be an immunologist to undertake hybridoma work, although it helps. . . . Hybridomas are rather fastidious cells and the chances of producing them and maintaining them are certainly higher if the worker has previous cell culture experience. . . . The most important prerequisite in terms of expertise relates to the antigen type to be used and the assay for antibody against the antigen. Hybridoma technology is secondary and can be learned, but it is essential to have experience working with the material which is the subject of the project, be it a virus or a peptide, a lymphocyte differentiation antigen or a pathogenic parasite. (Zola and Brocks 1982:7).

As the above quotation clearly indicates, the purpose of such manuals is to allow researchers from other disciplines to acquire the technique without necessarily coming to grips with the theoretical principles (and the practical consequences of those principles) that underlie it. The technique is thus attributed a secondary or peripheral status. It is mere technique, a tool for the furtherance of other disciplinary projects.

In other instances, hybridoma technique may be accorded a more central status. In such cases the technique is no longer the tool of a particular discipline but a vehicle for advanced knowledge as well as a manifestation of the practical mastery of that knowledge. As one immunologist noted (interview, fall 1985):

> There are different strategies to make hybrids very specific against what you want: More and more fine questions are asked and you then need more specific monoclonals. You may produce hybrids one by one, and keep looking, but the more specific you want your monoclonals to be, the longer it gets. Now, very few people understand how the immune system works and the best way to do hybrids. People who are not immunologists produce monoclonals by following instructions in the books, that is, very inefficiently.

This wavering between a disciplinary and a mere technical status is reminiscent of the fact/technique distinction discussed in Chapter 1 and will be further discussed in Chapter 3 in relation to the transformation of hybridoma technology into a generic tool, as well as in Chapter 4, in relation to the institutional arrangements surrounding the introduction of hybridoma technology into academic and industrial research centers.[16]

Not only are there different ways of objectifying the hybridoma technique, but the technique may be objectified or formalized to different degrees; the more the technique is formalized (or packaged), the more it tends to be seen as pure technique and thus less central to the scientific preoccupations of the discipline. Hence, it cannot be decided *a priori* whether the hybridoma technique is of a formal or artisanal nature or whether, in fact, it is "only" a technique. These attributes are determined through practice and thus can serve only as descriptions of the technique in relation to a particular work setting. The changing status of the technique, which may be described as *sociotechnical* (Callon and Latour 1986), appears furthermore to depend upon the shifting relationship between disciplines as well as industrial and academic institutions.

In contrast to the Materials and Methods section of scientific papers, laboratory manuals offer what attempts to be an exhaustive description of standard procedures, ranging from such mundane items as equipment requirements and addresses of suppliers to more technical items, such as cell culture and fusion protocols (see, e.g., Liddell and Cryer 1991). Some manuals, in an attempt to overcome the limitations of written descriptions of visual variables, have resorted to photographs. Figure 2.5, for instance, shows the use of a photographic series designed to help the researcher decide when to screen cells (see our previous description of this procedure in this chapter). The use of a time series, by in-

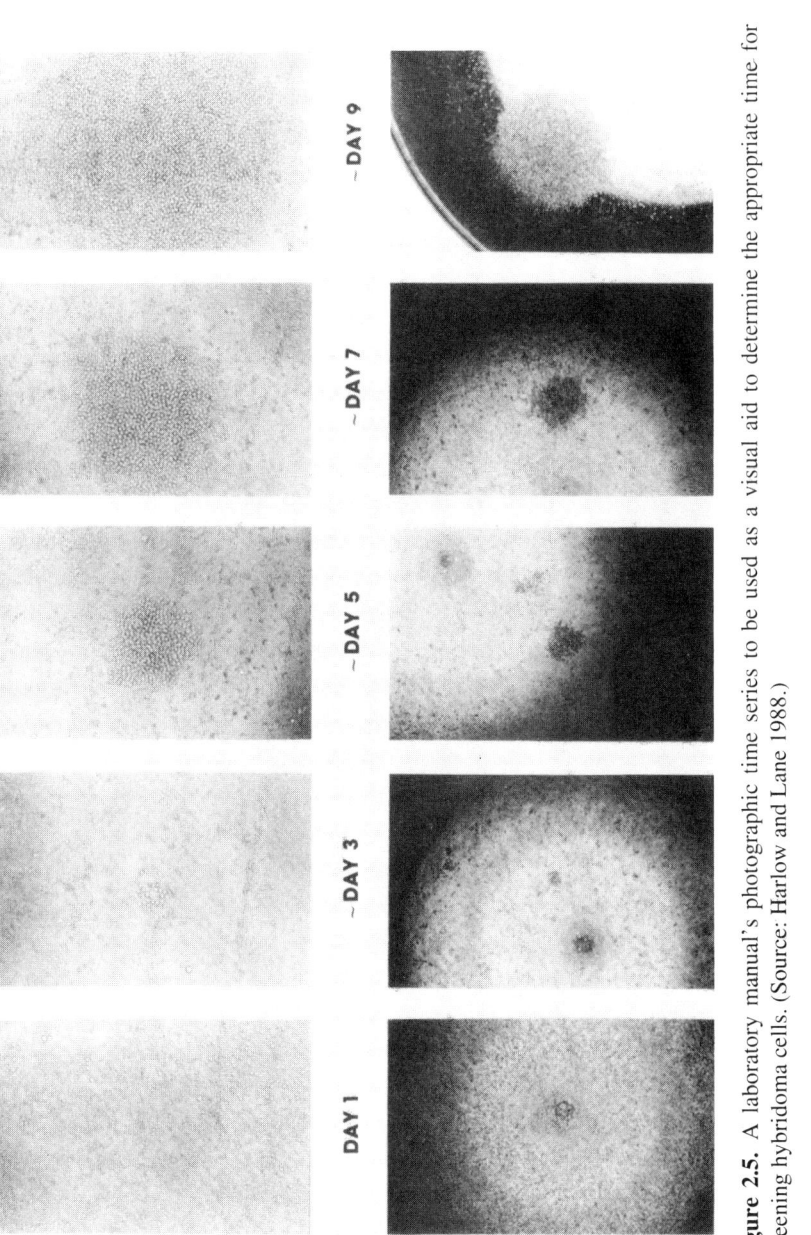

Figure 2.5. A laboratory manual's photographic time series to be used as a visual aid to determine the appropriate time for screening hybridoma cells. (Source: Harlow and Lane 1988.)

troducing a comparative dimension, is obviously meant to alleviate some of the shortcomings of photography, for instance, fixed depth of focus.

Some authors of manuals go so far as to seek a reconciliation between a merely technical and a theoretically informed description of hybridoma technology:

> I have written this book because I believe that previous accounts of the production, and particularly the usage, of monoclonal antibodies have been too dogmatic and inflexible. "Recipes" have been given which work if followed to the letter, but little attention has been given to the underlying principles. . . . I have therefore tried to emphasize the important variables which make for success or failure in the use of antibodies. . . . I have also tried to point out areas in which the literature gives misleading impressions. (Goding 1983:3).

Like the protocols produced for restricted diffusion, manuals represent a form of packaging and, consequently, a form of standardization such as that described by Fujimura (1987, 1992). Presumably, the proliferation of such manuals will result in the reduction of the importance of "golden hands" in the production process. As we have seen, however, not only are there different degrees of packaging, but the relevance of a standard technique varies according to a number of factors, such as the setting in which it is to be used.

"Improving" Hybridoma Technology

Articles bearing on specific features of the technique have appeared regularly in journals such as the *Journal of Immunological Methods*. While they complement the different kinds of publications discussed in the previous section, their stated purpose is not to teach but to propose modifications of the technique in order to make it more efficient. The status of these modifications is somewhat ambiguous for, as several researchers pointed out, alternative protocols are best confined to manuscript documents for internal use and do not in themselves represent much of interest. An academic researcher noted (interview, fall 1987) that, although his lab had done extensive studies on different aspects of the technique, "we never published that because we were trying not to put out too many papers on the small facts of lab work." Nonetheless, another researcher pointed out that one of his papers, which provided a detailed description of the optimal configuration of the various parameters (weight, age, and sex of the mouse; number of hybridomas injected; and so on) related to the induction of ascitic tumors in mice (and thus the production of high levels of monoclonal antibodies in the ascitic fluid) had gained much recognition, as measured by the over 1000 reprint requests he had received.[17]

The preceding indicates two things. First, the fact that hybridoma technology, as previously noted, is said to have remained basically unchanged does not mean that all laboratories are using carbon copy protocols; in other words, attempts to introduce modifications, both in the laboratory and in the scientific literature on hybridoma technology, are a common occurrence. Second, modifications are contentious, being highly valued by some researchers and dismissed by others. The term *modification* itself is more often than not ambiguous, insofar as it refers to various degrees of departure from Köhler and Milstein's original protocol(s), ranging, in the scientists' own dichotomous characterization, from minor variants to major improvements. Of course, scientists do not necessarily agree on whether a given modification should be classified as a mere variant or as a real improvement—scientists, in the course of a single interview, sometimes provide contradictory statements in this respect—but the variant/improvement dichotomy itself is maintained. In turn, the categorization of a modification as a variant or as an improvement underlies decisions such as whether to explore, publish, or adopt it.

To illustrate the distinction between variants and improvements, we can refer to the remarks of the codeveloper of hybridoma technology. Commenting on the early stages of hybridoma technology, Milstein (interview, January 11, 1988) noted:

> One recurrent issue, then, was solving problems and identifying those problems. Different people identify different things and then they publish on the technology. This boils down to, it doesn't matter if you do this or that way, but it works. [Dr. X] has a paper, one of the earliest papers if I remember, in which he says this is the way it works. Those papers I regard of very little consequence because usually what they meant was, eventually you make the technique work, and the other way it would work as well! At that time there were a variety of myths developing ... little recipes. Essentially that is unimportant. Later there are a number of developments that are more interesting trying to solve individual problems. But when you look back, the technique itself has remained essentially unchanged from the beginning, the early stages.

Having said this, Milstein immediately went on to mention what he explicitly considered, in opposition to the little recipes, important changes, namely, developments in the immunization of animals and the selection of cells, as well as actual developments of technology, such as the use of animals other than mice or the production of hybrid hybridomas. In the same vein, in a 1991 paper he noted that "[hybridoma technology] has been improved over the years, particularly by the preselection of antigen-binding B cells and by screening with antigen-coated filters" (Winter and Milstein 1991:293).

Various modifications qualified as improvements have been proposed over the years (see Figure 2.6 for a schematic illustration of the theme of improvement). Since hybridoma technology is a package of various objects and techniques, it is not surprising that no *a priori* consensus exists as to which of these elements or set of elements should be improved. Nonetheless, two modifications that were introduced very early and have become part of hybridoma technology are unambiguously, and retrospectively, recognized as improvements. The first is the already-mentioned substitution of a chemical fusion promoter (PEG) for the Sendai virus originally used to initiate fusion (Galfré et al. 1977).[18] The second is the use of myelomas that do not secrete their own immunoglobulins and that therefore do not interfere with the production of the required antibody (e.g., Kearney et al. 1979).[19] Other potential improvements, though widespread, are still subject to discussion and are not universally implemented; as a result, they are often classified as little recipes. Such is the case with the addition of feeder cells to hybridoma culture wells and the use of serum-free culture medium.

Other improvements have been rejected as dead ends or have only survived in some niche. Such is the case of electrofusion (i.e., the use of short electric pulses, as opposed to the use of PEG, to promote fusion), which, despite the many articles crediting it as a great advance in fusion efficiency (*Bio/Technology* 1983), has been adopted by few laboratories. Among the researchers who tried it out, some discarded it altogether, while others restricted its use to some particularly difficult task. A public health researcher, for instance, mentioned (interview, winter 1993) that he used it only in his attempts to produce human monoclonals, sticking to the conventional PEG fusion for murine monoclonal antibodies. Another researcher (interview, fall 1989), who characterized electrofusion as "a quite strong disappointment," accounted for its lack of success in sociotechnical terms: "What was lacking in the case of electrofusion was a couple of credible laboratories who would replicate the technology and say that it works well."

An interesting case is that of two modifications that were not widely adopted, in spite of having been trumpeted in the biotech literature as major improvements (Wilson 1981; *McGraw-Hill's Biotechnology Newswatch* 1982a; *Genetic Engineering News* 1984; Klausner 1984; *McGraw-Hill's Biotechnology Newswatch* 1984c), and despite having been published in prestigious scientific periodicals—*Science* and *Nature*, as opposed the *Journal of Immunological Methods*—thus laying claim to scientific, as opposed to mere technical relevance. The first modification is the above-mentioned Taggart technique, in which the selective system used to separate fused from unfused cells—the so-called HAT/HPRT system (see Chapter 1)—was replaced with another system (called APRT), leading allegedly to more stable hybridomas (Taggart and Samloff 1983). But replacing the HAT system was not everyone's priority. As a Stanford immunologist noted, "The HAT method is fabulous. A way of screening for the hybridoma producing the desired antibody is what needs improving—that's

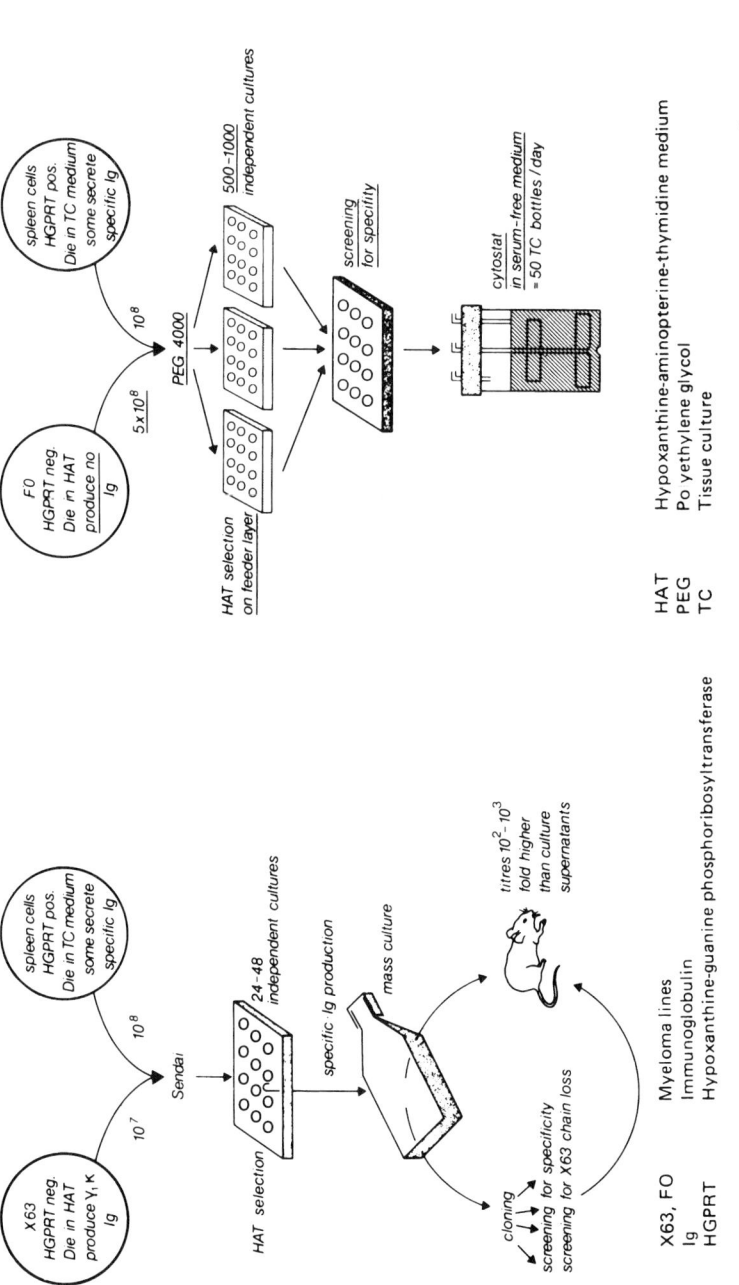

Figure 2.6. Hybridoma technology then and now: a schematic representation of various "improvements" made to hybridoma technology. *Left side*: Hybridoma technology in 1975. *Right side*: Hybridoma technology in 1983. "Improvements" are underlined. (Source: Fazekas De St. Groth 1985.)

where the assaying becomes difficult" (*McGraw-Hill's Biotechnology Newswatch* 1982a).

Similarly unsuccessful was the receptor directed system developed by a team led by Solomon H. Snyder at Johns Hopkins (Lo et al. 1984). In a letter to the authors (February 16, 1993), Snyder commented that although his technique "worked quite nicely" according to third-party evaluations, the standard technique was obviously "good enough for most peoples' needs," a remark that recalls March and Simon's notion of "satisficing." According to this latter notion, decision-making does not involve the discovery and selection of optimal alternatives but, rather, of satisfactory alternatives; hence, the definition of *satisfactory* is context bound.[20]

Similar arguments, this time from the point of view of potential users, were offered by researchers commenting that the conventional technique was so effective that the possible gains of adopting the new technology were offset by the time one would need to invest in order to implement it:

> [Hybridoma technology] is so effective.... With a good antigen, we can easily produce between 1000 and 2000 clones with a single fusion: so, if with all those clones you are unable to find the antibody you need, that means you've got a big problem!... [Major modifications] could be interesting for some very specific problem: antibodies against certain hormones, against small peptides. But in general the technology is so efficient ... that it's better to make four consecutive fusions in order to find the antibody you need than to reinvent the whole process.
> (Interview with a public health researcher, winter 1993).

> People prefer to sacrifice three times more mice than to spend six months trying to make a technical improvement.
> (Interview with an academic researchers, fall 1989).[21]

This did not prevent other researchers, such as Matthew Scharff, from wondering why only a few reports of successful fusions using improved protocols, for instance, so-called antigen-focused fusion, were to be found in the scientific literature (Pirovski 1990:7S). In the light of the satisficing quality of the more conventional protocols, one might as well ask the opposite question, namely, what justification researchers provide for proposing and/or adopting improved protocols. Given the contingent nature of scientific practice, the number of possible answers to this question is potentially very large; we shall limit ourselves to a few. A cell biologist (interview, fall 1989) noted that "[My concern was] to simplify as far as possible the technique for producing monoclonals. You know, the situation was similar to when motorcars were derived from horse carts. Aerodynamic studies were at first not a priority, but slowly people realized that, in the case of motorcars, an aerodynamic design was a plus, especially with the increase in car speed."

Elaborating on his metaphor, the researcher raised the following example. Köhler and Milstein's protocol had borrowed the use of the HAT selective medium, designed to eliminate unfused cells, from a previous cell fusion system developed in the 1960s in which both fusion partners were able to survive independently in a normal culture medium. In the case of hybridoma technology, however, only one of the unfused fusion partners, namely, the myelomas, needed to be eliminated because the other partner, the antibody-producing spleen cells, quickly die out in culture media. For this more limited purpose, the HAT medium was, in his opinion, overkill. The preservation of this remnant of previous work was all the less justified because the HAT medium was faulted for causing many problems in the hybridoma technology system.

In this particular case, the drive toward a more aerodynamic design was grounded in disciplinary differences. Training in cell biology and cell genetics, as opposed to immunology, was credited with providing both a reason and the means of improving the fusion aspects of hybridoma technology by bringing them in line with state-of-the-art practices in cell biology. In other instances, the line of work in which a given researcher's interest in hybridoma technology was expressed was used to account for his or her focus on improvements. For instance, in a service unit devoted to the routine production of monoclonal antibodies for the research purposes of other laboratories, the improvement of hybridoma technology became the creative and innovative aspect of what would have otherwise been a rather dull endeavor. Indeed, researchers were attracted to the service unit with the guarantee that 50% of their time could be devoted to work on the advancement of hybridoma technology (interview with an academic researcher, fall 1989). Finally, improvements of hybridoma technology are often related to the attribution of a research frontier status to the work performed in a given laboratory. Work on rare antigens, for instance, is said to make the use of highly efficient variants of hybridoma technology inescapable.

Hybridoma Technology and Its Variants

Independently of the dispute over improvements discussed in the previous section, numerous differences exist between the written procedures used in different laboratories; further, the practical use of these instructions within the same laboratory varies. This is a fact openly recognized in technical manuals: "There are a large number of fusion protocols in general circulation and most of them work. . . . It has been emphasized throughout this book that the number of variations in procedure is immense" (Campbell 1984:127–131).

An adequate description of this variation, as we already noted, would necessarily call forth both technical factors (i.e., the biological problem at issue) and social factors (i.e., the previous experience of the researcher). An individual's choice of procedure depends, more often than not on social factors relating to the origin of the protocol in question. "There are people who, if they see a protocol originating from an institution or an individual they don't consider to be prestigious, will not try that protocol; it could be the world's greatest protocol, but they won't try it" (Interview with an industrial researcher, winter 1986).

Variants of the hybridoma technique may be loosely classified in the following categories. There are, first of all, *formal* variations, which are duly noted in written protocols. If limited to the central phase of the fusion procedure, these variations would include such factors as the concentration of the fusion agent, the temperature, the means of sterilization of PEG (autoclave or filtration), and the precise duration of the fusion. Some of the variants are subject to controversy in the literature.

Feeder cells are a case in point. Consisting of a cell preparation, they are often added to cultured hybridomas in order to promote their development. Despite the term *feeder*, little is known of the mechanism of their action (Goding 1983:71). Some say they are useless, while others declare them to be a major improvement of the technique (Fazekas De St. Groth 1985:5). Still others maintain that while their benefits may be unknown, they certainly don't do any harm (Goding 1983:71; Zola and Brocks 1982:25).

There are, secondly, informal variants sometimes known as *shortcuts*. For example, rather than count B cells and myelomas under the microscope in order to obtain a given proportion, say 10:1, it is possible to simply compare the volumes of two pellets of cells. Given that myelomas are about 10 times larger than B cells, equal volumes of each gives the desired proportion. The result of experience acquired in the course of many fusions, these shortcuts do not appear in written protocols, not even those for internal use, and are transmitted orally.

Shortcuts of the latter type may be distinguished from the use of *sophisticated* techniques (sometimes also referred to as shortcuts), which may replace certain parts of the procedure. For example, rather than screening the hybridomas by searching for the required antibody in the cell culture supernatant, it is possible, with the help of DNA probes, to determine the presence of the gene coding for the sought-after antibody. Using such a technique allows one to screen a much larger number of hybridomas than would otherwise be possible.[22]

Within the private sector, sophisticated procedures of the type just mentioned are not often patented but are protected as trade secrets because to patent this form of intellectual property would result in diffusion of the knowledge without the ability to control its use. If a trade secret remains entirely secret, however, it sometimes loses part of its commercial value. Fully aware of this problem, Hybritech, the pioneering biotech startup company created to commercially exploit hybridoma technology, advertised the existence of a "secret" system allowing its employees to rapidly screen large number of hybridomas.

Finally, there are procedural elements that are perceived as the most immediate expression of local idiosyncrasies and that are categorized as magic in opposition to practical scientific know-how. The use of similar terms has been noted by sociologists of science. Lynch (1985:108–111) has documented instances of superstition, and Fujimura (1987) of black magic. According to one of our informants,

> I consider that the actual fusion has a lot of voodoo. There is a lot of things people do, they don't know why. I don't know why but I just copy what they do and they say: "If you do it differently, it will not work." They told me I had to spin the fusing cells with the top open. Why the top open? It doesn't make any difference, this is a small, desk-top centrifuge, it doesn't matter whether the top is open or closed I think, the history of it is (laughter) that you can't regulate the speed that well, so initially when people used to do it, they would open the top and see how fast it would spin. Now people know how to regulate the speed and they don't really have to look at it anymore, but they leave the top open! They told me I had to leave the top open. I am supposed to be a scientist. I don't believe the top has to be open. But I am not going to put it down, because if the fusion did not work, they would tell me it's because I left the top down.
> (Interview with an academic researcher, fall 1985).[23]

Some magic is written down, while other magic is transmitted through personal contact and thus circulates in the same manner as tricks of the trade. Still other magic circulates under the guise of reason. If a researcher is forced to spend 10 minutes on the telephone in the course of an experiment and if that experiment is successful, then it is possible that the subsequent protocol will contain the instruction "leave for 10 minutes." Magic, in turn, may hide experience. Such is sometimes the case with the optimization of experimental conditions: "We had to do experiments—with different kinds of feeder cells, with different kind of serum—that you never write out but allow you to go some place later and to become a wizard. At the end, you end up with a kind of voodoo ceremony with all these experiments you know make a difference, but you don't know why" (Interview with an academic researcher, winter 1986).

There is indication that with the passage of time and the concurrent transformation of hybridoma technology from a research-front technique into a background skill (see Chapter 4), many idiosyncratic elements of protocols lose their salience. For instance, a recent review of a book on immunological methods criticizes the advice given on the production of monoclonal antibodies for offering "many outdated phenomenological frills, making the process look much more complex than it is" (Campbell 1994). This does not necessarily mean that magic is no longer at work in everyday practice, where it may still be active in tacit routines, but rather that magic tends to disappear from or be regarded as an oddity in written accounts.

The Problem of Codification

Despite the fact that it is hardly possible to test all variables and their interactions, technical manuals and laboratory discourse sometimes propose the maximum reduction of experimental incertitude.[24] It is more often the case, however, that methods "become established as soon as they happen to work at all" (Fazekas De St. Groth 1980:1).

The decision not to codify a procedure is based on a variety of considerations. First of all, scientists argue that to the extent that a technique works, it is not worth the effort to clarify details that have no direct relation to research objectives. Discussion of the degree of necessary objectification is often related to prior social distinctions between university and industry, and between researchers and technicians. For example, some university scientists claim that in industry, where routine work is carried out by technicians, the researcher in charge will surely have written up protocols allowing a mechanical reproduction of the technique. This discussion is reflected in the literature as follows:

> Experiments to study all these variables are tedious and relatively uninteresting at a time when investigators are anxious to produce some useful antibodies, irrespective of the efficiency of the process. Thus, it is not surprising that successful procedures become entrenched, and that dogmatic statements about technical variables are accepted unchallenged. As the initial excitement wears off, it is to be expected that much work will be done on technical aspects and that the procedures will lose much of their empiricism and mysticism. (Zola and Brocks 1982:4–5).

The prediction advanced in the last part of the paragraph is far from being true for all researchers. While the move from art to science is indeed possible, so is the reverse:

> You can make different parts scientific. When we do experiments and record what the results were, in a sense we are making things scientific. But sooner or later, it goes back to art: We know the technique that works; therefore, we do it, even though the next generation has never tested it. So it becomes an art. The value of making it science is not necessarily high, the value of making it work is high. (Interview with an academic researcher, winter 1986).

Concern over recognition within the network of scientific relations may also militate against the pursuit and publication of technical improvements seen as minor or trivial:

> If you want to publish a technique, you do it in *Journal of Immunological Methods* or *Hybridoma*, but they are not prestigious journals, many scientists don't even get them. It's not worth your time to write papers for them, so you don't. If people want to know your technique, they just call you up, and if they have problems, they send somebody to see how you do it.
> (Interview with an academic researcher, winter 1986).

Moreover, optimizing experimental conditions (experimenting around) is seen as work suited mainly for doctoral students: "Postdocs have to start immediately to write papers. They don't have the time." (Interview with an academic researcher, winter 1986). Nonetheless, these perceptions are not universal and vary according to the prestige, centrality, and vocation of the laboratory. Recall, for instance, the previously mentioned case of the researcher who published in the *Journal of Immunological Methods* a paper on the induction of ascitic tumors; he claimed this was the success paper of his career.

Mixed considerations, including disciplinary training, determine attitudes towards technique. Some researchers once claimed that if PEG were purified by recrystallization, it would lose its fusogenic qualities, which apparently reside in the impurities contained in the commercial lots and not in the PEG itself. Other researchers argued otherwise (*Art to Science in Tissue Culture* 1983). The researcher who mentioned this controversy to us pointed out that while he was attempting to perfect his own technique, he had chosen to ignore this particular problem and the line of research it suggested. He explained: "I'm a cell culturist and not a chemist; that's how you choose." In other cases, reasons range from supposed contamination, to cells' preferences or ease of work:

> We had two different sources [of PEG] and some worked better and some didn't. The same was true of the molecular size of the polyethylene glycol. We used 6000 at the very beginning. Later on we switched to 1000. You can get as good fusions with 1000 as 6000. Some human cells prefer lower molecular weight. Mouse prefers higher molecular weight. The differences are really due to contamination and not really to molecular weight. It's much easier to work with 1000 because it's fluid and you can easily measure it instead of taking crystals and weighing it.
> (Interview with an academic researcher, fall 1987).

Artisanal elements of laboratory work are often held to constitute the style of a laboratory, which can be seen as either an obstacle to standardization or as yet another form of it. Researchers in two different laboratories within the same university distinguished between the two labs on the basis of equipment procurement and maintenance. One lab was characterized as possessing Gucci equipment ("You know . . . like Gucci leather"), while the other maintained less fancy apparatus:

> Spencer's lab is known for what they call their "Spencer grade": It's low tech, but it always works. If they have a broken piece of equipment, they say "it's Spencer grade." The way I interpret it is that their equipment is all very well used, they have nothing fancy, but everything is functioning, and it is an excellent place to learn hybridoma technology.
> (Interview with an academic researcher, fall 1985; Spencer is a pseudonym).

The decision to use more rudimentary equipment allowed researchers in Spencer's lab to display artisanal dexterity foreign to the Gucci lab: "When 'plating out' the fused cells I am of the old school, I use a pipette with the finger on it; some people use multiple pipettors, I don't trust them." (interview with an academic researcher, winter 1986). It has allowed members of the laboratory to trademark their style: "We have T-shirts: '100% Spencer grade.' The philosophy behind this is do as much as you can with as little as you can, use old instruments, that is, Spencer grade equipment" (Interview with an academic researcher, winter 1986).[25]

It may be argued that characterizing differences between laboratories, such as the choice of myeloma, in terms of style, itself conceived as a sort of epiphenomenon with regard to research, tends to eliminate the problem of the existence of different and sometimes contradictory prescriptions of the hybridoma technique. Questions of style, however, involve as much problems of content as they do of form (Goodman 1978:23). It is therefore worth asking how the researchers themselves account for variations in hybridoma technique.

Some researchers characterize protocols as the reproducible and effective, implying therefore that there are others that are idiosyncratic and futile. According to French et al. (1985:345), for example: "A number of fusion protocols use polyethyleneglycol to promote fusion. We have found the protocol described by Fazekas de St. Groth to be reproducible and effective." Even from a researcher's point of view, however, such a solution is not entirely satisfactory because it tends to remove the recognized role played by artisanal elements.

Other researchers prefer thus to distinguish between rigid protocols and minimal type protocols: "I have minimal type protocols. Hybridoma technology is mostly a question of instinct and experience. I look at cultures by their color, I don't do cell counts. I'm not a very rigid type, but I do know people who have very rigid protocols as far as feeding, splitting, manipulation of cells, etc. goes. I believe rigid protocols are overdone" (Interview with an industrial researcher, winter 1986).

In general, however, both scientists interviewed and texts surveyed tend to distinguish between *important* and *accessory* parts of research protocols. Important steps refer to those that are supposed to have a direct and determinant effect on the experimental results. As such, they are subject to careful experimentation with regard to the parameters they entail. Accessory steps exert only a secondary influence on the hoped for outcome and are therefore considered to be subject to the idiosyncrasies of the laboratory concerned. A similar distinction is also introduced with regards to the elements whose presence or absence defines the rigidity of a given protocol. The following quote deals with the possibility of including instructions concerning the transfer of cells within written protocols:

> We do that in some cases. The indicator cell line for the assay of T cells has to be passed every two days, given a supplement every two days; people who tried to stretch that ran into problems. For other cell lines, I haven't written it down. Some you write down, some you don't. Every cell line is different, so writing it down doesn't mean a lot. But for indicator cells it is important. If necessary, we do it. Most of the time it's not necessary. Some people are better at that sort of things than other people. Depends on how good a farmer you are . . .
> (Interview with an academic researcher, winter 1986).

When questioned about the lack of consensus as to the criteria for important and accessory, and the fact that laboratories using protocols differing in important steps still manage to produce hybridomas, researchers have recourse to finer distinctions. Hybridomas themselves are divided into ready to wear (i.e., directed towards extremely immunogenic antigens and thus, by definition, easy to produce) and sophisticated. Laboratories are divided into advanced ("We are a year and a half ahead of everybody else") and ordinary, or industrial and academic, or distinguished according to disciplinary affiliation, wherein the technique has central or secondary meaning for the problematic. As can be seen, the understanding of research protocols by scientists implies a distinction between the technical and the social which forms a part—call it a sociology—of the researchers' practical reasoning.

From Art to Science

The terms *science*, *art*, and *magic* have so far been used to describe different parts of the hybridoma technique. In this final section we examine how these categories have been applied to hybridoma technology as a whole.

From art to science is a common expression in areas such as immunology and cell culture (e.g., Schon 1983). It also appears regularly in the various essay reviews and technical manuals devoted to monoclonal antibodies. In spite of what has been said so far concerning the artisanal and sometimes magical character of hybridoma technology, the latter is often presented as a decisive step forward in the move from art and/or magic to science in the antibody domain, as instanced in the following quotations:

> Prior to 1975, the production of antibodies was considered by some to be a black art practised by immunologists. . . . The uncertainties about the specificity of individual antisera led to many prolonged and acrimonious debates. All that has now changed. (Goding 1983:1–3).

> Serology involving conventional polyclonal antibodies used to be an art bordering on science, and immunologists could be divided into those who believed in immuno-chemistry and those who believed in "immunomagic." While the latter school will always be with us, the discovery of hybridoma antibodies has done much to put serology on a firm scientific basis. (Goding 1983:40).

The theme of a move from art to science is not restricted to university researchers. It surfaces regularly in the advertisements of companies specialized in the sale of scientific equipment and reagents. A technical bulletin distributed by the HyClone company, purveyors of the Taggart Hybridoma Technology mentioned earlier, bears the title *Art To Science in Tissue Culture*. The Invitron company publicizes its cell culture products proclaiming that "The Art of cell culture has passed away. . . . The Science of cell manufacturing has arrived." According to Invitron, the art of cell culture was characterized by the use of "ascites fluid" and "esoteric protocols," whereas the new "science" requires the use of "computerized automation" and "bioengineering."

There are, however, different roads from art to science. In Invitron's case, it would appear that the route is entirely technical. Not only is the transformation accomplished through sophisticated technical equipment, but the vision of science advanced is one of a series of technical operations largely devoid of conceptual content. University researchers, on the other hand, tend to see the transformation conducted at the level of the concepts themselves. Arguing that the production of monoclonal antibodies has made many artisanal aspects of immunology scientific, Goding (1983:40) claims. "The old uncertainties of specificity and reproducibility have been replaced by the promise of unlimited supplies of standardized, monospecific antibodies. Terms like *titre* and *avidity* have become virtually obsolete. We can now talk about mass and affinity of antibody in a very precise way."

The degree to which an experimental practice is perceived as artisanal or scientific also depends upon the perceptions and self-perceptions of the discipline in question. The classification of a technique as either art or science, for example, not only determines how a given technique will be circulated but is often an expression of a hierarchy among the laboratories involved in the circulation of the technique. One researcher told us that it had previously been necessary to visit another laboratory in order to learn the hybridoma technique as applied to T cells. Now, however, his own laboratory had become a second possible port of entry into the domain. The classification of the technique may, in addition, serve as a means of promoting technical changes as improvements or stigmatizing changes as idiosyncratic variations of little scientific impact. In such cases the application of the label may serve to establish or disrupt the scales of credibility that distinguish researchers.

Disciplines, too, may be implicated in the process of classification. As the quotation at the beginning of this section suggests, immunology has often been taxed with having indulged in immunomagic. This often occurs when researchers trained in supposedly "harder" disciplines, such as biochemistry or molecular biology, reflect on what appears to them to be the more arcane or esoteric procedures in immunology. Having decided to devote himself to the study of immunology, a successful biochemist we interviewed found that his former colleagues viewed his newfound interest with skepticism bordering on hostility.

This conflict is reflected within immunology by the division between those, as Goding (1983:40) would have it, "who believe in immunochemistry and those who believe in immunomagic." Here, however, the dispute is exacerbated by the fact that the relations between science, art, and magic form the basis of the opposition between two schools of thought in modern immunology, the *system immunologists* and the *step-by-step immunologists*. The latter school is represented by researchers who restrict themselves to the sequential solution of problems dealing with a restricted number of variables. The system school, on the other hand, is represented by those concerned with providing somewhat indirect solutions to very general problems such as the causes of cancer. Because of the opposing views of the relations between theory and practice, evaluation of research becomes especially problematic:

> If there are two ways of looking at immunology, what do you do if you have a system immunologist who is a lousy scientist, you cannot easily verify his results, and he did a bad experiment? To account for his results, he usually invents a complicated theory.... Some of these people who are bad scientists and who build a house of cards can become very prominent. In immunology, bad scientists cannot be easily detected. (Interview with an academic researcher, fall 1985).

In such cases, judgments concerning the reliability of a researcher's results can only be based on an assessment of the researcher's long-term performance; this, in turn, raises the question of the experimenter's regress, as described earlier.

In the field of industrial production, the classification of experimental procedures as art, science, or magic is determined in part by the demands of commercial success as well as the guidelines of the various regulatory bodies governing activity in a given industrial sector. Comparing the relative merits of two recent techniques, DNA probes and monoclonal antibodies, on the basis of their possible use in commercial diagnostic kits, Nash (1985) noted: "Anything which involves a great deal of 'art' or extreme complexity will be relatively disadvantaged. Art particularly is anathema to rational production decisions and to the regulatory and supervisory mechanisms in the health care industry of most countries." The standardization of procedures using monoclonal antibodies has been described in the following mixed metaphor: "a jungle full of pitfalls" (Haaijman et al. 1984).

From the point of view of the university researcher, the perception of his or her practice of the hybridoma technique as art has certain advantages with regard to his or her relation with industry. First of all, it allows the researcher to distance himself from industry by projecting the routine aspects of hybridoma technology as industrial practices. At the same time, it allows the researcher to reaffirm a relationship of mutual dependence between university and industry in the domain of biotechnology. Given the fluid nature of the boundaries between industrial and academic institutions in this area (several biotech startups stress the quasi-academic climate of the firm), it is no surprise to find that the opposition between art and routine is also used within the industrial sector to distinguish one firm from another or different departments within the same firm.

Finally, the classification of knowledge has many consequences for patenting practices. It may be argued that the passage from magic to science in the area of antibody production has opened the possibility of patenting an antibody against a given antigen. As we shall see in Chapter 5, questions relating to the status and the mode of circulation of patentable knowledge have played a central role in the court battles that have engaged two pioneers in the commercial exploitation of hybridoma technology, Hybritech and Monoclonal Antibodies Inc.

Conclusions

In this chapter we have examined how researchers using hybridoma technology classify their knowledge and their activities using the categories of science, art, and magic. We have seen that in the establishment and diffusion of a scientific technique, which may be conceived of as an embedded system of practices, scientists have recourse to many forms of knowledge. The part that may be considered tacit or local depends upon the network of relations constitutive of the scientists' work. This network is comprised of a system of heterogeneous elements (theories, machines, patents, products). The articulation of these diverse elements occasions the emergence of the scientists' categories of knowledge.

Recent work in the sociology of scientific knowledge has attempted to construct similar classifications of scientific knowledge and practice using such categories as objective, declarative, procedural, tacit, and local knowledge. Despite the fact that the sociological classifications are presumably the result of a concerted effort of reflection and analysis, they are not, as we have seen, fundamentally different from the supposedly naïve, ad hoc typologies of the scientists. For although the sociological categories presume to describe dimensions of science overlooked by or invisible to scientists, they invariably make use of the scientists' categories to achieve this end. It is true that the use of these categories by scientists is not always consistent and that the boundaries between categories vary amongst institutions, practices, and interests. But the same may be said of the sociologists' categories. We have attempted an empirical demonstration of the inadequacy of these categories, considered fundamental by sociologists, and the need to relativise them. In particular, we believe that the existence of immunomagic (i.e., that knowledge and know-how that scientists have agreed to drop from discussion for a given period of time) shows that these categories are unable to account for the strategies employed by scientists.

As we have seen, while scientists often present ideal, algorithmic accounts of their work, they also recognize and work with tacit or local dimensions of knowledge, whether they be classified as art or magic. In many respects, the scientists' own description of the kinds of knowledge with which they deal on a daily basis are more precise and more comprehensive than the descriptions offered by sociologists. Not only are the scientists capable of describing the choices open to individuals and institutions, but they also recognize the many ways tacit and local knowledge, contrary to the sociological definitions of these terms, circulate among different scientific and technical cultures. Indeed, contrary to what some sociologists of science argue, a common culture is not a prerequisite for the emergence of a scientific network.

Equally important is to note that talk about local or tacit knowledge is not exclusive of but rather, and somewhat paradoxically, constitutive of standardization. In the next chapter we shall see how, to borrow O'Connell's (1993) felicitous expression, the circulation of particulars is constitutive of universality. The important thing is not to oppose local to universal, or tacit to standard—an exercise in reification—but to focus on the circulation of materials and statements. Indeed, it is precisely in relation to this circulation that actors' notions such as tacit, local, etc. exercise their regulatory role.

NOTES

1. Allan Jones is a pseudonym. The reader will have noticed that Jones cites as a source of information a personal communication from another scientist rather than MILSTEIN 75. It is noteworthy that Dr. Jones, working in London, should learn of the Cambridge-based work through a New York colleague.

2. In his initial letter Jones had not specified for what "work" he wanted the culture.

3. "We have been using, and sending away, the same P3 line that we sent you. Its correct name is X63Ag8, although we have also called it X67Ag8 and P3Ag8."

4. Milstein's problem was imputed to a toxic batch of HAT medium; Köhler's to a still mysterious, yet different factor; see Milstein (1986) and Tansey and Catterall (1994:326). The difficulties experienced by Köhler and Milstein temporarily called into question the reproducibility (and thus the significance) of their first, successful experiment (David Secher quoted in Tansy and Catterall 1994:326). More recently we interviewed a researcher who had a similar experience. After having successfully implemented hybridoma technology in his lab, during a six-month period he was unable to make it work. The reasons for this prolonged breakdown were never fully clarified, although toxic sera and a possibly defective CO_2 incubator were seen as possible causes. (Interview with a public health researcher, winter 1993).

5. The *locus classicus* is Collins (1985).

6. For a forceful critique of sociology as the unveiling of forces or interests unrecognized by actors, see Boltanski (1990), especially part 1.

7. See also Fujimura (1987).

8. Vincenti's (1984) typology of knowledge is also based on a dichotomy, this time between explicit and procedural knowledge. The former encompasses descriptive and prescriptive knowledge; the latter prescriptive and tacit knowledge. Prescriptive knowledge is a watershed between procedural and explicit knowledge. Tacit knowledge is only a subcategory of the main dichotomy. Collins's argument is directed against this kind of typology.

9. For an interesting debate on this topic, see Dreyfus (1992) and Collins (1992).

10. In addition to sociologists of scientific knowledge, sociologists of work and of medicine have discussed tacit knowledge in detail. See, for example, Jones (1983), Jones and Wood (1984), Kusterer (1979), Armstrong (1977), Gordon (1988), and Sadler (1978).

11. See also Ferguson (1992). Awareness of this fact prompted Vincenti (1984:574) to further restrict the domain of tacit knowledge to "implicit, wordless and pictureless knowledge essential to engineering judgment and workers' skills." To emphasize the fundamentally private and nontransmissible nature of tacit knowledge, Vincenti proposed a purely secondary function for verbal and nonverbal communication in the production of tacit knowledge: "Words, diagrams, and pictures can help suggest and promote tacit knowledge. The knowledge itself can come in the end, however, only from individual practice and experience." Note that for Vincenti, as well as Collins, knowledge in habits the individual. As such, their position differs from Lynch.

12. See also Calvino (1985:94): "Or rather: a silence can serve to dismiss certain words or else to hold them in reserve for use on a better occasion. Just as a word spoken now can save a hundred words tomorrow or else can necessitate the saying of another thousand. 'Every time I bite my tongue,' Mr. Palomar concludes mentally, 'I must think not only of what I am about to say or not to say, but also of everything that, whether I say it or do not say it, will be said or not said by me or by others.'"

13. For a similar argument, whereby the sociologists' attempt to define what skills and tacit knowledge are is replaced by a description of how actors define and use these categories, see Anderson (1992). For a historical example of the actor's awareness of these categories, see Lawrence (1985).

14. Materials for this chapter has been drawn mainly from three sources: a) published literature, for instance, technical manuals and methodological articles; b) laboratory observations in the Boston and Montreal regions; c) interviews with scientists (mainly from the United States, Canada, and France) in both academic and commercial settings. Some interviewees having requested anonymity; we have decided to extend it to all interview material in this chapter.

15. This point can be related to Vincenti's (1984:571) distinction between two different modes of circulation for innovations: *diffusion pattern* and *simultaneous pattern,* the difference between the two modes laying, among other things, in "the range of availability of the necessary aptitudes and expertise."

16. This can be compared with the controversy surrounding the introduction of molecular biology into an Australian research institute described in Stokes (1985). See also Mackenzie, Cambrosio, and Keating (1988).

17. This can be a time-consuming enterprise: It took two years to examine all the parameters and to devise an optimal configuration (interview with a public health researcher, winter 1993). The paper describing this work received 48 citations in the 1985–1990 period.

18. See Chapter 1 for more details.

19. Rajewsky, it will be recalled (Chapter 1), was among the very first recipients of Milstein's P3-X63-Ag8 myeloma cell line. The new myeloma cell line was a subclone of the cell line obtained from Milstein.

20. Snyder (letter to the authors, February 16, 1993) used the following analogy: "I suppose the situation is analogous to techniques for measuring protein levels. The classical Lowry technique was published in 1954, and surely there are many more sensitive and accurate techniques that have been developed subsequently. However, since the Lowry procedure generally was good enough for most peoples' needs, few have changed over to novel procedures." On "satisficing," see March and Simon (1970), March and Simon (1958), and March (1978).

21. Readers interested in the cultural aspects of scientific practice will have noticed how animals and equipment are here being used interchangeably. On the "sacrifice" of mice and rats, see Lynch (1988).

22. Compare with Vincenti (184:562).

23 For a literary discussion of this kind of magical practice, see the chapter "Cromo" in Levi (1975).

24. Manuals agree on the fact that uncertainty cannot be entirely eliminated. See, for example, Campbell (1984:70):

> This parameter [hybridisation frequency] varies quite widely among research groups and, within groups, among particular experiments. No detailed comparisons of all available cell lines against a single type of antigen are available and much of the evidence is anecdotal. Even of two halves of the same spleen from an immunized animal it is difficult to obtain a valid comparison since the two fusions must necessarily involve either two operators or a time delay between the two experiments.

25. See also Traweek (1984).

3

"From Immunofantasy to Monoclonal Reality": Building a New Tool

What next?   Milstein (1981)

In 1990 César Milstein summarized the momentous career of his and Köhler's achievement in the following terms:

> In 1975 a method was described for making cell lines that secrete a single species of antibody (monoclonal antibody) with the desired specificity to antigen. The technique—"hybridoma technology"—proved to be general, and a wide range of monoclonal antibodies have been made which bond to protein, carbohydrate, nucleic acids and hapten antigens, and which even have catalytic activities, leading to many practical applications for monoclonal antibodies in research and human health-care and to patent disputes. (Winter and Milstein 1991).

Sociologically speaking, the most interesting passage in the preceding quote is not, as conventional social scientists would argue, the allusion to patent disputes, but the following: "The technique—'hybridoma technology'—proved to be general." This sentence unintentionally glosses over a problem of wide-ranging importance, namely, how something that is local and contingent is made general and universal.

The question of how things are made general is indeed a crucial issue for the sociology of scientific knowledge. The universal, acontextual characteristics of scientific entities have often been held as evidence against a possible sociological account of the content of scientific practice. The answer to this objection has taken the form of detailed ethnographic accounts of laboratory work and of scientific controversies that bring into focus the local, contingent nature of scientific knowledge and practice. Pursuing this line of inquiry, the transformation of a local result into a universal fact or technique has been interpreted not as flowing from the intrinsic validity of the claim in question; rather, this transformation is represented as an ongoing process of construction of a given claim's generality through the progressive extension of the local situations in which it can be made to work. The process is not one of abstraction, whereby facts and techniques are stripped of their contingencies to reveal their universal core. It is an active undertaking whereby the network along which a given fact or technique circulates is progressively enlarged, thus increasing the domain of validity of that particular fact or technique. There is thus no inductive leap from the local to the universal but, rather, an accumulation of local instantiations.[1]

This line of reasoning draws upon various aspects of scientific practice that were often ignored or taken for granted in conventional accounts. Chiefly among these figure standardization processes. The establishment and enforcement of standards involves a great deal of work that ensures that laboratories around the world use procedures and material that are, for all practical purposes, identical, thus creating the conditions for the successful replication and daily implementation of other laboratories' results. The transformation of material practices, their ongoing modification in order to make things work, and not some magical correspondence between nature and scientific representations, accounts for the generalization of results.

From this point of view, hybridoma technology is no exception. In investigating its transformation into a tool, we did indeed find many instances of standardization, both of the procedure and of its constitutive practices. Monoclonal antibodies were made general, they did not just happen to be general. Standardization, however, is only a specific instance of a more general process, that of regulation. The term *regulation* is not used here in the restricted sense of government regulation and, thus, does not refer solely to the activities of regulatory agencies such as the Food and Drug Administration (FDA).[2] Regulation, as we understand it, is the (often unintended) outcome not only of explicit initiatives but also of tacit agreements. In general, it follows from the stabilization of practices. This is not to deny the importance of guidelines and regulations issued by official agencies but to stress that the latter are the tip of the iceberg in the sense that they often originate in and are predicated upon the existence of a larger set of technoscientific practices. These include the establishment of voluntary or *de facto* standards and the enforcement of definitions of *good* or *state-of-the-art* science.

Indeed, as we shall see, the transformation of hybridoma technology into a "powerful new tool in biology and medicine" (Yelton and Scharff 1981)[3] was coextensive with the regulation of its use and the redefinition of its characteristics. Some aspects of hybridoma technology became the target of what Laurent Thévenot (1984) has called "investment in forms." These aspects underwent varying degrees of standardization and, correspondingly, became the objects of investment by international organizations, official institutional agreements, etc. Other parts of hybridoma technology were left to more informal or ad hoc forms of standardization. In yet other cases, a high degree of indexicality characterized the implementation of hybridoma technology (see Chapter 2). The decision to standardize certain areas and leave others unstandardized was, of course, not the result of some form of central planning but, rather, an emergent accomplishment.

As we saw in Chapter 1, despite a final paragraph indicating the possible general applicability of the technique, the results reported in MILSTEIN 75 were limited to the production of antibodies against sheep red blood cells. The authors themselves pointed out that "it remain[ed] to be seen whether similar results [could] be obtained using other antigens." The exact meaning of "results" was not specified. To be sure, there was no mention of hybridoma technology in the 1975 paper, and the original purpose of the research was clearly not to develop such a technology. Not surprisingly, the 1975 paper was at first viewed as one among a number of papers that used cell fusion techniques to dissect the genetic control of antibody diversity.

At some point, around 1977, the production of monoclonal antibodies became an end in itself, no longer restricted to the initial immunogenetic network. This was the beginning of a process leading to the establishment of the generality of hybridoma technology and, correlatively, to the translation of monoclonal antibodies into "a powerful new tool in biology and medicine" (Yelton and Scharff 1981). *Generality*, here, can be taken to mean both that the technique was not restricted to a particular kind of antigen and that it was not restricted to a particular production site.

Scientists themselves have offered two quite different accounts of the diffusion of hybridoma technology. The first may be described, following Gilbert and Mulkay (1984), as *empiricist* and represents researchers as mere spokespersons for natural events and properties, which are considered the driving forces behind scientific and technological development. The second, which may be described as *contingent*, uses social factors to account for the evolution of scientific practices. For example, Milstein's remark that hybridoma technology "proved to be general" implies an empiricist diffusion model, whereby monoclonal antibodies' properties alone account for their spread through scientific and commercial spheres. These properties are seen as independent of human intervention. Researchers recognized the overwhelming advantages of monoclonal antibodies and rapidly adopted these "new powerful tools." The intervention of social factors is acknowledged only in the form of obstacles to the diffusion, such as scientific conservatism and market inertia.

Indeed, Milstein (1981:393) presented hybridoma technology as "a clear example of the artificiality of the dissociation between so-called basic and applied research," pointing out how a serendipitous discovery in a very esoteric field had resulted in unexpected and wide-ranging practical applications.[4] In the same vein, Köhler (1985) commented that his work was a paradigmatic example of "pure fundamental research," leading quickly to worldwide commercial application.[5] Because it attributes to hybridoma technology the power to rapidly and somewhat mysteriously spread to different areas, this argument is consistent with an empiricist diffusion model. Again compatible with this representation is the fact that both Milstein and Köhler claimed to have been surprised by the sudden transformation of their discovery into a biotechnological bonanza, a process to which, it would seem, they were largely extraneous.

However, Milstein has also resorted to a contingent model. While no doubt assuming that the generality of monoclonal antibodies was in the last instance grounded in some natural property, he has claimed, on occasion, that human intervention played a major role in establishing the superiority of monoclonal antibodies over alternative tools and, consequently, in ensuring their spread. In his Nobel Lecture, Milstein (1986) acknowledged that "for several years [he had] shelved the antibody diversity problem to demonstrate the practical importance of monoclonal antibodies in other areas of basic research and in clinical diagnosis." In practice, this had meant teaming up with researchers from other fields to produce monoclonal antibodies relevant to those domains. As a consequence, Milstein was able to *progressively build the generality of the technique*, showing that it could be applied in fields ranging from the clinical classification of leukemias, to transplantation, blood typing, neurobiology, and large-scale protein purification (Milstein 1981).[6] This ongoing activity was more than a simple demonstration, as instanced by the fact that as late as 1980 Milstein still only claimed that "the experience accumulated *tends to indicate* that the method [hybridoma technology] is general" (Milstein 1981:399, emphasis added).

On a number of occasions, Milstein has insisted that what we now see as obvious logical conclusions concerning hybridoma technology had in fact to be established through experiments designed to undermine received wisdom. In 1984, in the preface to a volume summarizing the results of the first international workshop on leukocyte surface antigens, he noted:

> That [monoclonal antibodies] were going to be a basic tool in studies of cell surface antigens was not as obvious in 1976 as it may seem today. Among many other unknowns, the specificity of antibodies was a matter of considerable controversy. The possibility that the specificity of antisera [i.e., polyclonal antibodies] was more the result of the heterogeneity of the polyclonal response than of specific molecular recognition was discussed many times, and was the subject of a major paper presented at a meeting held only 2 years earlier.... So it had to be demonstrated that [monoclonal antibodies] to differentiation antigens *could* be made and that when made they did not show signs of unexpected cross-reactions.
>
> (Milstein 1984, emphasis in text).[7]

Contingent accounts, in general, rely heavily on personal anecdote and narrative, whereas empiricist accounts, while not necessarily quantitative, often lend themselves to quantification in terms of the sums invested or the number of papers produced. In the following section we shall present quantitative material used to illustrate the empiricist narrative. In the subsequent section, interview material will be marshaled to elaborate a contingent version of the "same" events. We shall then argue that although only the second account leads to an ethnographic understanding of the generalization of hybridoma technology, the first captures important aspects of the monoclonal antibodies story, notably the speed of diffusion with which a contingent narrative must reckon. In other words, rather than oppose the two accounts, we claim both have merit.

An Empiricist Account

There are clearly grounds for comparing the spread of monoclonal antibodies to an effervescent diffusion process, too effervescent, it would seem, to be accounted for by anything other than the intrinsic superiority of monoclonal antibodies over alternative tools. Graphs are particularly effective devices for constructing and validating such a narrative. Figure 3.1 shows the annual increase in publications indexed with the terms *Monoclonal antibodies* and *Hybridomas* in *Medline*, the on-line version of *Index Medicus*. We can easily distinguish the characteristic pattern of the logistic curve, with a phase of exponential growth followed by saturation that has, however, yet to reach its limit. Those familiar with scientometrics (the quantitative study of scientific activities) since the early days of *Science since Babylon* (De Solla Price 1961) will immediately recognize in the logistic curve the icon of a major scientific breakthrough. Thus, not surprisingly, in a scientometric study of monoclonal antibodies, Rothman and Parkinson (1984) characterized the increase in the number of publications devoted to or making use of monoclonal antibodies as "dramatic."

Because publication data are not interesting per se but only as indicators, the following question arises: A dramatic increase of what? In the present case, Rothman and Parkinson went on to compare the empirically derived monoclonal antibodies curve to the theoretical logistic curve, which, according to sociologists of science,[8] characterizes the growth of new research areas. They commented that monoclonal antibodies had taken off and were now (in the early 1980s) in the central stage of growth, to be eventually followed by decline or displacement. They cautioned, however, that because monoclonal antibodies could be used as research tools, it was possible "that the field as a whole may remain in the rapid growth phase for a considerable time, for as research problems are solved in one area the possibility of new ones opening up elsewhere is high" (ibid.:C38), a claim that several additional years of hindsight and Figure 3.1

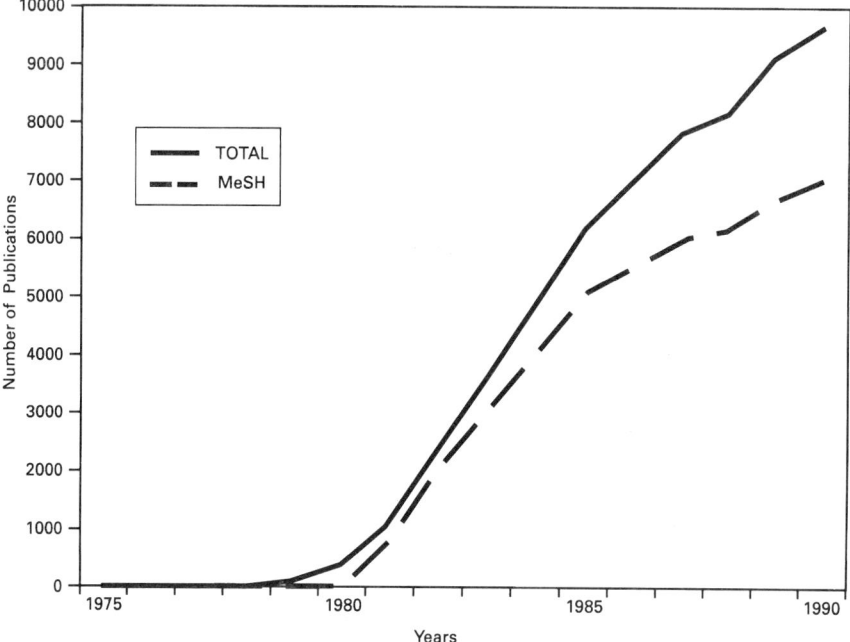

Figure 3.1. Number of publications indexed with the terms *monoclonal antibodies* and *hybridomas*. (Source of data: *Medline,* the on-line version of *Index Medicus.*) The terms *monoclonal antibodies* and *hybridomas* were added to the list of official descriptors (Medical Subject Headings or MeSH) in 1982. Before that date, we searched for the two terms in the title and abstract of articles. After 1982, the figure shows both the number of publications indexed by the two McSH terms (indicating the number of publications in which monoclonal antibodies play a central role) and the papers in which the terms *monoclonal antibodies* and *hybridomas* are present but not as a MeSH, thus indicating a secondary role for monoclonal antibodies.

could arguably support. Rothman and Parkinson's double characterization of the domain as both a technical domain and a scientific research area is of particular interest to us because it brings us back, through a quantitative detour, to our original question, namely, how a given entity, in this case monoclonal antibodies, acquires the status of a tool.

Further indications of hybridoma technology's dramatic growth may be obtained by counting citations of one scientific paper by others. Indeed, scientists themselves resort to these techniques. For instance, a graph of the rapid growth in the number of publications citing MILSTEIN 75 was featured in a review article as an indication "of the rate of spread of this technique and its implications" (Kennett 1981:1037). Citations can also be used to relate the growth of the field to Köhler and Milstein's original contribution. Figure 3.2, for example, shows

"*From Immunofantasy to Monoclonal Reality*" 87

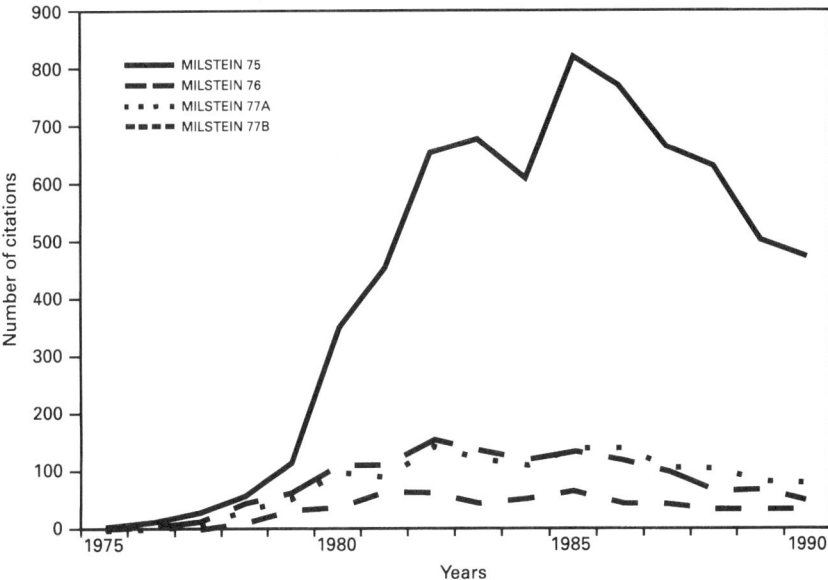

Figure 3.2. Number of citations received by hybridoma technology's four foundational papers. (Source of data: *Science Citation Index.*)

the number of citations received by hybridoma technology's four foundational papers (Milstein's tetralogy, as we called it in Chapter 1) and highlights the rise of MILSTEIN 75 to the status of ritual reference, with an impressively high and long-lasting citation count.

Figure 3.3, which combines the two previous figures, shows that between 1975 and 1980 the number of publications using monoclonal antibodies closely followed the number of citations to MILSTEIN 75. The fact that after 1980 the number of publications greatly outstripped the number of citations to MILSTEIN 75 can be explained in two complementary ways. First of all, authors started referencing their own publications rather than Köhler and Milstein's paper as a source of technical details concerning the production of monoclonal antibodies. Secondly, the latter became so widespread, a sort of background skill, that reference to the foundational paper, although it continued to enjoy a very high citation rate, was no longer deemed necessary.

The commercial end of the diffusion story can be embodied in graphs such as Figure 3.4, which shows, once again, the logistic curve as related, this time, to the increase in U.S. and world patents indexed by the terms *monoclonal antibodies* and *hybridomas*. Figure 3.5, in which the number of world patents is plotted against the number of publications, is the iconic expression of yet another recurrent trope of the science studies field, the time lag, in this case very short, charac-

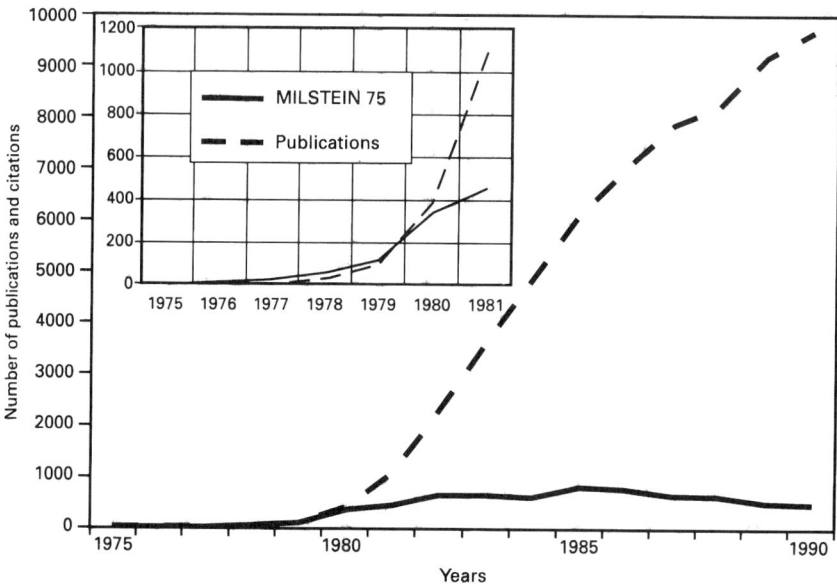

Figure 3.3. Comparative evolution of monoclonal antibody-related publications and citations to MILSTEIN 75. (Sources of data: see Figures 3.1 and 3.2.)

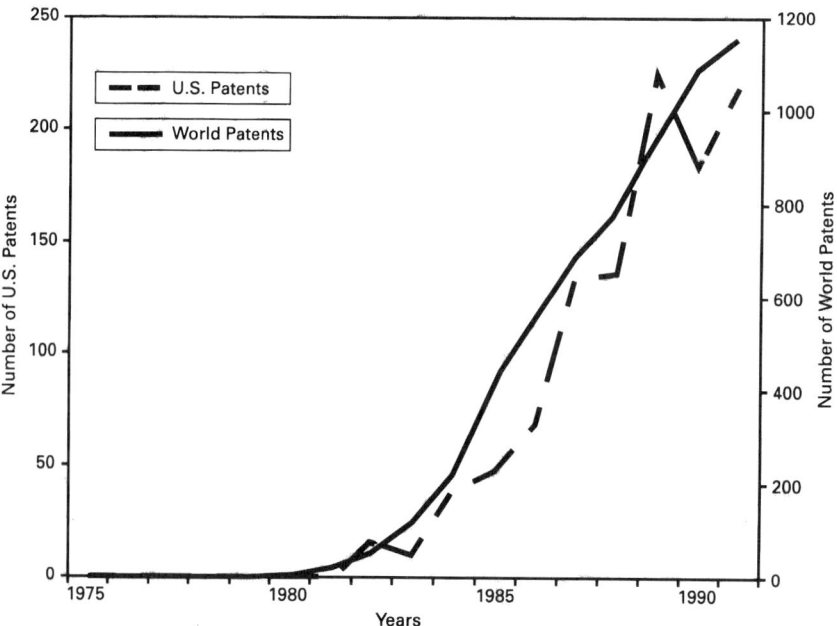

Figure 3.4. Number of U.S. and world patents related to monoclonal antibodies. (Source of data: *U.S. Patents Claims* and *World Patents Index.*) The striking overlap effect between the two curves has been produced by using two different y-axis scales.

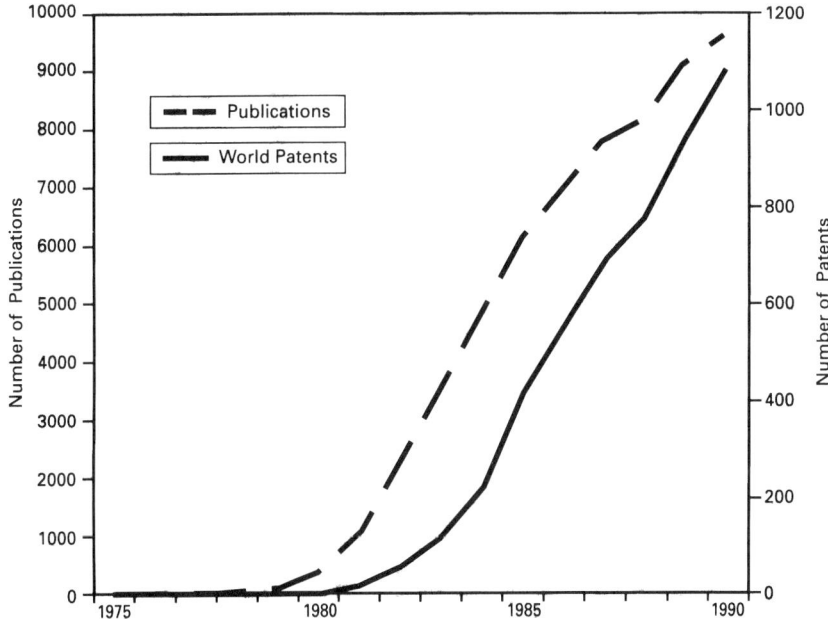

Figure 3.5. Comparing the growth of patents and publications. (Source of data: see Figures 3.1 and 3.4.) The graphic effect has been produced by using two different y-axis scales.

terizing the commercial application of scientific discoveries. So short, indeed, is the time lag in the case of monoclonal antibodies that it lends credibility to the previously quoted remarks by Milstein and Köhler that hybridoma technology demonstrated the absurdity of drawing boundaries between fundamental and applied research.

Finally, Figure 3.6, reproduced from Gosling (1990),[9] adopts a different format, the area chart, to represent the inroad of monoclonal antibodies into commercial immunoassays.[10] The choice of this format corresponds to the replacement of the growth metaphor, as embodied in the logistic curve, with a spatial metaphor: Monoclonal antibodies are shown to occupy more and more territory, pushing aside established approaches and, with them, the whole menagerie of rabbits, goats and sheep used to produce conventional (polyclonal) antibodies.

Commenting on his chart, Gosling noted that in 1990 (i.e., 15 years after the development of hybridoma technology) monoclonal antibodies had made an impressive inroad into the domain, insofar as over 50% of new immunoassays used this kind of antibody. It may equally be wondered, however, why, after 15 years, had only slightly over 50% become monoclonal. In other words, if monoclonal antibodies were such a superior tool, why were polyclonal antibodies still being

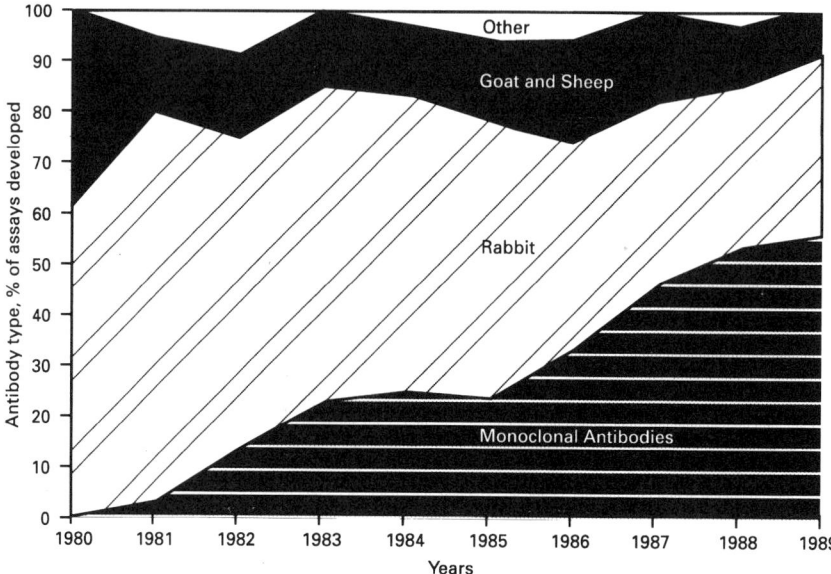

Figure 3.6. Monoclonal antibodies' inroad into commercial immunoassays. (Source: Gosling 1990.)

used to produce new assays? The demise of polyclonals and, correspondingly, what has been termed the *decline of the rabbit* needs to be qualified![11]

Indeed, textbooks on monoclonal antibodies often pointed out that "for many purposes, conventional antibodies will do the job adequately, with much less work" (e.g., Goding 1986:250),[12] while review articles cautioned that "because of the fundamental differences between [conventional and monoclonal antibodies], it is unsafe to assume one can automatically be substituted for the other" (Yelton and Scharff 1981:664). Enthusiasts, on the other hand, felt that these qualifications smacked of conservatism. This difference of opinion indicates not only the fact that the superiority of monoclonal antibodies over alternative serological methods was problematic but also, and more interestingly, that the characteristics of monoclonal antibodies were not defined in abstract terms but, rather, in opposition to other substances and techniques. Thus, their patterns of use were not given *a priori* but, rather, were the outcome of disputes over the merits or shortcomings of monoclonal antibodies as embedded in specific tasks and work settings. The point is not simply that the characteristics of monoclonal antibodies were negotiated but, more importantly, that by engaging in these negotiations researchers defined monoclonal antibodies as particular technoscientific objects, endowed, for instance, as in the quotation from Milstein that opened this chapter, with generality. In turn, as discussed in Chapter 2 with regards to tacit knowledge, this attribution of specific characteristics resulted in specific patterns of use in biomedical and commercial networks.

But how exactly did this happen? Can we go beyond the by now routine reference to negotiations and local settings? While empiricist narratives endow monoclonal antibodies with properties that allow them to perform dramatic feats, epitomized by logistic growth, contingent narratives endeavor to describe the socio-technical dynamics that led to the present place of hybridoma technology in the biomedical field. A good example of a contingent narrative was supplied to us by Leonard Herzenberg of the Stanford University Medical School.

A Contingent Account

Trained in genetics and biochemistry, Herzenberg had been working since the 1960s on the genetics of immunoglobulins as well as in cellular immunology, studying markers on the surface of lymphocytes. In the late 1960s to early 1970s he invested time and work in the development of an apparatus known as the fluorescence activated cell sorter (FACS), which was designed, as he retrospectively observed, "to meet a growing need for cell separation methods that would allow genetic and functional studies with viable lymphocyte subpopulations" (Parks, Herzenberg, and Herzenberg 1989:782).[13] In 1976–1977, during a sabbatical, Herzenberg traveled to England to work with César Milstein.[14]

There were several reasons for this choice. Milstein was a renowned scientist working in the same field as Herzenberg. Herzenberg had known him for a long time, and he hoped to improve his skills in molecular biology by working with him. In addition, Herzenberg also hoped to convince Milstein and other key British researchers to adopt the FACS, a commercial version of which was then being marketed by Becton-Dickinson.[15] Hybridoma technology had not been a factor in his decision to spend a sabbatical in Cambridge because his travel plans and fellowship applications had been made before hybridoma technology was developed.

The sabbatical year did not work out as expected, as there were tensions between Herzenberg and Milstein. Milstein, for instance, did not seem to share Herzenberg's enthusiasm for the FACS. However, the unexpected bonus of the stay in Cambridge was that Herzenberg learned about the newly developed hybridoma technology. He claims to have immediately recognized that hybridoma technology represented a solution to a problem encountered during his FACS research. Herzenberg very quickly articulated these two lines of work, so that the former became the solution, at least retrospectively, to the problems encountered with the latter. In effect, the FACS, it is now claimed, would have had only a limited success due to the variability of the traditional serological reagents used to detect the cell-surface antigens.

As Leonore Herzenberg, his wife and collaborator, pointed out (interview, March 27, 1988), "meeting after meeting after meeting there would be a fight with people because one would say my reagent doesn't do this and another would say my reagent does do this." Monoclonal antibodies offered the possibility of standardizing reagents and thus of standardizing the laboratories, making the data they produced comparable:

> Our first desire was to make [monoclonal antibodies] as available as possible because I saw them immediately as being very important standard reagents, where everybody could get the same results with the same antibodies. There was an unlimited supply of the very same reagents, so that immunology could become almost like chemistry, where people could use absolutely defined reagents for their work. I thought that was very important. Part of the reason that I thought it was important was because of our interest in the FACS, which we developed and used to develop many applications in immunology. The biggest problem we had was to have standard reagents for the FACS. So I was very interested in having standard reagents available for people working with the FACS-type technology.... The FACS was a tool which we wanted to develop. I wrote a paper called "Monoclonal Antibodies and the Fluorescence-Activated Cell Sorter: Complementary Tools in Cell Biology."[16] I gave a lot of seminars with that title because they were very complementary tools. It was just perfect. The [monoclonal antibodies] were needed for the FACS, and the FACS was one of the major applications of the [monoclonal antibodies].   (Interview, March 27, 1988).[17]

By their own account, the Herzenbergs were instrumental in launching two initiatives that contributed significantly to monoclonal antibodies' career in the United States. The first entailed convincing people of the potential usefulness of hybridoma technology and thus prompting them to adopt monoclonal antibodies over the more conventional antisera. The second was to actually make monoclonal antibodies available to the converted.

As far as the first line of action was concerned, Leonard Herzenberg took advantage of the fact that he had been nominated co-chair of the 1977 ICN-UCLA Symposium on Molecular and Cellular Biology to organize a workshop on hybridoma technology. He also managed to convince a somewhat reluctant Milstein to participate. The workshop, "T and B Cell Hybrids," attracted a large crowd (about 300 persons) and, according to Herzenberg, introduced the U.S. research community to hybridoma technology. Indeed, the workshop summary (Milstein and Herzenberg 1977) reveals a carefully orchestrated performance. Milstein first presented "a bit of the history and the current status of work in his laboratory," which provided an introduction to the topic. This was followed by speeches of various participants, who "told of making hybridomas making monoclonal antibodies to a variety of antigens." This was meant to demonstrate that "clearly the technique is widely applicable to the making of extremely useful serologic reagents of monoclonal specificity." The final comments restated the main message, that hybridoma technology provided an "enormous potential for characterization of the antigens coded by genes of the MHC of mice and other species, including Man."

At the same meeting, Herzenberg convened a workshop on "Cell Separation and Characterization," in which the FACS was presented as "clearly the most versatile and generally effective means now in use for specific cell purification and analysis," adding that "the obvious limitation in experiments with the FACS often is the failure to verify stringently the serological specificity of reagents used to attach fluorescent cell markers" (Herzenberg and Wofsy 1977). Although this was not spelled out in the summary of the workshop, the implicit lesson was that the solution to this problem was to be sought in the results reported in the workshop on hybridoma technology.

The ICN-UCLA symposium meeting paved the way for the first meeting devoted entirely to results obtained with hybridoma technology. Held in Bethesda, Maryland in April 1978, and sponsored by the National Cancer Institute, the workshop "Lymphocyte Hybridomas" assembled the majority of researchers who had so far produced monoclonal antibodies (Melchers, Potter, and Warner 1978).[18] In the proceedings of the workshop, a table listing the hybridomas produced by participants shows that most of the activity was still located in a few centers: In addition to Milstein's MRC laboratory in Cambridge and the Basel Institute of Immunology, to which Köhler had returned after his stay in Cambridge, the bulk of monoclonal antibodies originated from the initial recipients of Milstein's myeloma cell line: Klaus Rajewsky's team at the University of Cologne; Hilary Koprowski's team at Wistar Institute; Norman Klinman and Roger Kennett at the University of Pennsylvania, who had received the myeloma cell line from the nearby Koprowski with Milstein's agreement (Koprowski to Milstein, 19 November 1976; Milstein to Koprowski, 1 December 1976); Herzenberg's group at Stanford; and a group of French researchers associated with Gérard Buttin and Pierre-André Cazenave.

The second line of action involved making myeloma cell lines available to those who wanted to produce their own hybridomas as well as making monoclonal antibodies available to those who wanted to use the antibodies produced by other laboratories as, so to speak, off-the-shelf reagents. Let us note what Leonore Herzenberg (interview, March 27, 1988) said in this regard:

> [From the very beginning, the question of the public distribution of monoclonals] was a major issue, and for the most part when the first few were made it created a

> situation of haves and have nots. It wasn't a question of whether people wanted to use the antibodies. It was a question of whether they could. For the most part, everybody was playing very close to the bat. They gave their friends some antibodies, but they were not going to give the antibodies out. They were generally not going to make them publicly available. From our point of view, we thought very differently, and we discussed it in the lab. If you want to standardize the reagents in the field and if you want to have people doing research where you don't sit at the meetings and listen to them argue about my reagents or your reagents, then the reagents can be put out very quickly.

Sending out antibodies to anyone who requested them, however, soon became time consuming and expensive. Herzenberg thus decided to use a commercial company to perform this task:

> So I think that [the fact of] the companies being involved and making these antibodies was actually very important to the development of the whole field, because it was very difficult for one laboratory to develop a whole library or battery of reagents that it needs for its work. . . . The idea of hybridomas was that everybody should have the same specificity, reactivity, same amount of color, and reagents. So if everybody made their own . . . there was great difficulty logistically in everybody making their own. It also defeated the purpose, the great advantage of monoclonals. So I felt it should come from central sources. [Becton-Dickinson] agreed that I could train their people so they would be very good at making standard reagents and keep the quality up. (Interview, March 27, 1988).[19]

The agreement between Becton-Dickinson and the Herzenbergs did not simply result in the establishment of a commercial distribution network but also in the distribution of reagents that could be certified to be "the same." In other words, availability and standardization, and thus reproducibility of results among laboratories, went hand in hand:

> One of the things we did was to establish the criteria for quality control. In the contract that we made [when] delivering the original reagents to [Becton-Dickinson], we gave them standards for quality control, things that had to be done in order to be sure it was the same antibody. Those were incorporated and became the standard for the field in fact. . . . In addition, when [Becton-Dickinson] started distributing these—the mouse reagents and basically the reagents I was using in the lab—I spent some time with them and set up reporting sheets for what you should tell the investigator about the reagent as long as you're distributing it. That also became the standard. Now I notice that all the other companies do that. But those were key because without these kinds of reporting of the quality control, you couldn't use them for good research work. Now they do it standardly. Most of the people who see them probably don't even know what it means. But if you need to know about it, it's there. (Interview, March 27, 1988).

Herzenberg's narrative clearly makes room for human intervention in the diffusion process, but, more importantly, it allows one to postulate a mechanism for the generalization of hybridoma technology. On this view, hybridoma technology's generality depended on the establishment of centers of production and networks for the circulation of standardized monoclonal antibodies. This, in turn, effectively standardized work in laboratories around the world and thus transformed monoclonal antibodies into an "obligatory passage point" (Latour 1987) for the performance of state-of-the art research. We shall therefore take a closer look at the issue of standardization in the next section.

Building a Tool: Generality Through Standardization

The theme of standardization goes back to the very beginnings of hybridoma technology. It can be found, for instance, in the proceedings of a 1975 symposium organized by the Royal Society of Medicine Foundation (New York) and the Royal Society of Medicine (London), which was to our knowledge the first, and rather uneventful, public presentation of Köhler and Milstein's experiment (Milstein and Köhler 1977).[20] On that occasion, Edgar Haber (1977) argued, without referring specifically to Köhler and Milstein's presentation, that "The standardization of assays among many laboratories and maintenance of standards for a period of years has not been possible. A continuous supply of a single homogeneous antibody of precisely the right property would be most desirable; it would have a very large impact in the widespread application of [radioimmunoassays] methods." The standardization theme was picked up by Milstein and co-workers in a widely cited 1977 paper, which stated: "The established cell lines offer the further advantage of unlimited permanent supply of material, and the possibility of worldwide standardization." The paper further noted that the results it reported brought "the goal of producing standard permanent supplies of monoclonal antibodies for human tissue typing and other clinical uses one step nearer" (Galfré et al. 1977).

The insistence on the standardizing power of monoclonal antibodies was also a central and recurring argument in a programmatic document published by the National Institute of Allergy and Infectious Diseases (NIAID) in 1981 under the title *New Initiatives in Immunology* (NIAID 1981). Again we encounter the theme that figured so prominently in the Herzenbergs' narrative.[21] In its opening statement, the NIAID document ranked monoclonal antibodies among the "techniques and tools" (as opposed to factual findings) and (re)presented them as "reference reagents," which could be produced in "virtually unlimited amounts for indefinite periods of time." This would make them "available to all investigators or diagnostic laboratories needing them," where they could serve "as a reference reagent for as long as it is required." Past is the era, claimed the NIAID document, when the unpredictability and heterogeneity of the immune response made the production of antibodies more of an art than a science. Now antibodies could be produced that shared the standardized properties of chemical reagents and would result in the standardization of the results obtained by laboratories around the world. It is difficult to resist the conclusion that it was not because monoclonal antibodies were such a powerful tool that they led to standardization but, rather, that it is precisely because they were seen, from the very outset, as a potential vehicle for standardization that they became such a powerful tool.

Before exploring this process, let us note that the production of monoclonal antibodies as a standardizing tool was obviously dependent on the existence of a standardized biomedical infrastructure. The latter, although generally taken for granted, can become problematic when major breakdowns occur. One such instance—a "massive mouse mixup"—occurred when it became clear that shipments of BALB/c mice used in the production of monoclonal antibodies and distributed commercially in the United States by Charles River Breeding Laboratories were genetically contaminated. News of the mixup was soon followed by reassuring press releases from various monoclonal antibodies companies announcing that the potentially disastrous consequences of this event had been avoided (*McGraw-Hill's Biotechnology Newsletter* 1982c).[22] Independently of the outcome, this particular case points to both the work and arrangements necessary to provide scientists with a constant supply of raw materials, and to the artificial nature of the supposedly natural organisms on which experiments are conducted (Knorr-Cetina 1981).

The NIAID report discussed the creation of yet another layer of this biomedical infrastructure. For instance, monoclonal antibodies were to be provided to inexperienced investigators unable to produce them. The NIH was therefore requested to encourage the "development of shared hybridoma facilities as part of program or core grants." This would not, however, be enough, because the uncontrolled proliferation of locally produced monoclonal antibodies was certain to result in confusion; consequently, steps would have to be taken "to identify those monoclonal antibodies that are most useful and to see that the same antibodies are used universally." Additional steps in standardization and in the control of the standardizing tools called for by the NIAID report included the establishment of banking facilities and the publication of lists of available monoclonal antibodies. But here again, the use of "complex and individual terminologies" would have undermined the standardization effort. Thus, the NIH was asked to encourage workshops and exchange of reagents, namely, in the area of "antibodies directed against subsets of human cells."

These recommendations did not go unheeded. For instance, the call for workshops and exchange of reagents led to the establishment of the international classification of the surface antigens of human white blood cells, known as the *CD nomenclature*. By 1986, the number of laboratories participating in the ongoing production of this nomenclature had risen to 190. They performed more than 150,000 assays to characterize about 800 antibodies. The present-day classification of lymphocytes has thus as its precondition the constitution of a network for the establishment of identities between monoclonal antibodies produced by different laboratories (Cambrosio and Keating 1992).

The NIAID report's call for the promotion and standardization of monoclonal antibodies found its international equivalent in the initiatives taken by the World Health Organization (Houba 1984; WHO 1983). For instance, WHO organized or sponsored courses, workshops, seminars, and symposia in this area. Moreover, initiatives were taken in collaboration with the United Nations Development Programme and the World Bank to promote the use of monoclonal antibody technology in the study of tropical parasitic diseases, a domain also discussed in the NIAID report. In addition to promoting the diffusion of monoclonal antibodies, the World Health Organization adopted more direct measures to regulate and standardize the use of hybridoma technology. Three of these deserve mention here: first, the critical evaluation of the application of monoclonal antibodies in immunodiagnosis, and in the identification and characterization of antigens; second, the preparation of criteria for the standardization of the production of monoclonal antibodies, including quality control standards; and finally, the registration of monoclonal antibodies and the clones producing them.

The problem, as far as the latter measure was concerned, was to control the anarchic proliferation of monoclonal antibodies in various laboratories under idiosyncratic names.[23] In 1983, 50,000 hybridomas were thought to exist, and about 10,000 new hybridomas were being characterized annually (Bussard 1987b). Estimates in 1987 update to 20,000 the number of new descriptions of hybridomas that could be obtained each year through systematic searches of scientific journals.[24] Individual attempts to establish a simple registry had been tried in England and the United States, but these attempts were limited to narrow fields of application. Bulletins, such as *Monoclonal Antibodies News*,[25] listing and describing the available monoclonal antibodies were also of limited use.

Thus, a proposal to create a Task group on a Hybridoma and Monoclonal Antibodies Data Bank was drafted in 1982 by the Committee on Data for Science and Technology (CODATA) of the International Council of Scientific Unions. The World Health Organization decided to collaborate. In 1983 a decision was made to create the Hybridoma Data Bank (HDB) under the auspices of CODATA and the International Union of Immunological Societies (IUIS). The data bank's central office was located at the American Type Culture Collection (ATCC), with two additional branches in Europe and Japan (Bussard 1987b; Bussard, Krichevsky, and Blaine 1985).

The design of the Hybridoma Data Bank was based on the following requirements: The data bank had to be international (i.e., the input of data was to be done directly, without passing through regional and national registries), easily accessible, and inexpensive; that meant, of course, computerized. Hybridoma producers were requested to complete a data reporting form. Collaboration from individual researchers was, however, not as high as expected. This collaboration was critical for success since, as one of the initiators of the Hybridoma Data Bank had pointed out in 1983, "The success of the bank is related to the quantity of data collected relative to the amount of the total data existing" (Bussard 1987b). To overcome this problem, the Hybridoma Data Bank officials resorted to collecting data from published papers, commercial catalogues, and patent applications. Still, in 1989 the ATCC processed only about 2500 records (CERDIC brochure). According to the Hybridoma Data Bank officials' own criteria, this signified failure.

Two somewhat speculative and complementary explanations can be advanced to account for this. The first is that because scientific research is organized along informal research networks providing direct access to information and research materials, the detour through the Hybridoma Data Bank was redundant.[26] Indeed, those scientists who would be most likely to contribute information to the Hybridoma Data Bank would also be those least likely to need it. Those who were not part of a network, and who would thus need the Hybridoma Data Bank, would be most unlikely to contribute to the databank. Secondly, as shown by the example of the CD workshops, taxonomic and classificatory enterprises, including the establishment of standardized lists of available research material, seem to be more successful when they take place within a specific research domain, as opposed to a generic field, such as the one covered by the Hybridoma Data Bank. Thus, this episode points less to the absence of regulation than to its presence, which can, however, take different forms in different domains. Indeed, the limited success of the Hybridoma Data Bank was more than compensated for by the presence of informal modes of regulation governing the distribution and circulation of biomedical objects.

While information concerning the existence and availability of monoclonal antibodies was important, it had to be complemented by access to antibodies or to the antibody-producing cells. It was not merely a question of making monoclonal antibodies available to researchers but also of regulating the circulation of cells and cell products. This was a thorny issue. For instance, when the Herzenbergs decided to make their monoclonal antibodies available to all researchers who requested them, their decision was viewed with mixed feelings by fellow scientists, some of whom accused the Herzenbergs of forcing their hand. Leonore Herzenberg (interview, March 27, 1988) recalled:

> Well, I can remember . . . going to that meeting and announcing that we were making all these antibodies available and that anybody could have them and getting a tremendous positive response from the people at the meeting. There was almost a gasp when I said that all of these antibodies would be available. Then we got a negative response from people, who said that we had no right to make a unilateral decision because now everybody was forced to follow suit, and that was true. Up until that time, there were always discussions and decisions about [whether monoclonal antibodies] should be made public. And once we said we were giving five or six antibodies, at the time, as soon as that was done it forced the issue, and from then on most people gave their antibodies out.

As we saw in the case of the Herzenbergs, however, even the traditional mechanism whereby individual researchers sent reagents to fellow scientists who requested them was inefficient when viewed from the perspective of worldwide standardization. The Herzenbergs answer to this problem was to shift the production and distribution of monoclonal antibodies to a commercial company. Another solution was the establishment of centralized repositories acting as distribution centers. One such repository, which played a pioneering role, was created in a private research institution, the Salk Institute, by Melvin Cohn.

Cohn was already operating a cell bank containing murine immune-related culture and tumor cell lines that had been created in the early 1970s. Operating under a National Cancer Institute contract, Cohn had initiated a Myeloma Tumor Program using cell lines obtained from Michael Potter and from the Walter and Eliza Hall Institute (see Chapter 1). Although no hybridomas were listed in the third catalogue of Cohn's center, published in 1977 (Salk Institute 1977), by 1979 seven hybridomas figured in the fourth edition of the catalogue. The fourth edition also listed both the P3X63Ag8 myeloma cell line (used by Köhler and Milstein in their initial experiments), describing it as "derivative of P3" and "useful for fusions," as well as its nonsecreting variant NS-1 (Salk Institute 1979).

The budget justification section of the 1981 proposal to the National Cancer Institute for a contract renewal explained that "this new contract period reflects for the first time the shift in emphasis toward hybridoma technology." The proposal further noted that "the volume of work has increased disproportionately with the number of cells lines maintained and shipped because of the increased number of hybridomas in the library. Quality control procedures for hybridoma cell lines consume a considerable amount of time, as well as reagents." Similarly, in the progress report section, we read that "[t]he demand for cell lines and the number of cell lines in our inventory has grown substantially over the last year with the advent of many new hybridoma cell lines." The text further argues that the center was clearly "entering a new phase of work. In short we are becoming the *unofficial standard reference center* for hybridoma cell lines." The center was characterized as "the primary repository for the new hybridoma products that are revolutionizing many facets of biological research. Over the past year, more than 75% of our work has been hybridoma related" (Cohn 1981, emphasis added). From March to December 1980, for instance, the Salk Institute sent hybridoma technology–related mouse myelomas to 126 laboratories.[27]

An idea of the role and geographic range of centers like Cohn's can be gathered by consulting Figures 3.7. and 3.8. While we were unable to reconstitute a geographic map of the Salk Institute's shipments of *mouse* myelomas, Figure 3.7 shows the shipment of the first *rat* myelomas from Milstein's laboratory between 1979 and 1985. The situation is, to some extent, comparable because in both cases the new cell lines could be obtained only from a limited number of locations. The international reach of Milstein's shipments is apparent. As a comparison, Figure 3.8 shows the shipment of *mouse* myelomas from the ATCC between 1982 and 1985. At this late stage, myelomas were obviously available in many locations, both in national repositories and from individual researchers. As a result, ATCC shipments were concentrated in North America.

The role of Cohn's center was not simply to make cell lines available but also to provide researchers with essential, unpublished information, thus complementing the Materials and Methods section of published articles: "Often this information ... comes from other investigators who will call or write to our project manager." Cohn (1981) could thus claim that "A number of scientific investigations world-wide are directly or indirectly dependent on this program." That also meant providing a guarantee against losses, a reminder of possible "breakdowns": "We carry key lines from many laboratories guaranteeing that losses due to accident are minimized."

While Cohn's enterprise can be ranked closer to the more informal, decentralized type of regulation, more structured initiatives (public or semipublic) such as the previously mentioned American Type Culture Collection, soon took over the function fulfilled by his cell bank. For instance, the Hybridoma Cell Bank (not to be confounded with the Hybridoma Data Bank), supported by NIAID, began operation in October 1980, and the increased responsibilities of the ATCC in this field found a material counterpart in the construction of a new building at the ATCC headquarters in Rockville, Maryland (ATCC 1985:210).[28] Cohn's 1981 application for a renewal of the National Cancer Institute contract was denied, and ATCC personnel transferred the holdings of the Salk Institute cell bank to the newly created ATCC Tumor Immunology Bank.[29] In addition, as previously mentioned, commercial enterprises such as Becton-Dickinson or Ortho Pharmaceuticals also played an important role: By putting a large number of monoclonal

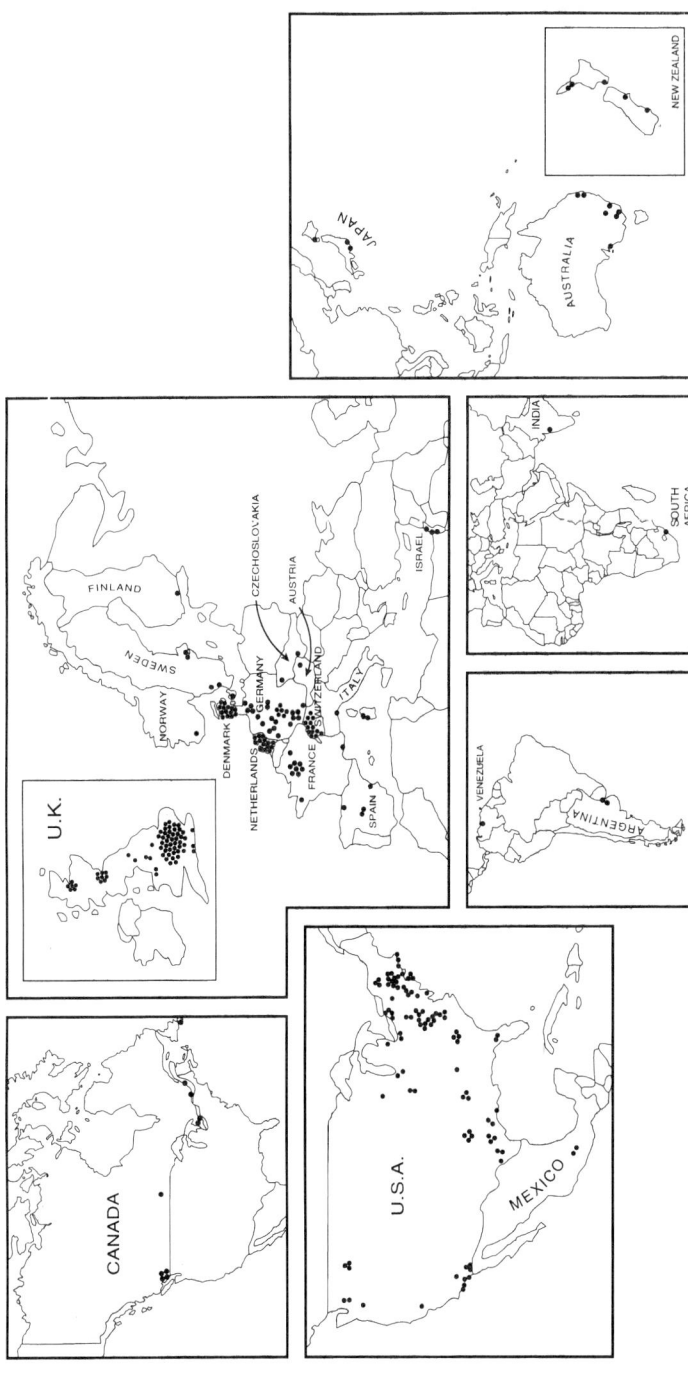

Figure 3.7. Geographical distribution of laboratories that received rat myelomas from Milstein's laboratory between 1979 and 1985. Each dot represents the approximate geographic location of a laboratory which requested and received at least one of the two available rat cell lines (Y3-Ag1.2.3. and YB213.0.Ag.20). (Data kindly provided by Dr. César Milstein; computer graphics by Richard Bachand.)

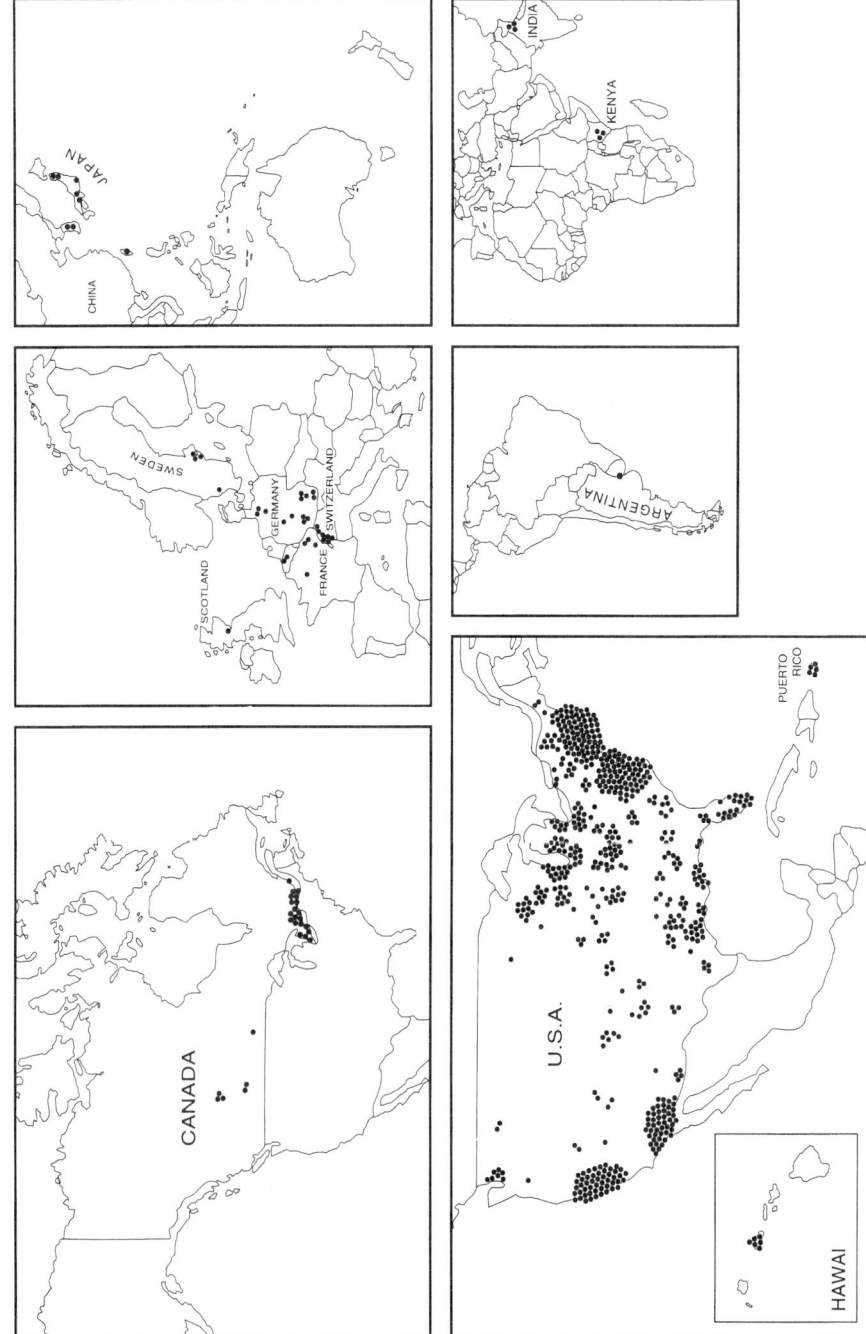

antibodies on the market, they not only ensured the circulation of those monoclonal antibodies, they also created a standard. Becton-Dickinson's Leu and Ortho's OKT series of monoclonal antibodies directed against human T-cell antigens are prime examples of this mechanism.

While the availability of monoclonal antibodies was obviously a condition of possibility for their adoption, their use in strategic sites of the biomedical research network was to constitute an additional step in their transformation into an obligatory passage point. The NIAID report, for instance, promoted the use of monoclonal antibodies "at least in the major reference laboratories that monitor viral disease throughout the world." Concurrently, a new monoclonal antibody–based rabies assay produced at the Wistar Institute and marketed by Centocor was being tested on suspect animals by the national centers that made up the international rabies monitoring network (*McGraw-Hill's Biotechnology Newsletter* 1981a). Monoclonal antibodies that had "pretty reproducibility in their use in different lab situations" were selected. Here, once again, we see two parallel mechanisms at work: On the one hand, the standardization of laboratories through the dissemination of monoclonal antibodies; on the other hand, the construction of monoclonal antibodies as a "pretty reproducible" tool, which, because it is reproducible, fosters its own dissemination.

Building a Tool: Generality Revisited

Let us reconsider Gosling's graph in Figure 3.6. The graph was used to represent the introduction of *new* immunoassays. Here, the term *new* has to be understood less as the upgrading of old assays (i.e., the replacing of polyclonal antibodies with monoclonal antibodies in existing products) than as the introduction of immunoassays in domains where the immunological technique was not being used. Thus, observers have likened the use of monoclonal antibodies to the "opening [of] new areas for physiological investigation that are still being explored," which in turn "provided the impetus for the enormous explosion in the application of immunodiagnostics" (Burrin and Newman 1991:48–49). Similarly, Yelton and Scharff (1981:677) had pointed out 10 years earlier that hybridoma technology had "overcome most of the practical, aesthetic, and conceptual objections to the applications of immunological techniques to basic and clinical questions,"

Figure 3.8. Geographical distribution of laboratories that received mice myelomas from the ATCC between 1982 and 1985. Each dot represents the approximate geographic location of a laboratory which requested and received at least one of the four available mice cell lines (P3X63Ag8, NS-1, P3X63Ag8.653, and SP2/0-Ag14). (Data kindly provided by Dr. William McKay, ATCC; computer graphics by Richard Bachand).

thus leading to the application of immunological methods to fields that had until then avoided their use.

Yelton and Scharff's statement can be read as recognizing the presence of extrascientific determinants of scientific practice, acting as obstacles to the diffusion of innovation. The claim we make is very different. Objections or obstacles are not passive barriers lying on a predetermined road to success; they make up the path that observers retrospectively perceive as having led to success. They are not external to the object—in our case monoclonal antibodies—they are part of it. Monoclonal antibodies' primary characteristics were defined in terms of their advantages and disadvantages over alternative tools.

The first of these characteristics was purity. Recall Herzenberg's claim, according to which hybridoma technology had succeeded in transforming immunological reagents into quasi-chemical ones: "There was an unlimited supply of the very same reagents so that immunology could become almost like chemistry where people could use absolutely defined reagents for their work." Recall also NIAID's claim that, thanks to hybridoma technology, antibodies could be produced that would share the properties of chemical reagents. Behind these statements and others lurk the notions of chemical purity and chemical reagent.[30]

Defined as "a fundamental concept of chemistry posing that substances are homogeneous when possessing reproducible properties under identical conditions" (Brock 1981a:352),[31] the notion of purity is related to that of reagent. The latter is defined as "any chemical used in a reaction although its specific historical meaning was a pure substance used to reveal the presence of another substance by the production of some striking effect." We further learn that "purity rapidly became an important criterion for reagents and 20th-century laboratory suppliers have marketed 'analytical reagents' (Analar) of specified homogeneity" (Brock 1981b). According to Gaston Bachelard (1953:71–81), "[t]he purity of a substance is . . . the work of man. It should not be taken for something given in nature. It retains the essential relativity of human works."[32] In other words, there is first of all no such thing as purity in and for itself; rather, there are purification processes.[33]

Second, these purification processes indicate more than the presence of human work but also the industrial nature of modern science. The complex and sequential nature of the various purification steps led to what Bachelard called the laboratory-factory. Third, purity also presupposes the existence of a coherent set of socially agreed upon, mutually defining reagents. Each scientific period can accordingly be characterized by a particular set of reagents, corresponding to a certain level of purification and to which a temporary privilege of purity has been granted. To sum up, paraphrasing Wittgenstein, there is no such thing as a private purity.[34]

Considered from this point of view, the notion of monoclonal antibodies as quasichemical reagents acquires an interesting twist. If chemical purity can be shown to bear witness to the "relativity of human works," rather than to some inherent quality of chemical substances, then the same analysis applies, *a fortiori*, to immunologic reagents. Monoclonal antibodies themselves have to be purified in order to be considered pure reagents: "Purification and characterization must be attained to take full advantage of these reagents. . . . Purified, well-characterized monoclonal antibodies can be called monoclonal antibody probes to differentiate them from the incompletely characterized hybridoma products" (Conway de Macario and Macario 1985:537–538).

But there is more. The very fact that a comparison is repeatedly drawn between monoclonal antibodies and chemical reagents shows that these two kind of substances are situated in an agonistic field where they are potential competitors. The claim that monoclonal antibodies correspond to a standardized and standardizing tool has to be understood as part of this ongoing dispute between immunologic and chemical reagents. It was only in the course of history that chemical substances came to be seen as pure substances and therefore as a kind of ideal standard against which immunological substances should be measured. Standardization is not predicated upon purity, it is not the outcome of the availability of pure reagents; rather, what counts as purity at any given time is the result of the regulation of clinical, laboratory, and industrial practices.[35]

A somewhat similar argument can be made with respect to yet another primary characteristic of monoclonal antibodies, their specificity.[36] As Bartal and Hirshaut (1987) pointed out: "[Y]esterday's 'sophisticated tools' are today's 'blunt instruments.'" The argument that immunologists faced a crisis in the 1970s when they were "forced to admit that polyclonal antibodies, although quite sensitive reagents, were not specific enough to answer many of the questions then confronting virologists and tumor biologists" (Bartal and Hirshaut 1987) has to be read as part of the evolving definition of chemical and immunological reagents. Specificity has long been used by immunologists to vaunt the superiority of their tools. To stress the difference between the specificity attributed in past writings to polyclonal antisera and the specificity now attributed to monoclonal antibodies, an expression was coined that has since become a regular feature of the literature on monoclonal antibodies: *exquisite specificity*.

However, specificity, as related to monoclonal antibodies, is a disputed notion, even within immunology. According to Yewdell and Gerhard (1981:203), for instance, the "designation of a monoclonal antibody as 'monospecific' is, in a strict sense, incorrect since an individual paratope [antibody-combining site] certainly has the ability to interact, though probably with different affinity, with a set of 'related' epitopes [antigenic determinants]."[37] Other researchers also noted that monoclonal antibodies crossreact with different antigens, adding that "crossreactivities found with monoclonal antibodies cannot be taken *a priori* to suggest a significant relationship between the proteins involved" (Nigg, Walter and Singer 1982). Thus, it is only by restricting the experimental system (i.e., by taking into account only, let's say, lymphocytes instead of an additional array of microbial and viral antigens) that one can claim that monoclonal antibodies are specific.[38]

From this perspective, conventional antibodies and monoclonal antibodies can be redefined as complementary tools as opposed to substitutes: "Observations made with individual monoclonal antibodies should always be evaluated in the context of the overall antigenicity as delineated by conventional antisera" (Yewdell and Gerhard 1981:205).[39] More importantly, the notion of specificity is displaced from monoclonal antibodies per se to monoclonal antibodies as the result of collective human activities: "Hopefully, the problem of restricted specificity will be minimized as the number of laboratories producing hybridoma antibodies increases"(Yewdell and Gerhard 1981:204).[40] Once again, we can resort to Bachelard and argue, as he did with purity, that specificity "retains the essential relativity of human works." If this is true, the exquisite specificity of monoclonal antibodies is better described as the result, rather than the cause, of their success.

In addition to purity and specificity, other characteristics attributed to monoclonal antibodies can be analyzed as the result of "reasonable agreements" grounded in shared practices. For instance, one of the qualities often used to promoted the use of monoclonal antibodies as a tool for worldwide standardization was that they could be made available in unlimited, permanent quantities. One no longer need to worry about the health of the rabbit producing some rare antiserum. However, as already noted in Chapter 1, the claim that hybridoma technology resulted in an "unlimited, permanent supply" of identical antibodies played on the in principle/in practice distinction: "*In principle*, an unlimited supply of a monogeneous antibody specific for almost any antigen can now be obtained. *In practice*, a number of technical problems persist that can be understood by examining the hybridoma experiments in a little more detail" (Yelton and Scharff 1980:513, emphasis added).

In particular, problems of hybridoma stability were raised by other observers, who noted that because of difficulties arising during the growth and maintenance of the hybridomas, successive batches of monoclonal antibodies would not be exactly the same (Clark 1986; Bussard 1987a). As Bussard pointed out, the question of stability could be tackled from a basic point of view (e.g., by arguing about the "microheterogeneity of proteins produced by one given set of genes" and the "stability of the structure of these proteins when they are synthesized for a long period of time through many generations"), or it could be tackled from a practical point of view. From the latter perspective the question was, for instance, whether purer monoclonal antibodies were obtained by growing hybridomas in vivo or in vitro. Bussard's statement of the problem is interesting insofar as it shows the transformation of the intrinsic characteristics of monoclonal antibodies into a matter of the regulation of their production practices.

Additional agreements concerning what should count as bona fide monoclonal antibodies had to be worked out in laboratory practice and in publication networks. The following quote illustrates this process:

> [Monoclonality] should be clearly established if the theoretical advantages of using monoclonal antibodies are to be claimed for a particular preparation. Unfortunately, it is not possible to prove monoclonality, only to demonstrate it beyond reasonable doubt.... This situation is not desirable, since it means that preconceptions of expected specificity determine the amount of evidence required to establish monoclonality beyond reasonable doubt. In practice, it is not unreasonable to accept that an antibody is monoclonal if: (1) it is produced by a hybridoma which has been put through a technically satisfactory cloning procedure; or (2) it shows exquisite specificity, which correlates with a preconceived classification.
> (Zola and Brocks 1982:38–40).[41]

Establishing such criteria[42] meant dealing with two problems: the assessment of what counts as a "technically satisfactory" procedure, which is in turn linked to the assessment of which laboratories count as reliable; and the problem of using a tool whose reliability was based on the correlation of its results with previously established classifications, as an "independent" tool for the establishment of new classifications (Collins 1985). The point in raising these issues is not to discount the whole enterprise but, rather, to re-present it as a practical accomplishment.

A final example can be provided with regards to the notion of reproducibility. First of all, reproducibility is, in operational terms, far more complex than some scientists, and certainly a lot of nonscientists, believe. For instance, in a review of a recent series on immunological methods, we read the following passage:

> Volume 1 ends with a lengthy 130-page section on optimization and validation of laboratory assays in term of precision and reproducibility. This should be compulsory reading for the plethora of research biologists who attempt to publish a single piece of immunological detection describing it as "reproducible" and "sensitive" without any understanding of the meaning of the words. (Campbell 1994).

More importantly, what counts as reproducible is what practitioners can reasonably agree upon as being reproducible, and these agreements can only be worked out in practice. A common misconception when discussing reproducibility is that it is always a yes and no situation: An experimental result is either reproducible or not. Reproducibility, however, is more often than not a matter of degree and involves the mutual adjustment of the different elements involved in an experiment or a diagnostic test. For instance, in commenting on the introduction of a theophylline monoclonal assay kit, a DuPont marketing manager noted that his company's automatic clinical analyzer was "widely accepted as the most reproducible around" (*McGraw-Hill's Biotechnology Newsletter* 1984a). Here, reproducibility was a matter of a comparison.[43]

In the case of the previously mentioned anti-rabies monoclonal antibodies produced by the Wistar Institute and marketed by Centocor, it will be remembered that they were tested in various national centers for the monitoring of rabies and declared to display "pretty reproducibility." However, it will also be remembered that reproducibility was achieved by selecting antibodies for reproducibility: Reproducibility was thus the outcome, not the starting point of that particular scientific activity. Furthermore, reproducibility required sustained effort. It involved, among other things, exchanging reagents and thus obtaining a "virtual pooling" of laboratories: "Well, you know, we have done this by sending our antibodies to Atlanta and the Pasteur Institute and to Tübingen, and they sent their antibodies to us. So there was a complete mix and swap of viral antigens and antibodies" (Wunner, interview, September 30, 1987).

The ongoing nature of the production of reproducibility is further illustrated by the continued reemergence of variation which has then to be explained away, by ascribing it to, for example, local incompetence in the handling of test conditions. In 1985, for instance, a University of California at San Francisco (UCSF) evaluation team found that a monoclonal 30-minute Chlamydia test marketed by Syva gave a relatively high rate of false positives and false negatives. Syva's Diagnostic's director of medical affairs disagreed with the readings of the UCSF team, and countered that "There seems to be an interpretive problem. In other places with more experienced technicians, the false-positive rate is much, much lower" (*McGraw-Hill's Biotechnology Newsletter* 1985d). Here we find the explicit acknowledgment that it is not the monoclonal antibodies themselves that guarantee reproducibility but the mutual adjustment of the various elements of the system in which the monoclonal antibodies are used. In the present case these other elements included, in addition to nonhuman components, the humans who performed the test.

We have seen thus far that one of the processes through which the generality of hybridoma technology was gradually constructed was the redefinition of monoclonal antibodies as tools. In turn, this successful redefinition was coextensive with the establishment of monoclonal antibodies' advantages over other tools; for, why should one adopt any new tool without some widely acknowledged advantages over previous tools? Once a tool has acquired an advantage, it is more than a question of taste whether or not to use it. In fact, as pointed out by Panem (1984:94), once a tool becomes recognized as state of the art, scientists who do not use it run the risk of "faring poorly in terms of grant review and in publication potential."[44] In other words, the tool becomes an obligatory passage point and its advantages acquire an institutional dimension.

Remarks concerning the advantages of monoclonal antibodies figure prominently in the literature devoted to monoclonal antibodies. They can be found in both scientific and commercial texts. In their Nobel Lecture, both Milstein and Köhler, for instance, discussed in some detail (adding tabular summaries of their claims) the advantages of monoclonal antibodies over traditional reagents. This was, however, problematic and the advantages and disadvantages of monoclonal antibodies became an issue in the biotechnology field. At a 1982 Battelle biotechnology conference, which highlighted the "slow paced conversion by the medical profession from conventional to monoclonal replacement products," a R&D vice-president of Cytogen, a biotech startup, remarked: "I don't see monoclonal antibodies as improving on conventional antiserum tests already in existence. Both would detect the same compound in the same way. What's the advantage of another system?" (*McGraw-Hill's Biotechnology Newsletter* 1982b).

Additional examples of the contingent nature of monoclonal antibodies advantages are easy to find. The vice-president of R&D of an established pharmaceutical company, Abbott, noted in 1983: "The mere mention of monoclonal antibodies these days causes investors' ears to perk up. We intend to introduce monoclonal-based products but regard them as just one arrow in our quiver.... Monoclonal antibodies haven't proven to be the be-all and end-all"(*McGraw-Hill's Biotechnology Newsletter* 1984a). Eric Ramberg, allergy marketing manager at Kallestad Laboratories, noted: "There is really no advantage to using monoclonal antibodies when you are dealing with a high-molecular-weight, heterogeneous protein like IgE.... Even in the constant region of the molecule there are subtle differences between individuals that make the specificity of monoclonals a disadvantage.... It's more a marketing issue—monoclonals sound very high-tech." To which Nick Harris, technical director of Allergenetics, retorted: "A polyclonal can be as good, but from a production and quality control standpoint monoclonals are preferable—once you have the right clone" (*McGraw-Hill's Biotechnology Newsletter* 1985a).

Philip Scuderi, vice-president and director of science of Carver Genetic Physics Corp., argued: "Monoclonals are great when you need to get rid of nonspecific reactivity. When that's not a problem, polyclonals are the tool of choice"(*McGraw-Hill's Biotechnology Newsletter* 1985b). David Milligan, vice-president for diagnostic R&D at Abbott noted: "With our reagents there have been few cross-reactivity problems, so the strategy has been to limit switchovers from polyclonals to those in which there is a distinct diagnostic advantage to increased specificity." William S. Knight, director of reagent development at

American Dade, commenting on the blood-bank testing area, concluded: "The economics [of conversion of existing serology testing to monoclonal typing] are hard to justify" (*McGraw-Hill's Biotechnology Newsletter* 1985c).

Fred Adler, product manager for infectious diseases at Ortho Diagnostics, made the point that choosing between monoclonal antibodies and polyclonals took careful testing. For instance, in the case of Ortho's new hepatitis direct-diagnostic test, "[w]e checked both monoclonal and polyclonal formats. The assay uses a microwell in which one antibody captures the antigen, and the second labeled antibody is the detector. After checking every possible option—mono-mono, poly-mono, poly-poly—we settled on polyclonals for both antibodies. The polyclonals showed greater sensitivity." A list of technical problems with monoclonal antibodies, drawn after five years of R&D, included the following: poor stability ("The dried [monoclonal antibody] just isn't stable. Polyclonals are such a mixture that if one's unstable, so what."), a not always optimal mouse immune response, low affinity, poor epitope coverage (monoclonal antibodies can be too specific for variable antigens), and production costs (often not close enough to polyclonals to justify the switch: "We'll think about it when our rabbit dies") (*McGraw-Hill's Biotechnology Newsletter* 1985c).

The point here is not whether these arguments were sound (refutations could be easily offered) but to show that assessments of monoclonal antibodies resorted to contingent comparisons of the advantages of monoclonal antibodies over alternative tools. It could be objected that the previous examples belong mostly to the commercial field, that they were mostly offered by corporate officers, and that they related to one specific domain, diagnostics. However, as previously argued, the relative advantages of monoclonal antibodies were also discussed in the scientific literature and, as we shall further see in the final section of this chapter, this trope was pervasive in that form of scientific literature known as the review article.

The Domestication of Monoclonal Antibodies

Given the preceding, it may justifiably be asked on what basis did the first users of monoclonal antibodies decide to adopt them. For, as has so far been argued, the defining characteristics of monoclonal antibodies were the progressive results of negotiations and not the immediate expression of some natural properties.

The early adoption pattern of monoclonal antibodies in the first local collectives to use them shows that they first occupied a niche within a given "experimental system" (Rheinberger 1992a,b) that was already occupied by other techniques. In other words, the first appearance of monoclonal antibodies was as a substitute and not as a novelty. This is clearly why the use of monoclonal antibodies has often been claimed to have been obvious. For, as an experimental system can be understood as a network of problems, statements, skills, equipment, and tools, it is precisely this network structure that creates a sense of obviousness when one of its components is replaced by another.

An example can be provided by one of the very first monoclonal antibodies produced outside Milstein's laboratory. Walter Gerhard, at Koprowski's Wistar Institute, produced anti-influenza monoclonal antibodies. Gerhard was interested in analyzing the antigenic variability of the influenza virus and, to that end, he had already used antibodies produced with Klinman's splenic fragment technique (see Chapter 1).[45]

So everything was already in place for monoclonal antibodies to function as part of the system, which meant not only that Gerhard knew how to deal with such technical issues as cell culture, antibody harvesting, etc. but, more importantly, how to attribute meaning to the new tool. To quote Gerhard (interview, September 28, 1987): "Many people, they may have said, it's nice but so what, what can we do with it? I didn't have to say that." Indeed, it became possible to argue, as Koprowski did (see Chapter 1), that monoclonal antibodies first arrived where they already existed. This actually meant that, knowing the influenza virus as he did, that is to say, intimately, Gerhard was able to assess his antibodies on the basis of the antigen, that is, to use the virus to judge the quality of the new technique.

A similar situation applies to anti-rabies monoclonal antibodies, also a very early product of the Wistar Institute. As pointed out by Dr. Wunner (interview, 30 September 1987), the Wistar people, including Koprowski and Tadeusz Wiktor, had been studying the rabies virus for almost 20 years prior to the advent of monoclonal antibodies. When monoclonal antibodies became available, they were integrated into a preexisting experimental system: "What monoclonal antibodies have allowed us to do, we have always wanted to do. It has simply helped accomplish the goal." We leave to the reader to gather additional examples by consulting the discussion in Chapter 1 of the early adoption of hybridoma technology by Bussard and Rajewsky and the discussion in this chapter of Herzenberg's quick conversion to monoclonal antibodies.

This is not to deny that researchers can take advantage of the opportunities offered by a new tool to develop new research directions or, to use Callon's terminology, to reconfigure local networks.[46] In fact, it could be argued (and indeed, this is what was argued during a patent dispute; see Chapter 5) that there is no such thing as a "mere substitution." Replacing one item in an experimental system modifies that system and often explicitly redefines the balance between the technical and the epistemic elements of the system. For the opportunities of a new tool to become apparent, however, the tool must first be domesticated within an existing experimental system.

These contingencies account for the fact that monoclonal antibodies moved through influenza and rabies viruses before reaching other viruses, and only later reached bacteriology and parasitology. Monoclonal antibodies, in other words, did not at first move easily into areas where polyclonals had only limited success. In the case of parasitology, some complained that immunoparasitologists had been "a little slow in recognizing just what a boost to the armamentarium of the experimental and applied investigator this technique offers" (Mitchell and Cruise 1981). Similarly, observers noted in 1985 that while immunology, immunochemistry, biochemistry, and virology had been "immediately invigorated by the use of [monoclonal antibodies]," the use of the new tool in bacteriology began later. A steady increase in publications in this field was noticeable starting only in 1983 (Macario and Conway de Macario 1985). When asked why this was the case, a scientist active in the field of bacterial diagnosis commented:

> Bacteriologists are ultraconservative people, and the bottom line is that a bacteriologist works with [bacterial] cultures. He [sic] grows bacteria, and bacteriology is grounded in the visual identification of bacteria, either by the gram technique or biochemical techniques.... As a consequence the confirmation, what is called the gold standard, is the isolation of the bacterium as such in order to make a final diagnosis. It was very difficult to convince those people that one could detect an antigen with a monoclonal antibody and believe what was being detected even if one could not visually inspect what was being detected. In virology it was easy. One never sees viruses; therefore, there were no conceptual or methodological problems. (Brodeur, interview, March 3, 1993).

The transformation of a technoscientific object into a tool can thus be taken to imply two distinct, though related, processes. The first is the use of that object as a technique within a given experimental system. A technique, in that sense, can only be of local interest—an idiosyncratic object among other idiosyncratic objects. The second process relates to the transformation of a local technique into a generic tool and thus involves a higher form of reification, one that leads to the attribution and stabilization of the characteristics (specificity, purity, stability, etc.) of the newly defined tool and to its standard use in different settings. At this stage, the advantages of the new tool have to be assessed in generic terms and represented precisely as generic advantages. This process, however, does not free the tool from its connections to other relevant elements. It provides more extended networks within which the tool circulates.

Two additional elements of the process of tool construction are worthy of discussion. The first concerns the establishment of equivalencies. We have argued that the new technique replaced another technique, mainly antisera, within a limited number of experimental systems, and that it was precisely the fact that monoclonal antibodies were inserted into a preexisting niche that prompted some scientists to comment in writings and in interviews that as soon as the technique became available, its use was obvious. The new technique, however, had first to be validated by the old technique. Rajewsky, one of the very first recipients of Milstein's myeloma cell line, commented after producing his first monoclonal antibodies against the mouse major histocompatibility complex: "The exquisite specificity of serological typing reaction thus *seems to be retained at the level of monoclonal antibodies*. This finding is important and suggests that monoclonal antibodies will play a key role in future histocompatibility typing" (Lemke et al. 1978:250, emphasis added).

Shifting now from local to extended networks, we find a similar approach in the World Health Organization program for the monitoring of viral diseases:

> For the past few years, [monoclonal antibodies] have been evaluated by the WHO Collaborating Centres for Reference and Research on Influenza in London and Atlanta for the identification of influenza viruses, *by comparing them with post-infection ferret antisera* [i.e., polyclonal antibodies]. At present, they are not used as a primary means of strain characterization, but selected preparations may be useful as an adjunct to specific animal antisera, particularly for the differentiation of very closely related variants.
> (*Bulletin of the World Health Organization* 1981, emphasis added).[47]

The process of establishing equivalencies is similar to that described by Pasveer (1989) in her analysis of the introduction of x-rays into clinical medicine, especially for tuberculosis. The significance of the x-ray pictures had first to be established by carefully constructing equivalencies between the x-ray images and the signs derived from established tools, such as the sounds perceived with a stethoscope and postmortem lung examinations. Only later was this relationship reversed, with x-ray pictures playing the primary diagnostic role.

A second consideration related to the shift from local technique to generic tool concerns the fact that monoclonal antibodies did not simply circulate along preestablished paths. They actually resulted in the establishment of new networks by joining previously independent practices. Monoclonal antibodies often profited from what we would call a *multiplier effect*: Because their use became synonymous with the introduction of immunological methods in fields previously untouched by them, they monopolized the generic advantages ascribed to those methods. Monoclonal antibodies became the link that established a connection between the network of immunological methods and various other networks of biological and biomedical practices. According to a Virginia Tech plant pathologist (Sue Tolin, interview, October 25, 1989): They [polyclonal antisera] have been sitting there unused.... Now all of a sudden people say ...: "Oh, we've got to have special projects so people can use monoclonal antibodies to detect plant viruses." If it was polyclonal, they didn't do a thing.[55]

This was confirmed by one of the very first recipients of Milstein's myeloma cell line, Gérard Buttin. Commenting on the fact that, although polyclonal antibodies had long been available, a number of researchers had been led to discover and/or adopt immunological methods only by the publicity surrounding monoclonal antibodies, he noted (interview, October 25, 1989, our translation):

> I think that monoclonals made enough noise to strengthen the interest for immunodetection approaches in various biological domains.... Suddenly, [antibodies] looked like a relatively clean tool, a reagent, and no longer the product of a more or less mythological strategy controlled by a restricted group of colleagues who were the only ones able to convince a rabbit to speak the right language.

Once translated into generic tools, monoclonal antibodies did not cease to function and to be assessed in relation to other elements of a given sociotechnical domain. In other words, the translation from local technique to generic tool corresponded to a shift from local collectives to extended networks. But how extended can these networks be? This is an empirical question, and its answer depends on the particulars under consideration. Consider the following example from the more extended side of the spectrum. A 1988 prospective study executed for the Organisation for Economic Co-Operation and Development postulated a close link between the redefinition of the health field towards preventive medicine and the extension of the diagnostic sector redefined by the use of, among other things, monoclonal antibodies (OECD 1988).

The OECD study also noted that the increase in the demand for diagnostic information resulted from the increased information available on antigens, such as viral or cell-surface proteins. Monoclonal antibodies have been used as a tool precisely to gather this kind of information, and thus there is a self-vindicating mechanism at work here. The OECD study added that the financial crisis of the health care system had led authorities to encourage various forms of self-treatment, including the use of over-the-counter diagnostic kits, a growing market sector epitomized by self-administered pregnancy tests. Simultaneously the popularization of medical notions concerning the role of viral antigens in cases such as human immunodeficiency virus (HIV) and Herpes provided a further stimulus for the demand of diagnostic services (Clark 1986).[48] The term *demand* should not be taken to imply a spontaneously expressed consumer need. The stimulation of this demand can be gathered from the importance industry spokespersons accord the education of consumers of in vitro diagnostics "about the need for testing" (Kolakowsky 1990:430–432).[49]

This situation can be nicely illustrated by First Response, a monoclonal antibody–based, over-the-counter diagnostic kit, designed "to predict ovulation in advance" [sic], thus allowing "accurate timing" of intercourse, leading, hopefully, to pregnancy. Marketed as an alternative to basal thermometer methods, the test did not enjoy the expected commercial success. A major limiting factor was found to lie in the existence of "widespread misconceptions about conception." A national survey sponsored by Tambrands Inc., who owned the First Response trademark before that trademark became the property of Carter-Wallace, Inc., allegedly showed that "about 90% of Americans [are] ignorant about the technics [sic] of conception," which included knowing how many days a month

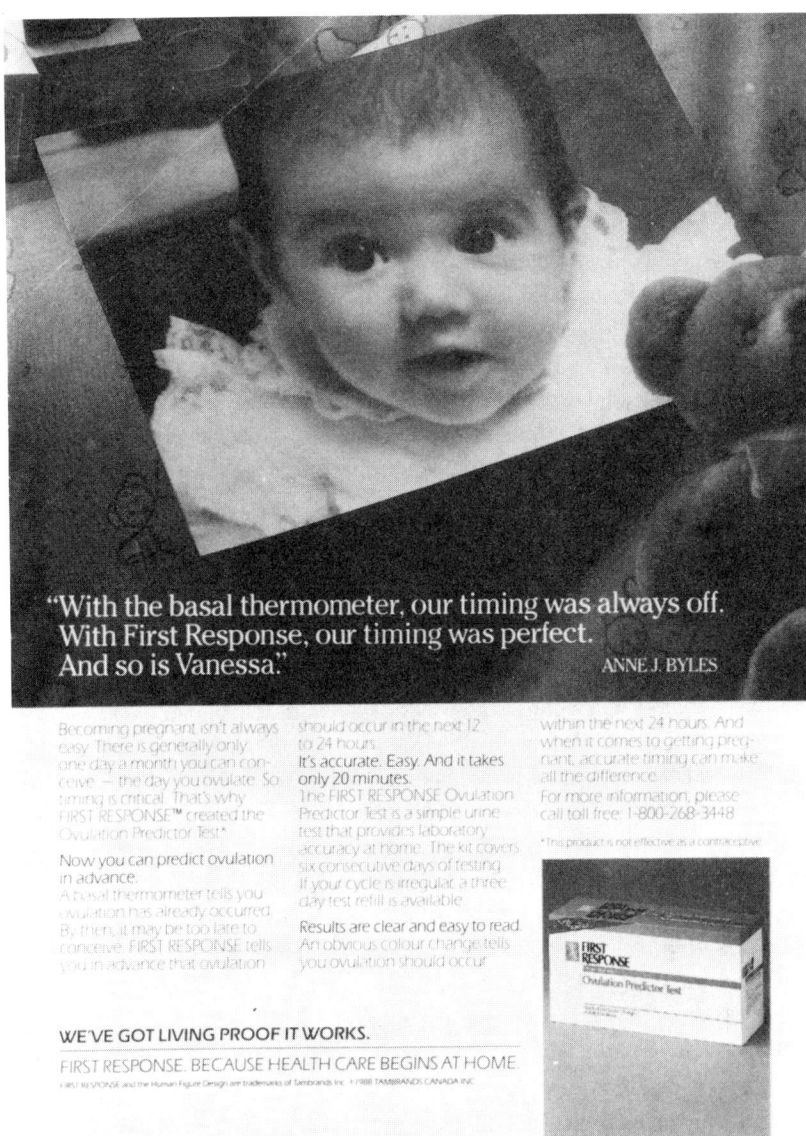

Figure 3.9. "Becoming pregnant isn't always easy ... so timing is critical." Advertisement for an over-the-counter, monoclonal antibody-based ovulation test.

a woman is able to conceive as well as being able to correctly define ovulation.

The General Manager of Tambrands' Diagnostics Division pointed out that while "many people think it's easy to conceive . . . conception actually requires delicate timing" (*BioEngineering News* 1986c). As a consequence, Tambrands Canada, Inc. embarked on a promotion campaign, with advertisements claiming that "becoming pregnant isn't always easy. There is generally only one day a month you can conceive—the day you ovulate. So timing is critical" (Figure 3.9).[50]

Providing Exoteric Interpretations

The drive to educate consumers was not restricted to lay people. Scientific consumers, ranging from fundamental researchers to scientists in clinical and diagnostic settings, also needed to be familiarized with monoclonal antibodies and their uses. In previous sections we have discussed how the promotion of monoclonal antibodies involved making them easily available and fostering their circulation by establishing repositories and shipping them to strategic research sites. While these conditions were certainly necessary, they were not sufficient. Something else was needed, namely, the development of "more exoteric interpretations"(Ravetz 1971:194–199)[51] that would ground the use of monoclonal antibodies in a shared understanding of their properties, possibilities, characteristics, and the consequences of their use. The difficulties experienced by a Wistar Institute researcher, Zenon Steplewski, illustrate this point.

Steplewski's attempts to publish results concerning anti-tumor monoclonal antibodies faced two problems. The first was one of disciplinary boundaries: Cell biology journals considered the results of work with hybridoma technology to be more appropriate for an immunology journal, while the immunology journals considered the results to belong to the domain of cell biology because monoclonal antibodies were only a tool, albeit an immunological one, used to address cell-related problems. Moreover, while papers describing the use of monoclonal antibodies in relation to known antigens fared well in terms of publication, articles on antibodies to unknown antigens such as, for example, those expressed on colon carcinoma cells had problems being accepted. As we shall see later, promoters of hybridoma technology had to press the point that hybridoma technology was so powerful that it had "stimulated investigators to use this technique to identify antigens that they are not certain even exist" (Diamond and Scharff 1982:3167–3168).

The second problem was one of clinical standards. According to Steplewski (interview, September 28, 1987),

> Again, if you wrote a paper on immunotherapy with monoclonal antibodies (these

were the early papers on toxicity and terminal patients) and you sent it to any of the medical journals, you got them rejected right away. Most of the criteria that we use for evaluation of the patients were immunological and were not the criteria that were used by chemotherapy—complete remission if the tumor disappeared in six weeks. Now we have seen patients in whom the tumor disappeared in seven months. You couldn't call it, according to their criteria, complete remission. It would fall into some sort of stable disease because the patient was stable for six months.

Reacting to what were perceived as preposterous criticisms by reviewers, researchers at the Wistar Institute initially discussed the possibility of creating a special section in an existing journal. At that point, however, Steplewski and Koprowski met Mary Ann Liebert, a New York publisher specializing in biotech journals (*Interferon, Genetic Engineering News*), who offered to finance a new journal entitled *Hybridoma*. First issued in 1981 with an opening article by Köhler entitled "Why Hybridomas?,"[52] the journal aimed at publishing papers "describing monoclonal antibody–defined antigens" as well as "papers on the application of monoclonal antibodies for diagnostics and therapy." The journal also published the abstracts of the "Annual Congress for Hybridoma Research," organized by a private firm, Scherago, in association with *Hybridoma* and *Genetic Engineering News*. In 1986, *Hybridoma* changed its title to *Hybridoma: A Journal of Molecular Immunology and Experimental and Clinical Immunotherapy*, to "reflect [the] constant developments in the field of hybridoma research," including the fact that the production and description of monoclonal antibodies, once the topic of Ph.D. dissertations, was becoming a technician's job.[53] Judging from the declining circulation of the journal (from an average of 1450 copies, including 850 mail subscriptions, in 1985 to an average of 879 copies, including 489 subscriptions, in 1991), it can be argued that the attempt to turn *Hybridoma* into the organ of the elusive field of hybridoma research has not been successful.

Indeed, in a recent interview a long-time hybridoma researcher pointed out that, while he had attended the initial hybridoma research meetings and consulted the journal, he no longer did so (Brodeur, interview, March 3, 1993). Two complementary reasons account for this. First of all, the very success of hybridoma technology made reports of its specific applications in the various biomedical fields easily acceptable to the more conventional disciplinary publications. Secondly, there has been a branching out of publications and conferences for leading-edge, highly specialized applications of hybridoma technology. Examples of this trend include the journal *Antibody, Immunoconjugates, and Radiopharmaceuticals*, created in 1988, and a 1992 Princeton conference on radioimmunodetection and radioimmunotherapy of cancer.

Clearly, hybridoma technology has not developed into a coherent research area with well-defined research problems. As the same researcher told us when asked about *Hybridoma* (Brodeur, interview, March 3, 1993): "I am not really interested in learning that a given researcher succeeded in producing a monoclonal antibody against, say, a protein from some insect. I am really not interested; but, on the other hand, a researcher who works on insects, well, it would be in his interest to publish this in an entomology journal."[54]

Hybridoma's demise can be seen as the result of the successful transformation of monoclonal antibodies into a generic tool. The creation of such a periodical can thus be seen as a temporary stage, certainly not the most important one, in the process of providing the more exoteric interpretations that made monoclonal antibodies familiar to almost every scientist in the biomedical field. Nonetheless, we would argue that a more decisive role, in this respect, was played by a peculiar genre of scientific literature, review articles.

Review articles ostensibly cover the state of the art in a given field. While review articles may adopt different rhetorical strategies depending on the kind of journal in which they are published and the audience at which they aim,[55] they at first seem to be factual summaries rather than prescriptive interpretations of recent work or, in other words, accounts describing the connections between the various elements of a given field, rather than plans for action charting future developments or guides to future experiments.[56] A closer look, however, reveals their prescriptive rather than exclusively descriptive nature, as shown by the presence of deontic ("ought to") modalities (Latour and Woolgar 1986:86). Indeed, review articles can more often than not be equated to manifestos indicating the direction future work should take.

The fluidity of the descriptive/prescriptive distinction can be illustrated by the following sentences: "[Hybridoma technology] should facilitate progress in many areas of biology and immunochemistry. In general, it will make possible advances in at least two areas: 1) analyses of the mouse B-cell repertoire and 2) production of monoclonal antibodies to be used as reagents" (Kennett et al. 1978).[57]

While this passage cannot be considered, *stricto sensu*, a description of the state of the art because it refers to future advances, researchers do perceive such statements as descriptions, insofar as the advances they chart are reasonable extrapolations: They logically follow from initial results. So reasonable they indeed appear to be that they were used and initially accepted during a patent dispute on monoclonal antibody–based immunoassays as a proof of the "obviousness," and thus unpatentability, of the contested invention.[58] The above-quoted passage thus exemplifies a self-fulfilling prophecy. The prescription of the areas in which advances must be sought, if accepted as unproblematic, that is, if read as a description of a logical path from the immediate past to the immediate future, will eventually lead to work in the predicted area and to the statement being retrospectively read as a factual description of the field.

All the review articles we consulted, even those devoting space to the conceptual rather than technical aspects of the development of the hybridoma technology,[59] presented monoclonal antibodies as a (new and powerful) *tool*. Their topic was not the establishment or the description of a scientific fact; it was the listing of the different domains in which the application of the new tool could be expected to lead to the production of previously unattainable results, or at least to easier ways of reproducing established facts. In other words, once you have a tool the question becomes one of the appropriate domains, projects, or objects to which it can be applied.

Review articles, then, converted monoclonal antibodies into tools by providing a list of domains and problems to which they should be applied, thus reinforcing the definition of monoclonal antibodies as tools waiting for new fields of application. In other words, this generalization of the object entailed its association with directions for use that simultaneously legitimized the object (Thévenot 1984). The upshot of this process was the understanding that a particular way of using monoclonal antibodies was what characterizes competent researchers.[60] Generalization, in this sense, is not restricted to review articles but is, for example, packaged into diagnostic kits that contain all the necessary reagents and devices, as well as detailed instructions on how the kit is to be used and how its results are to be interpreted.[61]

In order to further illustrate the role of review articles, let us examine a specimen of this literary genre whose title—"Whither Monoclonal Antibodies?" (Staines and Lew 1980)—clearly evokes its simultaneous predictive and descriptive status. The descriptive elements act as a condition of possibility for the efficacy of the prescriptive-predictive function, as in the following two passages in which future achievements are extrapolated from past realizations:

> The value of [monoclonal antibodies] *has been demonstrated* already in experimental immunochemistry and, *as yet to a lesser extent* in immunobiology. In situations where large amounts of homogeneous antibodies are needed, [monoclonal antibodies] produced in hybrid lymphocytes *will offer unparalleled opportunities* for laboratory experimentation and standardization and for clinical investigation.
> (Staines and Lew 1980:287, emphasis added; note the point on standardization).

> *It is clear* that [monoclonal antibodies] are highly effective in viral serotyping. . . . *Although less information is yet available*, [monoclonal antibodies] *would clearly be ideal* for serotyping bacteria. (Staines and Lew 1980:289, emphasis added).

This is also seen when monoclonal antibodies are represented as part of a long-term "drive" that makes their contribution predictable:

> *The drive* to characterize the antigenic components of the normal mammalian cell

> surface *has been given fresh impetus* by the development of [monoclonal antibodies] technology. *It is reasonable to expect* that HLA analysis will reach a new level of precision and that this *will aid further* the description of both the molecular basis of antigenicity and the genetic basis of HLA polymorphism.
>
> (Staines and Lew 1980, emphasis added).

In other words, the authors of this review article grounded their predictions/prescriptions in a continuum that went from "monoclonal antibodies are a better way of doing what we are already doing" to "monoclonal antibodies will allow us to do things we always wanted to do, but could not because of technical limitations." There is a tension here between continuity and novelty, and thus between description and prediction, that is part and parcel of the rhetorics of review articles.

Predictions and prescriptions are not only based on familiarity with previous work in the field, but also follow from the unique intrinsic properties ascribed to monoclonal antibodies, as in the following examples:

> The list of antigens that are poorly defined is endless. As a consequence of *the exquisite specificity of [monoclonal antibodies]*, it is possible to use them not only to define the epitopic determinants of antigens but also to isolate or identify antigenic molecules that have hitherto been elusive.
>
> (Staines and Lew 1980:288, emphasis added; note the expression *exquisite specificity*).

> *Because of their fine specificity*, [monoclonal antibodies] *may be used* to study the functions of pharmaco-physiological agents.
>
> (Staines and Les 1980:289, emphasis added).

The point here is to note that a) in highlighting this particular property—specificity—one is selecting among a range of properties that can be ascribed to monoclonal antibodies and b) specificity, as a property, can only be defined with regards to previous and concurrent laboratory practices.[62] The claim that monoclonal antibodies show exquisite specificity must be read against the background of the specificity of conventional antibodies, which, it should be added, had until then been perceived as very specific tools. As we have already mentioned, yesterday's sophisticated tools are today's blunt instruments. Indeed, there are signs that monoclonal antibodies themselves are beginning to slide into the category of blunt instruments. Evidence can be found in a 1990 review article's call for "novel approaches" leading to "more useful, less immunogenic [monoclonal] antibodies" (Pirovski et al. 1990).[63]

While "Whither Monoclonal Antibodies?" is particularly rich in expressions such as "will be solved," "will therefore prove to be of paramount importance," "will make possible," "may become valuable," "have the potential to become," "we may expect to see," as well as "there do not appear to be reasons to think that monoclonal antibodies would not . . . ," this is characteristic of review articles as a genre. Also not exclusive to "Whither Monoclonal Antibodies?" is the recasting of hybridoma technology as the outcome of a long-term endeavor. For instance, part of the title of the present chapter—"From Immunofantasy to Monoclonal Reality"—is borrowed from the title of another review article on hybridoma technology (Scharff 1984). Hybridoma technology was therein depicted as the embodiment of immunologists' long-standing dream, as fantasies made reality (Scharff 1981) or, to use yet another metaphor, as the "drive toward homogeneity" having "reached its orbit" (Day 1990:ch.8). As such, hybridoma technology, although described as a revolutionary and thus unexpected breakthrough, was also represented as a sort of prefigured disciplinary horizon and, accordingly, past events are reconstructed as a path leading to it.[64]

Yet another trope that figured consistently in review articles was the mention of persistent problems. At first this might seem contradictory. If one seeks to promote the use of a new tool, why stress its inadequacies? If our description of review articles as descriptive/prescriptive devices is correct, however, the presence of a section on persistent problems makes perfectly good sense. Not only does the article dictate the areas in which the tool is to be applied, it also dictates how the tool should be perfected. As we have seen in Chapter 2, the issue of improvement is indeed an open question.

The array of persistent problems discussed in review articles is interesting because of its heterogeneity. It shows how distinctions between cognitive and social elements are constantly blurred in scientific practice. So, for instance, the inefficient and labor-intensive aspect of hybridoma technology is contrasted with the difficulty of generating monoclonal antibodies to weak immunogens and to considerations of the affinity of the antibodies that can be produced. The potentialities of hybridoma technology will only be realized, it is claimed, when these persistent problems are solved (De Pinho, Feldman, and Scharff 1986). It is apparent that by defining the problems one charts the future developments of the technology.

But what proves that review articles have had any impact at all in shaping research practices? For instance, one could argue, as did the co-developer of hybridoma technology, Georges Köhler, that review articles play at most a secondary role in fostering the development of a new field, as they are far behind communications at meetings and personal contacts. Those directly involved in research do not need them, and those who do need them are, so to speak, end-users, unlikely to contribute to the scientific activity.[65]

In this respect, recall Fleck's (1979) distinctions between esoteric and exoteric circles and between journal and vademecum science that he used to describe the transformation of local laboratory results into stabilized facts. Fleck noted that the acquisition of factual status involved the circulation of a candidate fact between the esoteric scientific circle directly involved in its production and the exoteric circles that used it. This process involves, as argued by Latour and Woolgar (1986), the progressive removal of the modalities characterizing scientific statements. The crux of the matter here is that the establishment of factuality does not take place at the initial production site but, rather, involves the circulation of the fact within a network whose nodes include, among other things, laboratories involved in other domains, clinical settings, grant agencies, lecture halls, and textbooks. We are therefore not dealing with a unidirectional process, from the esoteric center to the exoteric periphery but, rather, with a complex pattern of interactions between various sites and modalities of technoscientific and clinical practice.

Fleck's argument can be applied not only to technoscientific items categorized as facts but also to those categorized as techniques. When a new technique appears in the scientific and/or commercial marketplace, its status, both epistemological and institutional, is uncertain. The question arises of how technoscientific objects acquire their status as innovations (i.e., come to be seen as new, both scientifically and commercially) as well as objects of daily use in the scientific and industrial laboratory (i.e., become banal or trivial). Review articles are not simply indicators of these processes; they are part of them. Review articles should be regarded not only as an important channel for the popularization of hybridoma technology but also as constitutive elements of the sociotechnical identity of hybridoma technology *tout court*.

Indeed, there are striking similarities between review articles and documents of a much more official and normative nature, such as those bearing the stamp of the major U.S. biomedical agency, the National Institutes of Health (NIH). In 1979, for example, the Immunology Study Group was established "to identify areas in which important developments are most likely to occur." One of the six areas selected for study was "hybridoma technology to produce monoclonal antibodies and the application of monoclonal reagents to biology and medicine." As previously noted, the report of the Immunology Study Group was released in January 1981, under the title *New Initiatives in Immunology* (NIAID 1981). The chapter on hybridomas was written by a panel co-chaired by Drs. Stuart F. Schlossman and Matthew D. Scharff. Dr. Scharff, during approximately the same period, co-authored several review articles on hybridoma technology.[66] Other members of the panel included such familiar figures as Koprowski and Herzenberg.

There are stylistic and substantive similarities between review articles and the NIAID report. Indeed, we would argue that the only important difference between them was that the report was issued by an agency with granting responsibilities. The NAIAD National Advisory Council recommended that research and training in all the areas covered by the document be significantly increased. Not only was more money to be made available, but it was to be channeled into specific areas. The process that led to the production of the NIAID document corresponded to a series of choices, from the initial selection of the areas to be explored by the panels to the final ranking of the recommendations drafted by each of the panels. It is our claim that review articles and the NIAID report were part of the same process that led to the stabilization of hybridoma technology as a new revolutionary tool.

As in review articles, the hybridoma section of the NIAID document contained prescriptive extrapolations grounded in a selective review of results. General claims that monoclonal antibodies had "launched a new era in immunological research" and that they promised "to revolutionize many aspects of biology and medicine," were followed by an examination of their "still unrealized extraordinary potential" in areas such as serology, virology, parasitology, tumor biology, autoimmunity, and clinical pharmacology. Confident, predictive/prescriptive statements such as "It is felt that hybridoma technology will permit [this or that]" were also applied to areas such as parasitology, where, admittedly, research was still in its infancy, as well as to areas where the basic premises on which predictions were made were, to say the least, doubtful, as in tumor biology ("It is believed that use of the hybridoma technology will lead to the identification of tumor-specific antigens, if they exist").[67]

As in review articles, a section was devoted to opportunities for future research (persistent problems), which included the excessive amount of work involved in producing monoclonal antibodies, the difficulty of producing monoclonal antibodies against poorly immunogenic antigens, and the difficulty of generating monoclonal antibodies in rabbits and humans. All these problems or opportunities were predicated upon the notion that hybridoma technology was a general technique in the sense that it could, in principle, be applied to the production of antibodies against all sorts of antigens. In turn, these problems and opportunities reinforced the notion that hybridoma technology was, indeed, a technique of general applicability.

Conclusions

The translation of monoclonal antibodies into tools was a complex, multilayered process. It implied a shift from local to extended networks, and thus was constitutive of and constituted by sociotechnical changes in laboratory, clinical, and commercial standards, involving, among other things, the establishment of institutions variously devoted to the production of the new tools and the creation and maintenance of arrangements regulating their use. The presence of an expanding network was not only a precondition for the circulation of cells and reagents. It was also, and more importantly, crucial to the constitution and maintenance of the properties attributed to those cells and reagents, such as purity and (exquisite) specificity. Last, but not least, the presence of a network was instrumental in the production of the new synthetic identity of the hybridoma specialist, who became a regular feature in the job advertisement section of scientific periodicals.[68] The emergence of such a figure was materialistically described as follows: "As a senior immunologist who has followed our discipline over the last thirty years, I am impressed to see how the modern tools of hybridoma technology have also generated a whole crop of young, and eager scientists" (de Weck 1987).[69] While some readers will no doubt subscribe to the metaphorical connotation of this quote, we would argue, on the basis of the material exposed in this chapter, in favor of a more literal interpretation.

NOTES

1. This topic is discussed from a philosophical point of view by Rouse (1987). The *locus classicus* for a discussion of this issue in the sociology of science is to be found in the work of Bruno Latour and Michel Callon; see, for instance, Latour (1987). Still in the sociological camp, but from a different perspective, the work of Thévenot (1984) provides a central contribution to this discussion. On standardization, see also O'Connell (1993).

2. The FDA did, however, intervene to regulate the production of monoclonal antibodies. The Office of Biologics Research and Review, Center for Drugs and Biologics of the FDA established a Hybridoma Committee, which in June 1983 issued a document entitled "Points to Consider in the Manufacture of *In Vitro* Monoclonal Antibody Products Subject to Licensure." An updated version of that document was issued in June 1987 under the title "Points to Consider in the Manufacture and Testing of Monoclonal Antibody Products for Human Use." The document was revised in 1992 by the Office of Therapeutics Research and Review of the Center for Biologics Evaluation and Research of the FDA; see Dutton (1993). For an overview of regulatory issues related to hybridoma technology in the United States see Bozeman (1982) and Kahan (1986:207–210). See also Merchant (1982), Hipolito (1982), and *McGraw-Hill's Biotechnology Newswatch* (1984b). For an example of state regulation of monoclonal antibodies in a European country, see Haase (1990).

3. Scharff used the same trope in the title of two other papers: Pollock, Teillaud, and Scharff (1984) and Spira et al. (1985).

4. An almost identical argument can be found in Newmark (1985:387).

5. Köhler quotes a predicted figure of 1 billion Swiss francs for 1987.

6. See also Table 2 in Milstein (1986).

7. See also Milstein (1990): "The most predictable and obvious of the applications of the hybridoma technology was the use of monoclonal antibodies as a substitute for antibodies in all sorts of immunoassays. . . . Not so obvious was the idea that hybridomas could revolutionise our understanding and knowledge of cell surface differentiation antigens. . . . Unless one is very familiar with the field as it was in 1978, this is not easy to appreciate."

8. Rothman and Parkinson (1984) cite Mulkay (1980:15–22).

9. Data originate from a sampling of the assays introduced in a leading journal in the field, *Clinical Chemistry*, from January 1980 to December 1989, and "were taken to be a reasonably representative

sample of all new immunoassays for clinical applications developed during the same period" (Gosling 1990:1412).

10. Immunoassays are a technique based on the use of antibodies, as opposed to chemical reagents, to reveal the presence of microorganisms or other substances of clinical and industrial interest in various kinds of specimens (see Chapter 5 for more detail).

11. Dubiski (1987) points out that the failure to induce rabbit myelomas prevented production of rabbit monoclonal antibodies, thus handicapping the usefulness of rabbits. Other authors have also predicted the replacement of rabbits by "lymphocyte hybridoma cultures"; see Melchers, Potter, and Warner (1978).

12. Having noted that the production of monoclonal antibodies involves a great deal of work, including the performance of hundreds or thousands of tests and the time-consuming activities involved in cell farming. Goding adds, "in comparison, the preparation of antibodies with nothing more than antigen, a rabbit, and a syringe, might be seen as a technological breakthrough!"

13. This is not the place to analyze in detail the development of FACS. This has been done in Keating and Cambrosio (1994). See also Cambrosio and Keating (1992).

14. The following reconstitution is based on the first of a series of interviews with Leonard and Leonore Herzenberg (Stanford, March 27, 1988).

15. For a description of this apparatus, see Herzenberg, Sweet, and Herzenberg (1976). Herzenberg profited from his stay in Cambridge to attend a meeting in September 1976 to which all FACS users were convened. At that time, about 20 FACS machines had been sold worldwide.

16. Herzenberg is referring to Herzenberg and Ledbetter (1979).

17. Other observers agreed:

Even though [the FACS and hybridoma technology] were discovered within an interval of three years, they were developed simultaneously. We should not forget how the cell sorters were used to enrich and to clone hybridomas and above all the essential role they played in the studies on the specificity of monoclonal antibodies directed against blood cells. Without their sensitivity to detect and their capacity to distinguish and purify minor cell populations, there would not be such a variety of monoclonal reagents for use in hematology today. In return, monoclonal antibodies have brought flow cytometry the keys to its success. Indeed, what can be done with an instrument for detection and measurement as sophisticated as the cell sorter, if the appropriate (that is, the most specific and best standardized) probes do not exist? Monospecificity, quasi-unlimited availability, easy use, physico-chemical uniqueness (individuality): these are the major characteristics which have made monoclonal antibodies the reagents without which the analyzers/cell sorters would still be curiosity pieces in a few rare immunology laboratories. (Poncelet and Roncucci 1984:2).

18. The Bethesda workshop was responsible for most of the 41 publications on monoclonal antibodies we were able to locate for 1978 in *Medline,* up from the seven found in 1977.

19. It should be noted that Herzenberg was not alone in shifting responsibility for the distribution of hybridoma technology material to the private sector. Milstein, for instance, confronted with the increasingly onerous task of furnishing cell lines to fellow scientists, turned over their distribution to Flow (interview with César Milstein, January 11, 1988). Panem (1984) discusses the crucial role played by the NIH in establishing standard reagents that allowed work on interferon to proceed in different laboratories and clinical settings.

20. Milstein and Köhler's paper was presented in a section entitled "Prospects for Cell Cultures in the Production of Antibodies," alongside other papers detailing other possible approaches to this task, including Klinman's technique (see Chapter 1). Sir James Gowans, Secretary of the Medical Research Council (quoted in Tansey and Catterall 1994:325) recently noted: "I don't remember being shattered, I think I was actually at the first meeting where César talked about his results and I remember being mightily intrigued. . . . One was not thinking at the time when one was in the lecture that there was a vast catalogue of diagnostic reagents just waiting on the horizon, or perhaps even therapy. The possibilities were certainly not mentioned in the lecture."

21. Herzenberg was one of the authors of the chapter on hybridoma technology in the NIH document.

22. The issue was originally raised in Kahan (1982), which was followed by a reply from two Charles River Breeding Laboratory employees: Foster and Balk (1982). The reply contains numerous remarks pointing to the various devices mobilized to construct and certify standardized BALB/c mice; they range from acquiring skills for biochemical markers to good laboratory practice regulations.

23. Often monoclonal antibodies were named after the coordinates of the well in a 96-well plate in which a particular laboratory had isolated the clone from which the monoclonal antibodies were produced. This is a particularly interesting conflation of local and general characteristics.

24. CERDIC (Centre Européen de Recherches Documentaires sur les Immunoclones) brochure, dated February 12, 1990. Since 1989 CERDIC has been publishing *Immunoclones,* a periodical whose purpose is to provide "a periodic survey of new hybridomas, other outstanding immunoclones and their products."

25. The first volume of *Monoclonal Antibodies News* was published in 1981 by the New York publishing house Mary Ann Liebert. In 1989, the periodical changed its title to *Monoclonal Antibodies.*

26. As a Canadian scientist put it: "We have very specific research projects, we know rather well the scientific literature in our domain, so we don't need to consult [the Hybridoma Data Bank]" (Bernard Brodeur, interview, March 3, 1993, our translation). Alain Bussard, the founder of CERDIC, commenting on the limited success of the Data Bank, noted (interview, December 13, 1992): "Our potential clients think they know [about the available hybridomas]. They are wrong."

27. Data computed from "Shipments under NCI contract # N01-CB-23886 from 3/1/80 to 12/31/80," kindly provided by Dr. Cohn.

28. On the occasion of the dedication of the new building, on June 7, 1981, the ATCC organized a conference on the "use, availability, and patenting of hybridomas and genetically engineered organisms." The papers delivered on that occasion have been published in the December 1981 issue of *In Vitro.* Construction of the new building was made possible by matching funds from the NCI and contributions from several pharmaceutical companies.

29. ATCC (1985:225); Rodney E. Langman (The Salk Institute), personal communication, July 2, 1993.

30. Hybridoma technology was credited with transforming serology from immunomagic into a discipline with a firm scientific basis, whereby "[t]he old uncertainties of specificity and reproducibility [had] been replaced by the promise of unlimited supplies of standardized, monospecific antibodies" (Goding 1986:40). In a section entitled The Case Against Antisera of a paper on monoclonal antibodies, Fazekas De St. Groth (1985) pointed out that the heterogeneity of antibody response had "dogged the use of antibodies as no two antisera are the same." He added that "[s]ince reproducible tests demand standard reagents, serious effort [had] been expended over the years to reduce this inherent heterogeneity, without much success," that is, until the advent of hybridoma technology, which became "the solution" to this problem.

31. On the emergence of institutions involved in establishing and maintaining chemical purity, see Brock (1992:173–176).

32. See also Tiles (1984). We are, of course, aware of the many essential differences between Bachelard's epistemology and the one expressed in this book.

33. Brock (1981a) cites A. Laurent (1807–1853), who once remarked that "chemistry [was] the science of substances which [did] not exist; for absolute purification [was] impossible to achieve."

34. We are, of course, alluding to Wittgenstein's remarks on private language. For a discussion of this issue, see Rhees (1970).

35. For a stimulating discussion, along similar lines, of the standardization of mice in cancer research and their comparison with the "normalized and standard chemicals bought from the chemical industry," see Gaudillière (1993a).

36. A sociological discussion of immunological specificity can be found as early as 1935 in Ludwik Fleck (English translation: Fleck 1979). For an extension of Fleck's analysis of specificity, see van den Belt and Gremmen (1990).

37. It should be noted that, in spite of this remark, the authors maintained that monoclonal antibod-

ies "achieve the highest degree of monospecificity available from immunological reagents" (p. 186). To differentiate between the specificity of a monoclonal antibody for a given microorganism (virus, bacteria, etc.) or substance of clinical or biological interest, and the specificity of a monoclonal antibody for a particular epitope that can be shared by several microorganisms or substances, Conway de Macario and Macario (1985:540) use the notion of "fine (molecular) specificity."

38. This point was recently stressed by Coutinho (1993). For a critique of the notion of monospecific antibodies, see also Hirschfeld (1980).

39. See also Conway de Macario and Macario (1985:535, our emphasis): "The two types of reagents, antisera and monoclonal antibodies, may be compared for their advantages and disadvantages, as well as specific uses. In some situations, one reagent is better suited than the other, and in others, *a combined, complementary utilization of both methods* yields better results than if one were used exclusively."

40. The authors, however, warn that "with the introduction of centralized hybridoma cell distribution centers, it is possible that all the workers in a given field will use the same, relatively limited panel of hybridoma antibodies. If this prevails, misleading results may be obtained and mutually reinforced because of the common use of a biased panel of antibody specificities." For a discussion of the specificity issue in relation to the antisera produced under the NCI Virus Cancer Program in the 1960s, see Gaudillière (1993a,b).

41. See also Conway de Macario and Macario (1985:538): "Removal of ambiguities from monoclonal antibody use is all the more imperative because it appears easy to fall into the trap of assuming that one is working with a truly monoclonal antibody probe [i.e., a 'well-characterized' monoclonal antibody] just because one has done a successful fusion and, perhaps, derived a cell line through a couple of clonings. This by no means ensures monoclonality or purity, nor does it provide results that can be interpreted without the hesitations inherent in serology with complex antisera."

42. This kind of negotiation can become explicit, as in the case of the consensus conferences organized by the NIH and discussed by Panem (1984).

43. Moreover, notice here that reproducibility was not presented as the inherent property of the monoclonal antibodies; instead, attention was called to the role played by another component of the kit, that is, the equipment used in the assay. This, in turn, highlights the tinkering involved in mutually adjusting the various components of a kit so that it becomes reproducible.

44. In 1979, for instance, 20–30% of the new grant proposals submitted to the NIAID in the field of immunology involved monoclonal antibodies; see Schmeck Jr. (1979). *State of the art* lies somewhere on a continuum between the unique, for example, the detectors described in Traweek (1988), and the standardized.

45. It is interesting to note that Klinman (1975) used the term *monoclonal antibodies* in referring to his technique before the advent of hybridoma technology.

46. On the notion of opportunities, see Rouse (1987:80–95); for a stimulating treatment of the notions of local and extended reconfiguration, see Callon (1994).

47. The memorandum was the result of a meeting held in Geneva in February 1981.

48. According to Edwards (1985), over-the-counter kits, and thus the gradual replacement of the laboratory, is a recent phenomenon, that goes back to the 1960s.

49. See also *Genetic Engineering News* (1993, our emphasis): "Marketing is critical in the pregnancy diagnostics and ovulation prediction markets, where products are similar in performance and price. Widespread distribution, packaging that catches the attention of consumers, and *advertising that generates product awareness* are keys to success in consumer markets."

50. First Response advertisement. The First Response trademark and the Human Figure Design used in association therewith are now trademarks of Carter-Wallace, Inc.

51. The Ravetz argument was adopted and developed by Rouse (1987).

52. The article compares hybridoma technology to other methods for immortalizing cells while maintaining their specific function.

53. This situation is similar to the one that characterized the evolution of DNA-sequencing activities. See Keating, Limoges, and Cambrosio (1995).

54. Similarly, commenting on why he had stopped attending the Scherago meetings, the inter-

viewee noted that "We went to those meetings, but we very soon realized that they were like a trade fair: We went there, everybody had developed some monoclonals. OK, they were basic tools, but they were often directed against things which had no interest for us." See also Köhler's comment (interview, March 15, 1992): "I don't know whether [*Hybridoma*] will continue to be a journal for a long time, because it seems to be a collection of who has made which specificity. That's not enough for a journal.... [When the journal was created] there was a lack of information, and there were so many people doing so many different antibodies. So there was a need of showing who had done what. I thought that was the idea of the journal. But now I don't think that's so important anymore."

55. Review articles on monoclonal antibodies range from texts written by scientists in a specialized field for researchers in that same field, to texts addressed to specialists from other areas who are likely to be end-users of black-boxed products, to even more general texts addressed to a general audience of, for instance, clinicians.

56. This distinction has been borrowed from Young (1992).

57. The reader will have noticed the dual structure (factual: analyses of the mouse B-cell repertoire; and technical: production of monoclonal antibodies to be used as reagents) of the quoted statement.

58. *Monoclonal Antibodies Inc. vs. Hybritech;* see Chapter 5.

59. See, for instance, Yelton and Scharff (1981); see also the chapter "Theory of Monoclonal Antibodies" in Goding (1986).

60. Compare with Ravetz's (1971:196–197) distinction between transforming things themselves and providing more exoteric interpretations of them.

61. Compare with Pinch's (1986) discussion of black-boxing as a way to function across different evidential contexts.

62. Specificity can be contrasted with other negative properties, which were, once again, assessed on the basis of their relation to laboratory practices. The NIAID report *New Initiatives in Immunology* pointed out that monoclonal antibodies did present some problems when used as routine serological reagents, namely, that they did not precipitate directly in agar and thus could not "be used in the routine Ouchterlony analysis, in radial immunodiffusion, or in immunoelectrophoresis." However, the document quickly added: "Since agar diffusion is not useful when automated immunoassays are being used, it is likely that their [monoclonal antibodies'] inability to precipitate directly will not be a major stumbling block" (NIAID 1981:104).

63. See also the call by the NIAID (1990:54) to "[d]evelop more effective and efficient methods for generating [monoclonal antibodies] and appropriate fragments of such antibodies; [and to] focus particularly on all-human, humanized, and chimeric monoclonals."

64. Consistent with this idea of the dream become reality, some review articles discussed pre-1975 attempts at producing homogeneous antibodies, which included the induction of myelomas in hyperimmunized rats, viral transformation of B cells, the use of simple antigens with small, repeating structural subunits, and Klinman's splenic fragment technique mentioned in Chapter 1. While it could be argued that monospecific antibodies have been the dream of many immunologists for long, one would have to answer the questions: What kind of monospecific antibodies? What for? This point can be brought home by the following quotation, according to which during the 1960s "immunologists [had] sought specific antibodies with molecular uniformity. It has been their goal to procure at will, and in a reproducible and predictable fashion, homogeneous antibodies to specific and defined antigenic determinants. But the prospects for achieving such a goal, until a few years ago, appeared bleak" (Krause 1970).

A post-1975 paper would at this point feature the standard line referencing the 1975 Köhler and Milstein's experiment. But the quotation is from 1970, and the text proceeded to argue that the quest for antibodies of molecular uniformity had led to the recognition that "immunization [of rabbits] with any one of several bacterial antigens might provoke antibodies with restricted heterogeneity." Thus, to the rhetorical question, "Are the means at hand to procure at will and in reproducible and predictable fashion, antibodies with molecular uniformity?," the author confidently answered, "All of the work summarized here suggests that this is so." The next question was, "If, indeed, rabbit antibodies with molecular uniformity are at hand, to what purpose can they be employed?" The answer read, "They should prove useful for at least three different lines of investigation. These are the structure-function relationship of antigens and antibodies and the topography of the antigen-combining site, the genetic control of the biosynthesis of the immunoglobulins, and the evolutionary mechanism responsible for their diversity." No trace, here, of "powerful new tools for biology and medicine."

65. "I think the spreading doesn't need reviews. Spreading is really mouth-to-mouth spreading. The reviews are the consequences of that, not the other way around." (Köhler, interview).

66. See, for instance, the following papers; Yelton and Scharff (1980, 1981); Scharff, Roberts, and Thammana (1981a,b); Diamond, Yelton, and Scharff (1981); Scharff and Roberts (1981). Dr. Scharff pursued his reviewing activity in this field in the subsequent years; see, for instance, Diamond and Scharff (1982); Pollock, Teillaud, and Scharff (1984); Spira et al. (1985); de Pinho, Feldman, and Scharff (1986); Pirovski et al. (1990). Some of these texts are more properly defined as popularization rather than review articles.

67. The jury is still out. . . . In a recent review of a book on tumor immunobiology (Manson 1994), we learn that "xenomonoclonal antibodies (mouse antibodies directed against human determinants) are probably not recognizing tumour-specific epitopes, but are mainly directed against species-specific carbohydrate epitopes."

68. A similar remark concerning the oncogene field can be found in Fujimura (1996). On expertise as a property of a network, see Cambrosio, Limoges, and Hoffman (1992).

69. This remark can be contrasted with and indirectly confirmed by Köhler's remark (quoted in Wade 1982): "Many people don't understand why I'm not making [monoclonal antibodies] against all kinds of antigens. . . . I successfully refused in the Institute to become the [monoclonal antibodies]

4

Monoclonals, Herpes, Hepatitis, and Other (not so Dangerous) Things

> It is possible to be serious, truthful, factual, thorough, scrupulous, referential—without claiming to be describing anything. Clifford (1990:68).

Authors' Note

Chapter 3 was a description of the spread of monoclonal antibodies into basic, clinical, and industrial laboratories. It does not, of course, qualify as a comprehensive description if by that one means a survey of all the different domains of practice where monoclonals were put to work. Rather, its claim to comprehensiveness is grounded in the description of the mechanisms by which monoclonals acquired generality. We have left it to the reader to extract those mechanisms from the substantive area(s) with which he or she may be familiar. It has not escaped our attention, however, that Chapter 3 is based, to a great extent, on local narratives, elicited through interviews. While the articulation of those narratives with a variety of other documents has led to generalizations, the original material is undoubtedly marked by the exigencies that presided over its production. From this perspective, Chapter 3 is a contingent, bottom-up construction, a combination of accounts that were first juxtaposed and then assembled on the authors' desks.

In this chapter we take a different tack, resorting to collage in order to describe the (re)production of hybridoma technology in two local settings. This allows us to use a new literary device: The story is told in the first person by two narrators, thus stressing the participant-centered nature of our approach. In the first case, the narrator is a fictional scientist, and the narrative mimics the transcript of an interview, with occasional comments by the interviewers. In the second case, the narrator is a laboratory ethnographer, and the narrative adopts the format of field notes. The speakers and their accounts are fictional only to the extent that they draw from different speakers and different sources, including observation notes, interviews, publications, and other documents (both public and internal) gathered in the course of several months of fieldwork in two different institutions. In the first text, the bulk of the material comes from a set of 25 in-depth interviews, complemented by informal exchanges that took place over several months in the fall of 1984 in a Canadian biomedical research institute. Additional material was gathered through subsequent interviews with scientists in Canada, the United States, France, and the United Kingdom. The publications and researchers referred to by the narrator are in most cases real, as instanced by the references in the footnotes. In the second narrative, the content is based on notes taken over an 11-month period of fieldwork (lab observations, attendance at team meetings, and informal interviews during coffee breaks and similar occasions) from the end of 1986 to the fall of 1987 in a Canadian biotech company involved in the production of diagnostic kits. The link between these two episodes will become clear in the course of the chapter. At first sight, Chapter 3 occurred in the abstract space of world science, where reagents and research materials circulate and are exchanged. Yet it resorted to local accounts in order to make its point. The local spaces evoked in Chapter 4 are replete with contingencies, yet it is because they illustrate generic features and events that they have been selected. The two chapters are obviously complementary.

RI Goes Monoclonal

The events recalled by the speaker occurred in a biomedical research institute (henceforth RI) not ranking among the elite and, more importantly for our purpose, not a major contributor to either the development of hybridoma technology or the application of monoclonal antibodies in the biomedical field. This choice of an average, as opposed to research-front, institution was designed to address the question of how such a center would integrate monoclonal antibodies into its daily work; it was our hypothesis that this stage corresponded to the transformation of monoclonal antibodies into a tool. We wanted to ask what was the status *attributed to hybridoma technology when it was first introduced. That meant looking at how* time *and* space *(both physically and institutionally) were allotted to hybridoma technology. We wanted to understand how monoclonal antibodies reshaped work patterns and institutional identities, and to bear witness to the transformation of monoclonal antibodies into a routine, background constituent of laboratory practice. The focus on an average*

> *institution does not mean that more visible actors are absent from the text; the speaker refers to them in the course of her account. In so doing, she revisits issues discussed in previous chapters.*

My name is Dr. Smith. I introduced hybridoma technology into this institute in 1979. At the time, RI's administrators defined the organization as a hybrid institution. They claimed that because the institute combined basic research, applied research, and some commercial activity, this definition was suitable. Financing from both public and private sources also tended to make RI a hybrid institution. The definition was first and foremost, however, meant to highlight their plan to engage in biotechnology-related activities.... Linguists call that a *performative definition*. We called it *hype*.

When I was hired in 1976 by the virology department, I was expected to study the antigenic determinants of influenza viruses, and that's what I did. I had done my Master's Degree in virology here in Canada and completed a Ph.D. in immunochemistry in a clinical research center in Britain. In the course of my Ph.D., I used what we would now call naturally occurring monoclonal antibodies that I isolated from the blood of patients suffering from an autoimmune disease. Needless to say, I was not aware of hybridoma technology, as it was just then being developed in Cambridge.

Back in Canada, I was given the opportunity to blend my virological and immunological skills. I first used conventional immunological techniques—polyclonal antisera—to study influenza viruses. I ran into an increasing number of reports praising hybridoma technology, however, so I decided to switch to the new technology. Why exactly did I do that? Well, as I said, there was the favorable reports, but there was more than that. For once, the new technology did not seem out of reach, both in terms of cost and equipment, and in terms of the necessary skills. As I just explained, my previous work with natural monoclonals had familiarized me with this type of material. I also thought that hybridoma technology would give me an edge over my colleagues here at RI and that a state-of-the-art technique would probably increase my chances of success in grant applications, which, in the end, it did. In addition, the institute was catching biotechnology fever.

> *This is congruent with Krimsky's (1991:32–33) claim that the growth pattern of new biotechnology enterprises entered an exponential growth phase in 1979, peaking in 1981.*

A major sign of the fever was a scheme, concocted by the administrators, called *internal priority grants*. They were supposed to attract researchers into commercially promising areas and to increase what was called *internal technol-*

ogy transfer between the basic and applied research. We didn't really need these incentives, as there was already great pressure to move into monoclonals. I guess this was common at the time; a lot of other researchers must have gone monoclonal for basically the same reasons. Take, for instance, the team at the Massachusetts General Hospital who developed monoclonals against hepatitis. They decided to learn hybridoma technology in 1979, the same year I did. And if you ask them why, they will tell you it was because of all the literature harping on the widespread applications and advantages of the technique, you know, the possibility of producing reagents of predefined specificity, of unprecedented purity, of increased sensitivity in virtually unlimited amounts, and so on.

> *We did ask them, and that is precisely what they said. Fujimura (1988) would attribute this to a bandwagon effect.*

Actually, the story is more complicated. It wasn't just a matter of changing technology to do the same thing. When switching from polyclonals to monoclonals, I also moved from influenza to the herpesvirus. I felt that using an innovative technology was not enough and that I also had to reposition myself with regards to my disease model. I'll come back to this later. First, let me explain how I came to master the technology.

I began to learn hybridoma technology using the descriptions available in the literature. As I already told you, hybridoma technology requires relatively simple devices that are found in any standard virology lab. The manuals I consulted made that very clear. Galfré and Milstein (1981:3–46) said:

> The essential requirements [were] common to ordinary tissue culture laboratories and include[d] 37° incubators with and without a controlled atmosphere of CO_2 and humidity ... sterile workbenches, inverted and ordinary microscopes preferably with phase contrast, water baths and/or hot blocks thermostatically controlled, centrifuge, liquid N_2 storage, plastic and glassware. Other items of equipment range[d] from highly desirable to luxurious.

In our lab, as in all virology labs, we also had the required expertise in cell culture. That was the bottom line: Without cell culture expertise you soon ran into trouble! Going from the published hybridoma technology protocols to the lab bench, however, was trickier than I thought it would be. Examples? Well, basically the things you described in Chapter 2: coping with the unexpected behavior of the cells (myelomas, hybridomas), mastering various tricks to improve fusion efficiency, that sort of thing. Hybridomas are not normal cells; you're dealing with monster cells that have been grown in culture for generations, stuffed with extra chromosomes, and so on.

After two months of tinkering with hybridoma technology, we still did not have a functional protocol, so I decided to spend a week at the Fred Hutchinson

Cancer Research Institute with Bob Nowinski. I also paid a short visit to the Pasteur Institute, not to learn about the technique, but to find out what they were doing with the monoclonals: I just wanted to make sure that I was getting the most out of the technique. It's not just a matter of knowing how to do it, you also want to know what to do with it! I should maybe add that I regularly attended meetings on the production and use of hybridomas. The first meetings—I am speaking of the 1979–1981 period—focused on the technology itself: the difficulties and how to overcome them, and so on. Later, the focus shifted to the application of hybridoma technology: Who had done what in cancer diagnosis, in therapy, and so on. Technically speaking, there was nothing radically new to be learned.

What I found, and still find, interesting was that, though I had to visit another lab and learn by doing, I only had to spend a week there. You see, the skills required by hybridoma technology were widely distributed, I basically had them all; it was just a question of a few missing links. Once they showed it to you, you could pick it up immediately, provided you already had some background in cell culture. Almost immediately after coming back from Seattle, I was able to act as a source of expertise for other teams. My lab was among the very first, possibly the first lab in Canada, to successfully produce monoclonals. I taught the technique to a colleague who was setting up the Hybridoma Section of the Canadian Laboratory Centre for Disease Control, and I gave university courses.

Why did I pick Nowinski's lab? I was interested in a place that had experience with hybridoma technology, not only in terms of the amount of time they had been working with it, but also in terms of the spectrum of antigens they had used. People I knew on the East Coast told me that Dr. Nowinski—I did not know him personally—was the one to see. I was not the only one to go through his lab. If you look at the "Acknowledgments" section of papers published in the early 1980s, you'll find several notes of thanks to Dr. Nowinski for his help in setting up hybridoma technology. By the way, Nowinski later became a founding member of Genetic Systems, a biotech startup specialized in monoclonals against sexually transmitted diseases (Teitelman 1989). So, we both ended up producing anti-herpes monoclonals.

Spending a week in Seattle was instrumental not only for mastering the technique but also for obtaining a myeloma cell line, a nonsecretory one—nicknamed NS-1—which had replaced the secretory one originally used by Milstein. This is a story that should be of some interest to a sociologist.

Block those stereotypes!

Today, you can get myeloma lines from the ATCC (American Type Culture Collection), but back in 1979 it was not clear who owned what, and, after what I heard had been a period of free circulation, it became difficult to get access to myeloma lines unless you were a well-known researcher; I mean by that, a well-connected one. Just look at papers from the period: It's not uncommon to find a note saying that the myelomas used in the experiments had been obtained from lab XY after permission had been granted by Dr. Milstein, from whom the line had originated. My guess is that Milstein's liberal distribution policy became more restrictive after Koprowski filed the patents you describe in Chapter 5. You know, those patents basically hijacked Milstein's invention . . . at least that's my opinion. Whatever the real story is, I had to write Milstein to ask for permission to obtain NS-1 from Nowinski. Permission was granted under the routine conditions that I not redistribute the cell line to other labs without written authorization.

So, after all, it was not such a big deal to get those myelomas . . .

When I got back from Seattle, the first thing I had to do was to adapt Nowinski's protocol to my lab. This involved a lot of fine-tuning. Being able to work with sterile techniques is essential. I gave priority to training technicians. A technician, depending on her previous experience, can take anywhere from six weeks to three months to learn sterile handling techniques. I didn't try anything fancy. I didn't try to improve the basic protocol I learned in Nowinski's lab. I wanted to have something operational, quickly. What do I mean by improvements? Well, electrofusion is an example: It would have taken two to three months to become familiar with it, not to speak of the cost of the apparatus (about $15,000 Canadian). And for what? For what we were planning to do the basic protocol worked just as well. Also, I felt that the more sensitive aspects of hybridoma technology did not concern the fusion per se, but the stability of the clones resulting from the fusion. Stability is a key issue: If your cell lines are unstable, then the work is wasted.

I can show you a summary report of the initial fusions done in my lab to produce anti-herpes monoclonals. You'll get a sense of the waywardness (Fazekas De St. Groth and Scheidegger 1980:5) of the technique. After each fusion—we did a total of five—we distributed the cells into 96-well plates. I say "we" because the work was done with a doctoral student. Look at this table. As you can see, in the first fusion, six wells out of 96 had anti-herpes hybridomas, but we lost them because of contamination. The second fusion produced no positive wells. In the third fusion, 36 wells out of 96 contained hybridomas; 13 wells contained anti-herpes hybridomas, and a total of nine type-specific anti-herpes clones were derived from two of these wells; others were lost because they stopped growing or secreting antibodies.

In the fourth fusion, all the wells tested positive for anti-herpes hybridomas, but no clone survived, although I was unable to find traces of contamination. Finally, the fifth fusion, for which mice were immunized with another viral strain (HSV-1 instead of HSV-2) and in which cells were distributed in a larger number of 96-well plates at a lower concentration of cells/well, 426 wells out of 576 tested positive. Out of these, we kept 119 hybridomas (22 type specific); 12 were cloned and seven were eventually kept for further testing. Of the several hybridomas produced in the third and fifth fusion, nine were selected for testing against clinical isolates and 3 were good enough to make it into the diagnostic kit we eventually produced and marketed.

Sorry about all these numbers. Basically, we obtained highly variable results. For obvious practical reasons, it was important to understand the origins of this variability. But it wasn't easy because of the number of variables. I asked the Ph.D. student to look into that, and here is what she says in her thesis: "details of fusion protocols vary from one lab to the other"; and look here: "*it seems* that the exact proportion of splenocytes to myelomas is not very important." As you can see, information on these variations more often than not bordered on hearsay. Of course, in our case we were tempted to write off the differences in yield between our first fusions and the last one to the change in viral strain used to immunize the mouse. There was a paper by McMaster University researchers, however, that argued against the existence of strain-related differences in immunization or hybridization outcomes (Killington et al. 1981). They had a lot of experience with herpesvirus, so we couldn't contradict them. In other papers, increased yields was attributed to changes in immunization methods, length of contact with PEG, the final dilution of the sensitized cells, the preparation of the antigen for immunization, and so on. Basically the "right" combination was a matter of trial and error.

That's about it. Well, actually it's not the whole story. I also had to spend a lot of time trying to convince people, both inside and outside the institute, that monoclonals were the right thing to do, that I should get more resources, that my lab should be reorganized into a special unit . . . basically that hybridoma technology should get the status it deserved, in all senses of the word: scientific, technical, institutional, and so on. I'll tell you about that later. First, I should fill you in on the herpesvirus monoclonals.

The Herpes Challenge

As I told you, I changed both my technique—from polyclonal to monoclonal antibodies—and the virus I was studying—from influenza to herpesviruses. I was probably not alone in this. I heard that at the Royal Free Hospital in London, somebody working on leukemia diagnosis with traditional immunological techniques decided to organize a hybridoma group to develop monoclonals for human lymphocyte subsets. So he asked another Royal Free scientist, a biochemist who had been working on cell fusion. Together they had the necessary skills. Shortly after getting together, they dropped the initial plan and went after hepatitis and Factor VIII, the one for hemophiliacs. They knew researchers at the hospital who could give them easy access to the viral and clinical material, and those targets had market potential, which at the time everybody knew.

Now, let me explain why I chose herpes. The influenza virus that I had worked on since coming to RI had always had special status at the institute. In the early days it had symbolized the alliance between science and public health. More recently, it has become a sign of the close ties between science and industry, you know, all that talk about the hybrid nature of the institute. We did basic research on the virus, which is known for its rapid mutation rate, and we also produced a flu vaccine that each year had to be adjusted to the latest viral strain. These two activities fed each other, or at least they were supposed to. Even though the institute was not making a lot of money, it could at least claim bioindustrial expertise—based on in-house scientific skills—and, in turn, this gave us credibility for future commercial undertakings. So a virus was not just another virus. I am trying to say that if you ask me why I picked herpes, you should ask me what were the characteristics of HSV at the end of the 1970s and not just the biological or medical characteristics, but also the social and commercial ones. I know this sounds like sociology ... but those things—social, clinical, and so on—were also important, and I was aware of that.

Your AIDS-era readers probably don't remember all the fuss about herpes in the early 1980s. After all, nobody, well, almost nobody, was dying of herpes. But just look at the articles published in popular magazines such as *Time*. I remember this one in particular because my student quoted it in her Ph.D. thesis. Herpes was going to undo the sexual revolution; it was nicknamed the *scourge*, the new Scarlet Letter, the V.D. of the Ivy League, and—I like this one—Jerry Falwell's revenge (Leo 1982). People talked about a full-fledged herpes epidemic. And the herpes scare was more than just some journalist looking for a new sensation. In the United States, there was a national self-help organization, the Herpes Resource Center: In the early 1980s they had more than 40 chapters and about 30,000 members (Leo 1982; Nahmias 1980).

It was not simply a question of some unpleasant biological manifestations—I mean, genital ulcers. I remember a paper by a leading herpes expert, Dr. Nahmias (1980), published in *The Yale Journal of Biology and Medicine*, in which he argued that the herpes epidemic was having devastating psychological effects: broken marriages, malpractice suits in the case of babies born with herpes, which led to an increase in the number of un-necessary cesareans, and he spoke of the sense of hysteria then pervading the public, the press, and the medical and nursing professions. In 1983 the U.S. Public Health Service included herpes genitalis in its *Annual Summary, Morbidity and Mortality Reports.* I still have the data. Between 1966 and 1983, according to the 1984 report, there had been a 16-fold increase in the number of consultations for herpes genitalis, from 28,000 to 423,000 (Kampmeier 1993:774).

As you can see, it was a social issue. But, at the same time, the technical-diagnostic problem was presented as the key to the social problem. The relations were explicit in both journalistic and scientific reports. If you look at the *Time* magazine article, it contained a lot of anecdotal information on the effects of the herpes scare on sexual behavior, but it also explained that researchers in the sixties had isolated two types of herpes, HSV-1 and HSV-2, the first having "above-the-waist" effects (typically cold sores on the lips) and the second, "below-the-waist" consequences, namely, genital herpes. It also explained that the two types were mobile: HSV-1 could be transferred to the genitals by finger or mouth and result in a venereal disease.

The problem was, as far as I was concerned, that because of widespread public knowledge about the viral strains, patients were asking their doctors for detailed diagnostic information, and physicians simply didn't have that information. Test methods were needed to assist patients, who kept asking the "who-gave-it-to-who" question, and to help doctors identify subclinically infected pregnant women at the time of delivery, or clinical epidemiologists who were trying to establish a link between HSV-2 and cervical cancer. Nahmias (1980:50) said something like, "we desperately need such tests," referring to virus identification tests that could be used routinely in the hospital laboratory for the rapid detection of HSV infections.

That was the bottom line; if you want to develop monoclonals and put them in a kit to identify and type herpes, you have to come up with reasons why the kits are needed in the first place. You can't wait for someone to show up and say, please, I need a herpes kit, make one for me. You have to develop something you expect to become essential, even if there is no immediate need. Just ask anyone in marketing. For sure, Nahmias had said there was a need for a rapid identification test. But there were also more qualified—should I say cynical?—arguments. A colleague said to me, "Let's say you develop an assay that can be performed in every doctor's office in a few minutes, and it gives you an 80% chance to be right and a 20% chance to be wrong. Then the doctor has to decide if he wants to be wrong 20% of the time, given the nature of the disease. For example, there is a lesion on the penis, the physician thinks it's HSV and does the test; if the test is positive, it's OK, the diagnosis is confirmed; if the test is negative, it could be a false negative, but so what? You can't treat it anyway." The lesson here was that it all depended on the market you targeted. In the fairly sophisticated American market, people wanted to know exactly what they had. Things were different in the European market. There was no point in even trying to market something like a herpes diagnostic kit in the United Kingdom, for example. Sales there would have been almost infinitesimal because these tests were done only in a public health lab, not in a doctor's office.

Now, given the situation, one way of consolidating the need for a test was to tie it to some other medical procedure so that the two would become mutually reinforcing. Let's say you develop a test that not only identifies HSV but also differentiates HSV-1 from HSV-2. Then you have a test that is not simply diagnostic for herpes in general, it also types the virus. Because we thought monoclonals could outperform other techniques in typing, this was the kind of test we decided to develop. A typing test, however, might appear even harder to justify than a simple identification test because knowledge of type did not at the time have any direct clinical value. One way to establish its utility was to link it to the use of anti-viral drugs with different therapeutic indications for HSV-1 and HSV-2.

The problem was that back then these drugs were not fully developed. Still, you could always argue that they were on the verge of being developed. That's what Nowinski did. I remember reading in a biotech newsletter (*McGraw-Hill's-Biotechnology Newswatch* 1981b) that one of his company's strategic products was a monoclonal kit capable of typing HSV "in hours, not days or weeks," and that, according to him, this was a decisive advantage over competitors because very soon a highly efficient drug—acyclovir—was going to be approved to treat herpes infections.[1] This was not just the Americans. Our Canadian colleagues at McMaster introduced their anti-HSV monoclonal antibodies, saying, "Presently, effective therapy for herpetic lesions is not available. However, the application of successful treatment modalities will require methods for rapid and accurate diagnosis" (Balachandran et al. 1982b).

As you can see, HSV was a hot virus in the early eighties and it offered a number of opportunities. To take advantage of those opportunities, I had to look seriously at the biological and serological tests then available. I soon discovered that the name of the game was to differentiate yourself from the others. No matter how subtle the distinction, there had to be a distinction. And because this was an ongoing game, you built distinctions on previous distinctions. You needed a map of the field to know where you were standing. It might sound strange, but at some point you and your monoclonals become the same thing. If you characterize your monoclonals and are able to show what makes them better or different from those produced by other labs, you are also showing that your work is distinct or better than that of other scientists. In the end, you are only as good as your monoclonals.

I switched to monoclonals because the literature credited them with many advantages. But I had to find out what those advantages would be for herpes. I didn't start from scratch. The literature had predicted that rapidity and specificity would give monoclonals a decisive edge in herpes diagnostics. In principle, rapidity could be used to discriminate against conventional tests, in which the virus first had to be grown in cell culture for several days or weeks. But would this work in practice? Would the monoclonals be sensitive enough to pick up a few virus particles directly from a lesion?

Specificity, on the other hand, seemed more straightforward: Conventional antisera produced ambiguous results when used to distinguish HSV-1 from HSV-2. This was a golden opportunity to boost monoclonals' superiority as diagnostic tools. I was not the first or the only one to have noticed that: The exquisite specificity of monoclonals, their ability to tell the two viral strains apart, was a feature stressed by all makers of anti-herpes monoclonals. Another advantage was that a self-contained monoclonal-based kit would be instrumental in shifting diagnostic work from the clinical laboratory to the general practitioner's office and, who knows, the over-the-counter market. We are talking about a lot of money. But don't get the wrong impression. The game was not restricted to monoclonals and polyclonals. There were other contenders, like the genetic engineering technologies, such as nucleic acid hybridization and DNA restriction endonuclease analysis, which threatened to replace serological techniques altogether.

I think the best thing to do now is to examine the publications my student and I thought relevant for our work: our map of the field. We ignored some of the research in this area and concentrated on the main contenders. Basically, we planned our work around those publications. You'll see what I mean shortly.

Let's start with the claim to have produced anti-herpes monoclonals. Contrary to what you might think, it was not enough to have produced them. You had to provide detailed results, which is a way of saying that without those results you didn't know what you had produced, if anything at all! Almost everybody agreed that the first anti-HSV monoclonals were produced by a British group at University College in London (Howes et al. 1979). The Wistar Institute team led by Koprowski had, however, already announced in 1978, at the first important meeting on hybridomas, the production of monoclonals against HSV-1. This was part of a more general paper—an important paper, by the way—reporting the production of monoclonals against different kinds of viral and tumor antigens. As a consequence, only a few lines were devoted to the anti-herpes monoclonals, basically stating that results similar to those obtained with other viruses had been achieved with HSV (Koprowski et al. 1978). The British paper credited Koprowski for having shown that the production of anti-viral monoclonals was possible, but it claimed priority for the first fully documented herpes monoclonals, and they apparently got away with that.

What strikes me today is that those so-called detailed results did not include the characterization of the specific proteins against which the monoclonals had been raised. I remember they admitted in the paper that their attempt at antigenic characterization had been unsuccessful. Antigenic characterization became, of course, the central topic of subsequent articles by other teams. Also, their monoclonals did not differentiate between HSV-1 and HSV-2, which is where the superiority of monoclonals lies. They left a lot up in the air. Moreover, they did not offer a rationale for the work. They merely speculated that anti-herpes monoclonals might become useful in serological typing, the identification and purification of specific viral antigens, the definition of tumor-associated minor antigens, and the evaluation of antigens important for protection against HSV. In other words, the point of their paper was the production of monoclonals per se, leaving the question of their future use open.

This was different from the strategy used by the leaders in the field of anti-herpes monoclonals. Let me take you through the literature. Here is a second paper announcing the production of anti-HSV monoclonals (Zweig et al. 1979). It appeared in 1979, the same year as the British paper, and was signed by a group of NCI researchers from the Frederick Cancer Research Center. This was the first in a series of papers by the same team that filed for a patent in 1980 (Hampar et al. 1980). As you can see, they followed the British by crediting Koprowski and coworkers for having demonstrated the possibility of producing anti-viral monoclonals. You will also notice, however, that their claim is more detailed than the British claim: Their monoclonals targeted a particular protein (p40) that defined a major component of the virus' nucleocapsids.

This placed their contribution within a specific line of work, namely, the definition of the antigenic structure of the virus. Their monoclonals also differentiated between HSV-1 and HSV-2, so they felt they were entitled to claim to have demonstrated what previous studies had only been able to suggest, that the p40 proteins of the two strains were different. Here is the next step: They claim that their monoclonals, inserted into an immunoassay "should allow rapid typing of virus isolates" for sero-epidemiological analysis or, in other terms, be of diagnostic value. Several subsequent papers (e.g., Zweig et al. 1980; Showalter, Zweig, and Hampar 1981) went along similar lines, reporting the production of other panels of monoclonals leading to the identification and characterization of viral proteins.

For the next group of papers, we move to the West Coast, where researchers led by Leonore Pereira reported the production of anti-HSV monoclonals in 1980. Initially hired by UCSF, Pereira later moved to the State of California Department of Health Services, where she co-authored a series of papers describing monoclonals for typing the virus. I immediately liked her style, direct and to the point.

Dr. Smith might also have been impressed by the networking evident in

> *Pereira's papers. Although the diagnostic work originated in the California Department of Health Services, Pereira used her monoclonals to conduct collaborative projects with researchers in other locations. A 1981 paper, analyzing the variability of HSV antigenic sites, was written with researchers from the University of Chicago and Copenhagen (Pereira et al. 1981).[2] A 1982 paper, once again dealing with the antigenic structure of the virus, marked the beginning of collaboration with the East Coast team and researchers from the University of Pennsylvania (Eisenberg et al. 1982).*

Look at the first paper. It starts with an attack on conventional antisera, arguing that they work poorly, if at all, when typing, and that they are difficult to produce and of low potency (Pereira, Klassen, and Baringer 1980). Here in a later paper she argues that because of crossreactions, antisera transform what should be *qualitative* diagnostic tests into complex *quantitative* estimates of reactivity (Pereira et al. 1982).[3] Monoclonals, obviously, are the solution to the problem. Both the East Coast and the West Coast papers, by the way, follow a similar path: They start from the antigenic characterization of the virus and proceed to the diagnostic-serological use of monoclonals, which they present as a sort of spin-off of basic research.

Pereira was important for us because she paid attention to diagnostics. And, involuntarily, she offered us the possibility of standing out in the field when she showed that monoclonals' specificity was a double-edged sword: It provided them with a decisive advantage over conventional antisera, but it also made them too specific. Even within the same viral strain you often found slight intratypic variations. There are often small differences in the proteins that differentiate HSV-1 from HSV-2. If your monoclonal targeted a protein with this kind of variation, it would be unable to recognize all the members of a single strain. Pereira was convinced that this was a real problem and that the solution lay in the production of a cocktail of monoclonals, each directed to a different type-specific antigenic determinant site.

> *Interestingly enough, the problem of antigenic variability convinced Hybritech—the leader of the biotech startups specializing in monoclonals—to leave the field of viral antigens, and specifically hepatitis, where they had hoped to make their first breakthrough. Hybritech's scientists openly acknowledged the existence of technical difficulties related to the polymorphism and complexity of the target antigen and speculated that monoclonals, given their specificity, would be better suited to detect simple molecules, like drugs and hormones, instead of complex organisms, like viruses and bacteria. Moreover, when confronted with the apparently suc-*

cessful production of an anti-hepatitis monoclonal assay by scientists from the Massachusetts General Hospital, Hybritech's scientists were initially skeptical as to the value of the assay in detecting viral subtypes (David et al. 1981). Dr. Smith will comment on that later.

In her 1982 paper on diagnostics, Pereira repeated the conclusions of the 1980 paper, claiming that the specificity of monoclonals had been vividly demonstrated but that because of intratypic variation, "the effectiveness of [monoclonals would] be considerably enhanced by the use of mixtures of type-specific antibodies." What I thought at the time was that if we could produce monoclonals with the right specificity—specific enough but not too specific—then we could beat her at her own game: Why make cocktails when you can use a single monoclonal! Of course, there was no way we could control the exact specificity of the monoclonals we were going to produce; we needed luck.

Let's switch to our Canadian colleagues at McMaster. Their team was led by William Rawls, a herpes specialist studying the relationship between HSV-2 and cervical cancer (e.g., Rawls 1977). Their first publication on the production of anti-herpes monoclonals goes back to 1981 (Killington et al. 1981). It appeared in a methods journal, and you will notice that the original finding, their distinguishing feature, was an immunization schedule resulting in a significantly higher yield of hybridomas. Rawls and his group then published a series of papers, similar to the papers by the East and West Coast teams, except that in keeping with Rawls' interest in HSV-2's role in cancer, the main target of the McMaster group remained that strain (Balachandran et al. 1981, 1982c). They also followed the path laid out by the two other groups in applying their antibodies to diagnostics (Balachandran et al. 1982b).[4]

Now, if you look at their diagnostic paper you'll see something interesting. For that paper they teamed up with a group of researchers from the University of Puerto Rico. To understand why, you have to know that in the serodiagnostic field the value of a given reagent can't be established by experimental demonstration. It has to be repeatedly tested against as many and as varied clinical isolates as possible and by comparing the results with those obtained by conventional tests, some of which count as the gold standard. Even if you do this, the possibility remains that additional clinical samples might prove the reagent to be inferior to other reagents, or even simply inadequate. Thus, the use of specimens from Hamilton and San Juan, two geographically and epidemiologically different regions, clearly added credibility to the paper's main message, which was that monoclonals could "be used to accurately identify and type isolates of herpes simplex virus."

The Massachusetts General Hospital team criticized by the Hybritech sci-

entists went to great lengths to ensure the credibility of their test: They collected and purified Hepatitis B surface antigens from the Philippines, Japan, the Middle East, France, the United States, Australia, and South Africa.

The McMaster paper also raised another important question that demonstrated that monoclonals were not the whole story. One had to show that the diagnostic system—in this case, immunofluorescence—was able to compete with and outdo other diagnostic techniques. Now, in the diagnosis of herpes, immunofluorescence, when used in association with polyclonal antibodies, was known to have serious limitations. Rawls' team, however, was able to argue that monoclonals not only overcame the shortcomings of immunofluorescence but gave it the ability, unlike other techniques, to identify and type the virus directly from smears of lesions. Also noteworthy was how Rawls and co-workers used a recent genetic engineering technique, endonuclease restriction. First, they promoted it to the status of a new gold standard and then showed, on that basis, that conventional approaches were deficient when compared to results obtained by the monoclonals-immunofluorescence duo. Because monoclonals were a lot easier to use than the endonuclease test, they were able to show that monoclonals were the quick and cheap solution for the diagnostic laboratory.

As far as I was concerned, these were the major players, and you can see how their monoclonals were dual-purpose tools. They were being used to dissect the antigenic structure of the virus—you could call them tools for basic research—and they were also being used for diagnostic purposes. Therefore, they were not only research tools but also potential products. As you know, I had no previous investment in herpes; the monoclonals provided easy access, but it was a restricted one. I was confined, for the most part, to clinical diagnostics, which the other players in the field presented as mere spin-offs of their research. In this respect, I was cornered because I was not going to be able to use one line of work as a springboard for the other. Still, I did manage to publish two papers on the topic.

The first appeared in 1983. It was a short article, and, in addition to publicizing the production of our monoclonals, it reported that they had been successfully tested against 198 clinical isolates. The second was published in 1984, but it had already been presented at a 1983 symposium. We used both herpes and Pereira as a target. As you remember, she had argued that monoclonals were too specific and had promoted the use of a monoclonal cocktail. We argued that this was no longer necessary because we had succeeded in developing type-specific monoclonals able to recognize all HSV strains in spite of intratypic variation.

The ability of our monoclonals to detect a comprehensive range of herpesviruses had to be convincingly documented. By comprehensive I mean biologically comprehensive, that is, different viral strains and substrains; geographically comprehensive, that is, viruses from different countries; and clinically comprehensive, that is, viruses recovered from lesions at different stages of infection. As far as the biological aspect was concerned, we argued that while only a few type-specific monoclonals were able to recognize the totality of corresponding clinical isolates, Pereira's monoclonals showed a more limited range of recognition than ours; or to put it the other way round, ours had a particularly large recognition range. In other words, we had been lucky.

We approached the geographical problem by using clinical isolates from public institutions, such as the Laboratory Centre for Disease Control (LCDC) in Ottawa, the Cadham Provincial Laboratory in Manitoba, and the diagnostic laboratory we had here at RI. These places had already done the job of centralizing diversity in a few places, and the only thing we had to do was to get access to that pool. It was, however, geographically limited; as a result, our claims were at first restricted to clinical HSV isolates circulating in Canada. This was not as bad as it might look because we are a country of immigrants, and people travel forth and back to distant geographic locations. We thought, however, that we could do better, and we did so by using our connections in a French laboratory to claim that our monoclonals had been assessed by that lab against clinical isolates from different European countries.

Finally, there was the question of the capacity of our monoclonals, and of monoclonals in general, to detect infected cells taken directly from a lesion, that is, without previous viral amplification in cell culture. Remember, this was important because it made rapid screening possible. Because the number of infected cells that can be recovered from a lesion is different at different stages of infection, this became a question of how much we could boost the sensitivity of our system. Notice: I said system. That means that it was no longer a question of monoclonals per se, but, rather, of the diagnostic system in which you used them. There were a number possibilities. We started with so-called indirect immunofluorescence; while this system required prior viral amplification in cell culture, it also allowed us to use the bare monoclonals, because the fluorescent reagent was added separately. As a result, we were able to make a kit quickly available. With the direct immunofluorescence method, we improved our kit by linking the fluorescent dyes directly to the monoclonals, using two different dyes for the anti-HSV-1 and anti-HSV-2 monoclonals.

The user, however, still had to go through the cell culture phase and still needed a fluorescence microscope. To get rid of these constraints, to develop a test that could be performed directly in a doctor's office, we felt the best bet was to operate with a so-called solid-phase system combined with an enzymatic method. The idea was to trap the virus present in the clinical isolate by using monoclonals linked to a plastic surface, such as the walls of a microwell, a tube, a bead, or—and this would be the top as far as simplicity is concerned—a dipstick. The virus would then be concentrated in a small area—with no need for virus amplification—where it could be detected by an enzyme system undergoing a color change, like in those over-the-counter pregnancy tests: "If it's blue, you're pregnant" kind of thing. Just imagine, you would take a little plastic stick, touch the lesion with one of its tips, dip it into a solution, and get the result!

> *About 10 years after Dr. Smith's interview, we learned that "simple, commercially successful antibody dipstick kits . . . are available at any high-street chemist for the cost of one issue of* Immunology Today—*the principles behind these are widely known, and home diagnosis of this type, with its potential to detect infections in everything, from the aspidistra to the goldfish, is a rapidly expanding market" (Campbell 1994). Other writers present a more nuanced assessment of this process. For instance, after having noted that in the past decade the laboratory diagnosis of viral infections had advanced in a quantum fashion, with immunofluorescence analysis of directly obtained specimens from the skin and other sites having replaced the time-intensive cell culture methods, one author claimed, "However, this idealized scenario has not been actualized in many medical centers that are attempting to implement viral immunodiagnosis. . . . Indeed, this situation reflects the reality that the 'technology explosion' of the 1980s has created, in some cases, as many problems as it has resolved" (Wick 1990).*

This may sound easy, but in practice the development work was long and painstaking: the kind of plastic you use, the format (beads, dipsticks, etc.), all these things make a difference. And there is the interaction between these components and the monoclonals. As one of the top scientists at Hybritech, then the leading biotech startup in the monoclonal area, noted, with polyclonal antibodies the system you use selects the appropriate class of antibodies out of the mix. In the case of monoclonals, you have to make that selection yourself (David et al. 1981). Most academic scientists who had produced monoclonals with commercial potential simply transferred them to companies who took charge of the kit development. That is what our colleagues at McMaster did. We sold our monoclonals to an American company who used them in a kit. But I also felt that I should be able to develop my own kit and to have it marketed by our production branch. This would have been a way of boosting the status of monoclonals within the institute, and thus my own.

The Institution of Hybridoma Technology

To be honest, I recently found out that my herpes articles did not receive a single citation in the five years following their publication. Before this interview, I asked a student to take the *Science Citation Index* and to count the citations received by the papers I just discussed with you, in particular the diagnostic ones. She gave me Table 4.1.

In addition to the papers we have discussed, the table shows citations to two papers published in 1983 by the Nowinski team. One of these papers (Peterson et al. 1983) appeared in the same journal as one of ours, but a few months later. They used the same arguments the McMaster team and we had made to justify the production of yet another battery of anti-HSV monoclonals. The 1983 Peterson et al. paper was singled out in a review article as a "most impressive demonstration" of the diagnostic potential of monoclonals (McDade 1985:143).[5]

Why that particular paper? Why that particular team? The answer is simple: money and power. The two go often together. If you check the second paper, also published in 1983, it lists among the authors' addresses Genetic Systems Corporation, Nowinski's biotech startup. So the commercial intent is evident. To top it all off, in 1983 the Genetic Systems group published a third article in *Science* reviewing the use of monoclonals for the diagnosis of human infectious diseases. The paper contained a section on the anti-HSV antibodies they planned to

Table 4.1. Number of Citations Received by a Selected Sample of Anti-HSV Monoclonals Papers in the Five Years Following their Publication, Self-Citations Excluded

Papers	Diagnostic focus	Number of citations
British		
Howes et al., J. Gen. Virol. (1979)		16
East Coast		
Zweig et al., J. Virol. (1979)		27
Zweig et al., J. Virol. (1980)		20
Showalter et al., Infect. Immun. (1981)		102
West Coast		
Pereira et al., Infect. Immun. (1980)		86
Pereira et al., PNAS (1981)		48
Pereira et al., Infect. Immun. (1982)	X	90
McMaster		
Killington et al., J. Virol. Methods (1981)		22
Balachandran et al., J. Virol. (1981)		41
Balachandran et al., J. Virol. (1982b)		63
Balachandran et al., J. Clin. Microbiol. (1982c)	X	38
Genetic Systems		
Peterson et al., J. Clin. Microbiol. (1983)	X	35
Goldstein et al., J. Infect. Dis. (1983)	X	54
RI		
Dr. Smith (1983)	X	0
Dr. Smith (1984)	X	0

Source of data: *Science Citation Index*.

commercialize as part of a diagnostic kit brand-named Micro Trak (Nowinski et al. 1983). Clearly, they had been able to concentrate on commercial-diagnostic work and, at the same time, attract scientific recognition.

Now, you might think that all this must have been very frustrating, and I won't deny it. But you have to understand that citations aren't everything. My audience was not just some abstract scientific community. I had other sources of recognition, such as local and national institutions, public health laboratories, provincial and federal diagnostic centers, and clinical and commercial institutions, not forgetting the community here at RI. I appealed to those audiences, and with respect to those audiences, the anti-herpes monoclonals brought me considerable recognition.

As far as people at RI were concerned, I have already told you that in the early 1980s management redefined its mission as both academic *and* industrial. In reality, this meant pushing the industrial side. One of the things they did was to establish a system of institutional priorities that functioned like an internal grant agency. I always did well with that committee. They consulted the priorities set out in the biotech reports published by various governments and organizations at the time: like the Brossard report in Canada (Government of Canada 1981), the British Spinks' Report (1980), and the Institut Pasteur report of the same year (Pelissolo 1980). Monoclonals were always among the priorities set out in those documents, and this, obviously, was to my advantage. I think you could say that it was not so much the case that the hybridoma unit was created within the context of the institute but, rather, that the hybridoma unit contributed a new context for the institute!

This doesn't mean that I just had to ride the wave. I had to fight for space for hybridoma technology. Money was scarce, and when I introduced monoclonals some colleagues were ambivalent; was it science or was it just a technical trick? You have to remember that our institute had university status; as a result, researchers and professors had a large degree of autonomy. The decision-making process was extremely democratic, which meant decentralized. So I had to take into account everybody's feelings and opinions.

I think it was important that the production of anti-herpes monoclonals also resulted in a Ph.D. thesis, because a thesis is recognized as a scientific, not simply a technical, exercise. At the same time, I did not hide the fact that the production of anti-HSV monoclonals had a clear diagnostic purpose and was not part of a broader research program. I made it clear that while I did not want to become a diagnostic kit maker, and while I was primarily interested in basic research, a product had become available and I was determined to exploit it. After all, we were a biomedical institute with a public health mission. We were not supposed to do research for the sake of research. As our director said, RI had evolved "in spite of and against all those who despised and still despise applied research."

In any event, I was glad Köhler and Milstein won the Nobel Prize. That sort of established the scientific status of hybridoma technology. I remember pinning a newspaper clipping of the Nobel Prize announcement outside the door of my lab. It was a way of saying we were doing science, not merely technique. No doubt, some continued to think that while the development of hybridoma technology was a real achievement, its routine application was, well, routine. One of my colleagues was very direct. He told me he could not understand why a Nobel Prize had been awarded for the development of a mere technique. That was kind of rude. Maybe he was over-reacting to the biotechnology hype at RI.

Many researchers here at RI, and I include myself among them, were genuinely excited by the possibility of pursuing basic research and yet, at the same time, being able to find commercial outlets. I remember the somewhat ambivalent feelings of some of my colleagues who rushed out to buy books about patenting in biotechnology but then hid them on the top shelf of their office library. As already mentioned, there was a lot of talk about internal technology transfer; a new R&D unit was created that was supposed to take over promising developments. This was slightly absurd because amidst all the talk about the disappearance of the boundaries between research and industry, management kept inventing new boundaries between more or less imaginary units. I mean, they kept splitting up—on paper, at least—the same old units, the same people and resources, and then felt entitled to talk about technology transfer between those units. You end up producing monoclonals in the same lab, but sometimes this would be R&D, sometimes basic research, and sometimes oriented research, which is what we were all supposed to be doing anyway in a biomedical institute like this one.

I learned to play the game. I knew I had to create a niche for monoclonals within the institute. The alternative was either hybridoma technology was going to be treated as just another technique, implemented on an individual basis by each scientist in his or her lab, or it was going to be centralized in one unit. I pushed for the second solution, banking on the highly specialized status of the technique and the commercial potential of monoclonals. The second approach, however, led to further complications. Some argued that the hybridoma unit should be split in two, a commercial and a scientific section, under separate control. I lobbied for the creation of a single hybridoma unit.

Towards the end of 1980, I sent a memo to the directors of the various research departments, asking if, given the increasing importance of hybridoma technology in research, scientists in their unit now needed or would be needing monoclonals. I presented my initiative as a response to the needs expressed by researchers, but I have to admit that I sometimes had to convince colleagues that they had needs they ignored. In January 1981, following the first memo, I convened potential allies to define the usefulness of hybridoma technology for interested researchers and to create a committee to draft a proposal to the institute director. Several researchers supported me, mostly virologists and immunologists. Other researchers refused. Interestingly enough, bacteriologists as a group claimed that none of their present or future projects would be needing hybridoma technology.

I also held several separate meetings with those in charge of the R&D sector of the institute, which existed mainly on paper. Some researchers thought the creation of an R&D unit was just a ploy to gain access to industrial research grants. The R&D staff thought they were developing some kind of commercial organization. As far as I'm concerned, the situation was that while the administration supported the establishment—once again, on paper—of the R&D unit, they didn't have the resources to hire experienced staff. I was the only hybridoma expert, which meant that I was negotiating from a position of relative advantage. This helps to explain why the proposal to the institute's director endorsed my position of creating a single hybridoma unit, and not two, as the R&D people would have preferred.

Building an R&D Unit, Tackling Hepatitis

I should say a few words about the R&D people as our stories overlap. While I was still busy developing anti-herpes monoclonals, I was asked to do some work on anti-hepatitis monoclonals as part of a project run by the two researchers trying to develop the R&D group. Notice I didn't say the researchers from the R&D group, because, as I just explained, the group was largely fictitious. Their idea was to use the hepatitis project to build an R&D infrastructure. Monoclonals were going to be an institution-building tool. I guess you could say the same thing of my herpes venture, with the difference, perhaps, that in their case there were more ambitious plans, more strategic thinking, and, as it turned out, more room for miscalculation...

Since the early 1970s, following the 1964 discovery of a hepatitis-associated antigen, the screening of blood collected by the Red Cross for the hepatitis B surface antigen (HBsAg), had been mandatory in many countries, including the United States and Canada. Consequently, a relatively large market had developed. The study of hepatitis itself had become a separate discipline (Farr 1981). For anybody aware of this situation—and here I mean the scientific or clinical aspects as well as the market situation—the decision by such a small group as the one at RI to tackle hepatitis must have seemed rather astonishing. But those aspects that worked against this decision also made it attractive. As a target, hepatitis was tempting because of its importance in terms of market and the relatively low development costs. Other promising markets, like cancer diagnostics, looked more difficult.

As in the case of herpes, monoclonals offered a point of entry, a possibility for outsiders to work around the competitive advantages created by established players like Abbott who dominated the North American market. The team here at RI calculated that monoclonals would allow them to solve two long-standing problems. The first concerned the lack of infrastructure for the large-scale handling of blood contaminated with hepatitis. Contrary to polyclonals, once good hybridomas were obtained, there was no further need to manipulate infectious material.

Secondly, the kit needed a competitive edge. One possibility was to play with the kit format. Abbott used beads, which could be easily washed. Organon had countered with a microwell format, which enabled one to read several samples at once. Using a new format or a new kind of plastic was not a realistic source of novelty for a small producer like RI who could not count on economies of scale. Monoclonals, however, were a source of novelty that did not depend on economies of scale. The plan was to use Organon's format—which, back then, was the only one using enzymatic, instead of radioactive reagents, and thus simplifying the handling of the test—and to substitute monoclonals for polyclonals.

The R&D people here at RI were not the first to use monoclonals in the hopes of breaking into the lucrative hepatitis market. Hybritech, for instance, had also targeted hepatitis for its first diagnostic product. But, as you previously pointed out, they changed their plans and dropped hepatitis. Although I was only marginally involved in the hepatitis project, the Hybritech decision couldn't be ignored so I consulted the commercial and trade literature to see what had led to the change of mind. Hybritech scientists had indeed presented HBsAg as their "entry into the monoclonal antibody experience" (David et al. 1981a). In 1979, Hybritech officials had even publicized a plan to go to market with the company's first product: "an antibody to diagnose hepatitis" (*Business Week* 1979). According to a company official, the plan was subsequently dropped, "because of competition out there," by which, no doubt, he meant Abbott. However, a biotechnology consultant argued that "Hybritech's test was simply not up to snuff" (Hall 1984). I concluded that the plan was dropped for both reasons.

As far as I could make out, there had been two kinds of technical difficulties. First, the monoclonals were supposedly too specific. We have already discussed this problem in relation to the herpes virus. With hepatitis the situation was worse, and, apparently, this had led Hybritech scientists to abandon the possibility of producing diagnostically reliable anti-viral monoclonals. Second, it is my impression that the Hybritech team, led by an immunochemist, paid too much attention to the immunochemical characteristics of the monoclonals per se, instead of concentrating on the behavior of the monoclonals within the kit system.

Whether the problems were technical, market related, or a combination of both, the net result was that, while Hybritech had been the first company planning to market anti-HBsAg monoclonals, another small startup, Centocor, reached the market first. A team at the Massachusetts General Hospital (MGH), which I have already mentioned, developed the monoclonals and the initial assay system for Centocor. The MGH team was not the only successful one. Anti-HBsAg monoclonals produced by a group of scientists of the Centre National de Transfusion Sanguine in Paris ended up in an kit marketed by Institut Pasteur Production under the suggestive trademark MONOLISA; those produced at the Royal Free Hospital in London were also marketed as a kit.

Even admitting that a kit could be made, how could RI hope to compete with a giant such as Abbott? This is where the Canadian connection intervened: The Liberal government, then in power, had made economic nationalism or self-reliance the cornerstone of its economic policy. Industrial research grants had been provided to local companies to develop products for a protected Canadian market. It was therefore possible to develop a product line that would not be stifled by United States–based competition. Monoclonals would add an element of glamour to what should have been the initial product of that line, the hepatitis diagnostic kit. Well, you know what happened next. The Liberal government was replaced by the Tories and their free-trade ideology. And, because the kit project had suffered serious delays caused by various organizational and structural problems, the comparative advantages were quickly eliminated. The economic rationality of the endeavor was called into question, which led to the abandonment of the project. This, by the way, was one of a number of events that led to a reassessment of the hybrid status of RI and, eventually, to a return to a more academic focus. As a result, other commercial ventures, including my pet herpes project, were dropped.

Hybridoma Technology: A Service Unit

The 1981 proposal to the director of RI to create a hybridoma unit emphasized three internal objectives: a) the production of monoclonals for fundamental and applied research, b) the production of industrially relevant monoclonals, and c) the design and development of technical improvements; and two external objectives: a) to play a consulting role at the provincial, national, and possibly international levels, and b) to achieve credibility with grant agencies. It was agreed that, because of the institute's budget, staff would be kept to a minimum, but this did not stop me from imitating management and drawing a flow chart (Figure 4.1).

> *This game corresponds to the replacement of a continuum of loose exchanges by a set of bounded units among which relationships can be posited or projected. Lakoff and Johnson (1980) speak, in this respect, of*

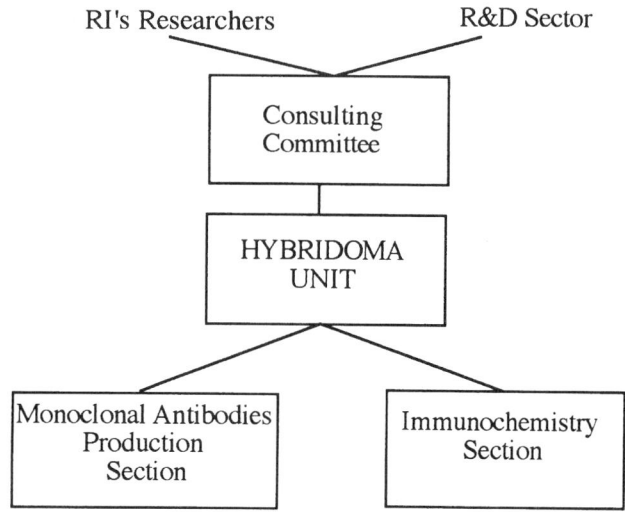

Figure 4.1. Flow chart of the Research Institute's proposed Hybridoma Unit.

the establishment of ontological metaphors.

This certainly added a sense of materiality to the hybridoma unit, even if it did not result in a serious increase in our budget. We obtained some additional money, but not enough to hire a supertechnician or to add major equipment. Still, the establishment of the unit allowed me to apply for grants in the name of the unit (and no longer as an individual researcher); individual applications by other institute members were also strengthened by referring to the unit as a locally available and reliable source of expertise. I was obviously put in charge of the unit, but, initially, I could only count on one or two technicians; later that number was increased to four. I repeatedly requested a research associate to take charge of routine activities, but got nowhere.

As a result, I had to personally supervise the technicians, which meant that I had to be available whenever important decisions had to be made. This was rather frequent as we were handling cells with highly individual behavior. We had to decide when to reclone them, when to freeze them, and so on. To do so, you have to understand the cells' life, a skill that takes time and experience to acquire. The person responsible for the viral diagnostic service occasionally helped, and I could also rely on the immunochemist heading the immunochemistry section, which was charged with antibody purification. That section disappeared, however, when it became clear that the other institute researchers tended to do purification in their own labs. It was also partly because the immunochemist had been unable to obtain small-scale automatic equipment. So he was stuck with artisanal purification methods, which defeated the purpose of having a section devoted to this task.

Now, you may think that this was a little crazy. Had we nothing better to do than to play around with organization charts, units, and sections? Well, the very idea of creating a hybridoma unit was something that was very much in the air in other institutions as well. For example, at the Royal Free Hospital in London, they seriously considered establishing a hybridoma unit to service local researchers. The hybridoma people, however, finally decided that there would be little scientific credibility to be gained by producing monoclonals for other scientists, not to speak of the fact that it would have taken time away from other, more research-oriented activities. As far as their first reason is concerned, I had a different attitude. I guess it depends on where you stand, which audience you are aiming at. I agreed with their second argument, however, and that's why I kept complaining about the understaffing of the unit.

At the Pasteur Institute in Paris the introduction of monoclonals led to the creation of the so-called Hybridolab (those French always come up with flashy names!). I visited them and I remember that, according to the original plans, the unit was not only to produce monoclonals for research and commercial purposes, but also to engage in technological innovation. I had similar plans, admittedly on a smaller scale, but I had to give up the innovation plans because of a lack of personnel. I think they also had problems on the innovation side. I spoke recently with a former director, who complained that the Hybridolab had become a mere monoclonal-production machine for the Pasteur Institute and the French public research network, the CNRS, doing as well as other institutions but no better.

I don't know if he was right or not, but the point is that you are caught in the middle of a service function and an innovative role. A research director from an Ontario company told me recently that their hybridoma unit had become just a service, like immuno-affinity chromatography, which means, among other things, that one doesn't need a gung-ho aggressive researcher as director or, to put it differently, that there is not a lot of scientific visibility to be gained there anymore.

> *This is reminiscent of the introduction of molecular biology into an Australian immunological institute. Newly hired molecular biologists wanted to create a separate scientific department, whereas the immunologists wanted to use the molecular biologists as technicians, spreading them among the different labs. They reduced molecular biology to a set of techniques (Stokes 1985). The analogy used by the Ontario research director, however, is different: He compared hybridoma technology to equipment, such as electrophoresis equipment, that was once sufficiently complex to require a special section, but that today is sufficiently simple that it can be found in every lab (Kay 1988).*

When a new approach, a new technique, in our case hybridoma technology, comes along, it's not clear how far it will go. How much will people be ready to invest in it? To what extent will it change the way we do things? With hindsight you can see how, in the case of hybridoma technology, previously disconnected areas were suddenly interfaced, because people in those areas now needed each others' skills. People in different domains of activity, I'm thinking here of academic and commercial institutions, started looking for better ways of communicating. New institutions were being created and older ones, like ours, redefined. But you can't really be sure that this will indeed work out. You go about it step by step, reassessing the role and importance of the new technology, its characteristics and potentialities. This is not an abstract process. It involves down-to-earth negotiations. For instance, would there be a separate hybridoma unit, how many people would be needed to staff the unit, how many rooms would be made available, what kind of daily work would be performed in that unit, what would be the status of the unit with regards to other units, and so on. In the end decisions like these settle the scientific status of a technique.

In the beginning, the unit was financed from the annual budget of the internal priorities program; in other words, it was considered a research project that would lead to definite, short-term results. The unit was soon transformed, however, into a research support service unit. The rationale for this was that we had evolved into a service—a good one at that—for the local research community. Over a four-year period, from 1980 to 1984, we worked on 20–30 different systems (by *system* I mean a set of monoclonals against a viral or bacterial strain, or a type of cancer cell), producing between 10 and 100 hybridomas for each system, which were stored in our in-house hybridoma cell bank. A computer technician developed software for managing the cell bank that, by then, contained about 2000 hybridomas, which had to be periodically thawed, recloned, refrozen, and so on. Having a service unit status assured us a regular budget. However exciting this might have appeared to me at the time, retrospectively I think that it also made our operation somewhat routine.

After we had succeeded in creating a hybridoma unit, we applied to the provincial government for recognition as an Advanced Training Unit (ATU). The ATU scheme was part of a larger biotechnology support program to promote the diffusion of key technologies by establishing training centers, each for a different technology, where, say, graduate students or industrial researchers could learn the latest skills. There was not a lot of money to be gained: Training costs were reimbursed, and there were funds for minor equipment costs. What you got was visibility and credibility, at least at the provincial level.

The competition did not specify techniques or topics. Research groups could apply by designating the domain of their proposed ATU. The decision to accept or reject the proposal was taken by a committee composed of academic and industrial researchers, and government representatives. My proposal, which of course focused on hybridoma technology, was rejected as by then—it must have been 1983—hybridoma technology had allegedly become a standard technique. I was told that several universities had submitted hybridoma technology proposals—all had been rejected—and that this proved that such expertise was readily available. We had only ourselves to blame for that: We had trained a number of hybridoma specialists in the universities. Also, some institutions had recruited postdocs, who had learned the technique in the United States. On top of all this, I was told that hybridoma technology was no longer considered among topics suitable for strategic grant support. I realized that my competitive base was being eroded and that it was no longer enough to produce monoclonals. The technique had become a service, which any reasonably staffed institute had to have.

Well, this brings the story to a somewhat uneventful end. I guess this is how a lot of things end. As the initial excitement faded, hybridoma technology drifted into the background and became routine: essential but invisible. Nonetheless, to end on a personal note, I would not be what I am today, for better or for worse, were it not for monoclonals.

Notes on Fieldwork at Bio-Bucks

A couple of years after collecting the information on RI, we undertook a period of observation in a Canadian biotech company—let's call it Bio-Bucks—which was involved in the production of diagnostic kits. What follows are excerpts from a fictional field diary.

Today is my first day at Bio-Bucks. I am doing focused ethnography (Law and Whittaker 1986). My goal is not to understand Bio-Bucks's cosmology, its overall culture. Rather, I'm interested in monoclonals. Two years ago, Dr. Smith had taken leave with some remarks about the routinization of monoclonals: I want to learn how things stand now. Unlike my experience at RI two years ago, I am stationed in a real commercial R&D institution, one that is not trying to be both academic and industrial. As I have learned from a somewhat formal introduction provided by one of the directors for R&D, Bio-Bucks has many different sections. I have specifically requested, and been given access to, the diagnostics section, which is composed of two groups: a microbiology team, working on diagnostic kits detecting bacterial and viral antigens, and an endocrinology team, working on kits for various hormones. I will be based mainly in the microbiology section: This will make comparisons with my previous fieldwork at RI easier. The head of this subsection—Dr. K—is also responsible for the lab producing monoclonals, which services both teams.

The diagnostics section is not very large. There are four main labs (plus a few additional rooms for animals, liquid nitrogen storage, etc.). One of the labs is known as the monoclonal lab. In addition to Dr. K, the monoclonal lab is staffed by two technicians: a senior technician (henceforth Senior), who was trained in hybridoma technology in a major university, and a junior technician (henceforth Junior), who is learning hybridoma technology from Senior. Senior and Junior are in charge of the day-to-day work with monoclonals, which, in addition to the production of new fusions, includes hybridoma maintenance work (storing in liquid nitrogen, periodic thawing, recloning and refreezing). The screening of monoclonals takes place in another lab.

The microbiology section is involved in the development of several diagnostic kits, but, right now, all energies are focused on one particular kit that is experiencing serious delays in its development schedule. There is an obvious division between the researchers in the monoclonal lab and those working on other kit components. The monoclonal lab looks more and more like an external module that has been stuck on the kit development group. There are various indicators of this, including architectural evidence. The monoclonal lab has its own room and is flanked on both sides by the microbiology kit lab and the endocrinology kit lab. In the back there is a fourth lab, called the assay lab, where radioimmunoassays and enzyme immunoassays are performed and that thus functions as a sort of service unit for the three front labs (see sketch in Figure 4.2).

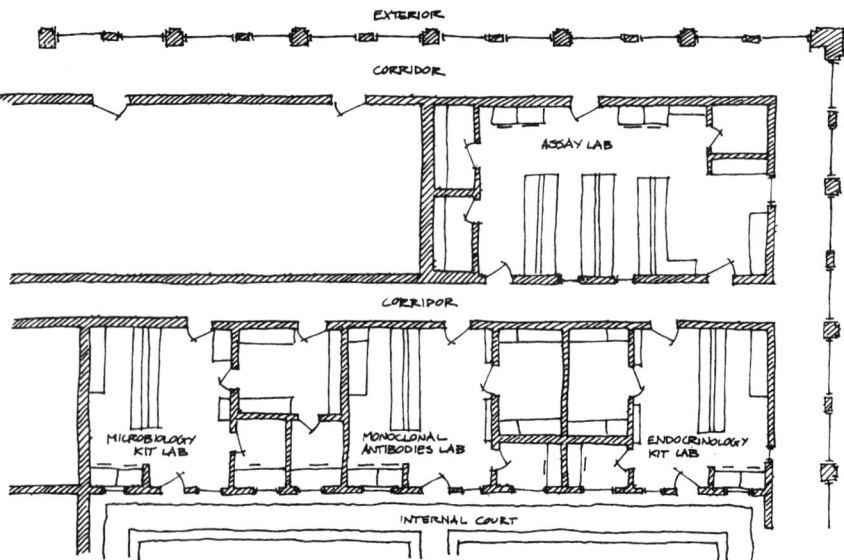

Figure 4.2. The ethnographer's sketch of Bio-Bucks's diagnostic section. (Drawing by Conor Sampson.)

Dr. K provided further evidence for the separate status of the monoclonal lab when he described the work involved in developing a kit. He drew a flow diagram in which the production of monoclonals (the initial fusion, the screening, and, eventually, the bulk production of the monoclonals to be used in the kit) was divided into one set of boxes and the various activities leading to the production of the kit into another. The two sets of boxes interacted only insofar as the monoclonals emerging from the first set were to be grafted onto the line of work represented by the second set. Actually, things were slightly more complex. In addition to monoclonals, the kit people also used polyclonals; when Dr. K added to each box the name of the persons working on that particular task, I realized that the kit work, *including* the production of the polyclonals, was being performed by an integrated team of seven persons, whereas work with monoclonals was entrusted to an entirely different team. Dr. K admitted that there was a structural gap between the two teams. They worked side by side, rather than together.

....

Today there was further evidence of a gap between the monoclonal lab people and the kit people. An urgent meeting was called to discuss the question of which format should be chosen for the kit that had run into delays and the monoclonal lab people were not invited. I decided to look further into this matter by inquiring into the origin of the monoclonal lab.

Bio-Bucks's officials had first planned to obtain monoclonals by purchasing them from academics who made them available as spin-offs from research projects. They soon became convinced, however, that an in-house hybridoma capability would prove to be an asset (it would, for instance, repackage the company into a high-tech firm) and provide a sort of safety net. So, they devised a scheme whereby, with the help of a government grant, money for purchasing hybridoma equipment and training personnel was made available to a university team with well-established expertise in hybridoma technology. The equipment and the newly trained personnel were then transferred back to Bio-Bucks. Senior is the main product of that operation. As I learned from Dr. K, she does not have a Ph.D. but she is very skilled in her area, which, to use his words, "implies not the planning or performance of experiments, but the production of things." She is a supertechnician.

Bio-Bucks's strategy for purchasing hybridoma technology expertise reminds me of a similar strategy adopted by another Canadian biotech firm in which I conducted interviews. In the early 1980s, after deciding that they had to get monoclonal expertise, the company offered a fellowship to a university team to train a postdoctoral student in hybridoma technology, with the understanding that he would subsequently join the firm. The postdoc, however, eventually accepted a job at the university, jeopardizing the firm's strategy. I am tempted to believe that Bio-Bucks, by providing not only money but also equipment, was able to recover the personnel by recovering the equipment. Moreover, in Bio-Bucks's case, the persons involved were technicians, not postdocs; this might have made the transfer less problematic. This also says a lot about the changing status of hybridoma technology in the space of a few years. So, basically, the monoclonal lab is a sort of self-contained unit, which was transferred as a whole—people and equipment—from one setting to another and is expected to continue performing a specialized task.

What qualifies the monoclonal lab work as specialized? I gained some insight into this question by chatting with Senior, listening to her exchanges with Junior, and attending a presentation she gave to the microbiology team. Two themes emerged. The first is one I am familiar with from my previous fieldwork: the importance of sterile techniques and the fear of contamination. Contamination stories are indeed a recurrent theme of Senior's conversations with Junior. As parables, they play an obvious pedagogical role. The second theme had, until now, escaped my attention: the obsessive care needed to keep track of the thousands of hybridomas distributed in different kinds of containers, ranging from flat culture bottles to microwell plates and frozen tubes. Not that I was not aware of the existence and importance of this kind of work: Latour and Woolgar (1986:245) referred to it in a amusing passage of *Laboratory Life* in which the ethnographer cum technician botched an experiment by losing track of the test tubes in which he was transferring solutions. I had not realized, however, the extent to which this activity could become a defining characteristic of a full-time hybridoma technician.

During her presentation to the microbiology team, Senior showed several overheads of schematic illustrations of a series of 96-well plates, each corresponding to a stage of the cloning process. Using those drawings, she explained how the positive wells (and thus the hybridomas they contained) were named so as to keep track of the origin of each clone. In general, hybridoma specialists use the coordinates of the plate: one side of the plate is inscribed with numbers (1–12) and the other with letters (A–H), so that B7, for instance, refers to the seventh well of the second row.

Senior used a more complex system, one which I had difficulties understanding and which I am not allowed to detail here (a mini trade secret?). I was relieved to learn, from the puzzled questions by members of the kit lab, that I was not the only one to be confused; but they soon gave up questioning. After all, this was not part of their job. Later, Senior told me that her system was not an international system; it had been devised in the university lab where she had been trained. Thus, learning hybridoma technology had also involved learning a sort of bookkeeping: not only how to label microwells and bottles, but also which information had to be included and/or overlooked. She was convinced that her bookkeeping technique was a superior tool for the control of the inevitable proliferation of clones (one single fusion I was able to witness a few weeks ago produced more than 2000 hybridomas), but at the same time it mobilized a lot of her energy: "I keep dreaming about it."

....

My previous observations about the labeling system prompted me to look more closely into the local dimension of hybridoma technology. In this area, I am reaching what qualitative sociologists call saturation: The same or similar elements appear over and over again, pointing to the fact that the topic has been exhausted. Some elements, however, came back with renewed vividness. One is the extent to which fusions and maintenance work had settled into an established routine. Senior explained to me that the fusion protocol she was using and transmitting to Junior had been fine-tuned in 1983 at the university center where she had received her training. For almost four years she has now been using it without modification: "It's an infallible method!" The reliability of the protocol allowed her to take charge of everything related to fusions. Dr. K did not even look in on the lab during last week's fusion.

Yet the attitude toward the list of instructions making up the protocol is sometimes quite relaxed. Senior acknowledged the equivocal origin and status of certain steps, which she sometimes followed and sometimes not. An example of the latter was her decision to no longer sterilize the bottles and the pipettes used to transfer a solution known as DMSO, since "[she had] heard that the solution [was] strong enough to kill the bugs." Examples of the former situation were the continued use of feeder cells despite her claim to have noticed that "they [did] not make any difference," or the calculation of the number of cells being handled, in spite of her remark to Junior (who had run into calculation problems) not to bother, because "after all, this [was] not really important." As an external observer, I perceived a sense of arbitrariness in these decisions, which juxtapose the macroscopic handling of containers and solutions with calculations and considerations involving invisible or even theoretical entities. I felt the presence of a sort of liminal space, where the visible blends with the invisible and in which experiential choices are made (see Cambrosio, Jacobi, and Keating 1993).

Senior's skills are often hard to dissociate from the equipment she uses. For instance, Senior claims to be able to estimate the number of cells in a given solution just by looking at the color of the medium (which contains an indicator sensitive to pH changes); however, this capacity is highly dependent on the incubator in which the solution was stored. All these elements conjure up a highly ritualized performance, that, when passed down to Junior, takes the form not of theoretical, but of experiential statements, very often uttered in terms of cautionary tales, such as the already mentioned "contamination stories." Senior's reaction to the possibility of introducing a robot in the monoclonal lab is very interesting in this regard. During the coffee break after the demonstration of the robot (which was not purchased), Senior came to me and said bluntly that "[she didn't] like that thing." First of all, it would take her place and force her into a routine, but it would also endanger the production of monoclonals: The robot could break down and, most importantly, it would constitute an increased danger (once again!) of contamination.

....

I have to gain a better understanding of what is going on in the kit lab. I originally intended to look mainly at monoclonals, but what I found in the monoclonal lab was ritualized routine. The action is in the kit lab. A few weeks ago, a postdoc from the kit lab came back from the American Society for Microbiology meeting, and he presented a summary of the new kit technologies introduced at that meeting. This week, the R&D director came back from yet another meeting, "Advances in Solid-Phase Technology," and also gave a presentation. The question of the format of the kit seems to be the most important question right now. Fresh information from meetings and from trade literature and methods journals is constantly brought in. The final decision concerning format, anxiously awaited by the kit lab personnel, has to be taken by the company's high level officials.

In the meantime, at the lab level, most of the experiments being performed consist of testing various formats. This activity includes the reverse engineering of other company's formats but mostly experimenting around with various membranes, blocking solutions, colored plastic beads, and so on. Speed and ease of use and interpretation of the test results are the qualities most expected to make a difference. This is a good example of how not only the final design, but also the development phase of a kit, is co-determined by commercial and technical considerations (Bibard 1991a,b). The author of a book review was right on target when she claimed: "the central issue of commercial immunoassay are antibody affinity, simplicity of readout, and no patent costs" (Campbell 1994).

Speaking of antibody affinity, what about the monoclonals? They are just another element of the kit, at the moment not the most important one. Neither Dr. K nor the postdoc seem to think that their use in the kit would result in major problems that need to be worked out in advance. What counts, so they claim, is the overall package, not a single component. The kind of diagnostic test they are developing—Dr. K explained to me—is not really qualitative (in the sense that the presence of a single microorganism would result in a positive reaction) but semiquantitative: It can only detect a given minimal quantity of microorganisms. The test's validity range must thus not only be determined to the satisfaction of governmental agencies, but the kit's behavior in that respect has to be made reproducible.

This results in a lot of tinkering, whereby trade-offs are made between the variables (speed, sensitivity, ease of use, and so on) that characterize the test. Complications might arise at this level if the delicate balance of the various components, achieved after much work, is altered by the replacement of polyclonals with monoclonals, or of a given monoclonal with another. But the overall impression I get from Dr. K is that he does not think that this will be a real problem. The antibodies, in other words, do not appear to him to be the most problematic component of the kit, at least for now.

....

I cannot avoid comparing my fieldwork at Bio-Bucks with my experience at RI, where monoclonals seemed to be the beginning and the end of almost everything. Right now, the people in the kit lab are working with polyclonals rather than monoclonals, although the latter are available. Dr. K told me that, with a few exceptions, such as the exquisite specificity of monoclonals that could lead to crossreactions, he didn't really see a big difference between developing a monoclonal or a polyclonal kit, and his job is to come up with a marketable kit. The main technician in the kit lab even seems to have cultivated a negative attitude towards monoclonals. He is heavily into testing various membranes and blocking solutions, and is exasperated by the possibility that the system he has put together might work with certain monoclonals and refuse to work with others. The main reason the experiments are now being performed with polyclonals is that the available monoclonals are said to have stability problems when attached to the so-called solid phase. But Dr. K does not seem overly preoccupied with developing new ones. According to him, it is even possible that the first marketed version of the kit will be entirely polyclonal. Future versions will certainly involve monoclonals, even if only in a mixed polyclonal-monoclonal system, to avoid infringing a Hybritech patent (see Chapter 5). I have no reason to doubt Dr. K's commitment to the use of monoclonals. After all, in the last months he has been spending hours every week testing two different models of bench-top bioreactors to be used in the bulk production of monoclonals, and he has also invested time in an attempt to improve the production of monoclonals in ascites. So, he clearly foresees an important role for them, but just as an element, among others, of the kit.

....

When I am not sitting in one of the labs, watching and listening as people go about their job, or at the cafeteria, chatting with them, I station myself in Bio-Bucks's library, writing up field notes and observing the lab personnel make use of the facility. Actually, the library goes to the labs as often as researchers and technicians go to the library. Recent issues of several journals are routinely circulated among laboratory heads, not to speak, of course, of the borrowed books that sit on laboratory desks. So, it's not surprising to learn that the written literature is a common resource in lab bench discussions, as when Dr. K. told a technician: "Don't try it with potassium, it's hearsay; try ammonium, at least you got literature on that"; or when he answered a technician's query by pointing to an open journal on his desk and saying, "Part of the answer may be in that paper." More importantly, perhaps, tables and graphs from books and journals are photocopied and pasted in the laboratory notebooks, side by side with locally generated numbers and curves. The adequacy between the outside world and the lab starts in these notebooks, where correspondences are carefully crafted in an ongoing process of trials and retrials. That's what they mean by reproducibility.

My regular visits to the library also allow me to survey biotech newsletters. By doing that I realized that the flashy headlines once reserved for the production of monoclonals are now pointing to a second generation of antibodies. For instance, an article entitled "Stage Set for 'Immunological Star Wars'" gives details on so-called chimeric, bifunctional, and bispecific antibodies, while another article introduces the term *quadromas* (Klausner 1987a, b). These developments (and others to come; in a few years I will learn about ways of bypassing hybridomas, thanks to genetic engineering, and there will even be talk of bypassing the animals)[6] concern methods and approaches that were never mentioned or even vaguely evoked in my presence as part of Bio-Bucks's plans.

This is not to say that Bio-Bucks is not interested in collaborating with outside scientists who develop new approaches. I observed a visit by a university scientist during which concrete technology transfer plans were discussed. But, as previously noted, the main input from the external world, in addition to the published literature, comes in the forms of reports from trade meetings and conferences, where the focus is on the overall product—the kit as a package—rather than on individual components.

A kit, as Bibard (1991b) has noted, is a complex representational device, in both senses of the word: Some specific antigens are targeted as representatives of a given microorganism on which they happen to sit; antibodies binding to those antigens will stand for them. Radioactive, enzymatic, or fluorescent labels will speak for the antibodies by making them, in principle, visible. The items that are collectively referred to as the format of the kit interact in transforming that potential visibility into an actual one, introducing, by the same token, a variety of parameters (ease of use, speed, degree of readability) that will identify a given system as distinct from another. Finally, the system must be idiot-proof, a goal that can be reached by black-boxing into the kit its conditions of use. All these elements are in a sort of steady-state equilibrium, so that difficulties in one part of the system can be worked around by modifying other parts. Moreover, the system is open; items ranging from marketing considerations to regulatory issues or the sudden availability or disappearance of certain embodied skills (a postdoc unexpectedly joined Bio-Bucks . . . and unexpectedly left) all make a difference. As Dr. K once said, when I pressed him on monoclonals: "We've got to see things in perspective . . . "

....

For some time I have been noticing a growing sense of uneasiness vis-à-vis my presence, especially from the once friendly R&D director. Bio-Bucks is navigating through some rough waters, a radical restructuring of the company looms ahead, and I have the feeling that my fieldwork will soon be over. This is not a major problem: I have seen what I wanted to see. So, it's a good time to draw some conclusion from my observations. What about the following one?

> *Monoclonals certainly contributed to the repackaging of Bio-Bucks as a high-tech company: This is apparent from reading their annual reports, although not so evident in their product line. But, in turn, monoclonals were repackaged as a component of a collective of humans, equipment, and devices that coalesced into the development of a specific line of products. It is not so much that monoclonals became marginal or secondary; after all, a lot of time and money were devoted to the production and maintenance of hybridomas. Rather, they became part of a sort of unproblematic background—much like microcomputers in a service sector company—against which other aspects of the overall task, such as formatting, came to occupy the foreground.*

NOTES

1. As argued in detail in Teitelman (1989), Nowinski's strategy, and thus the argument used to back it up, did not work out: He had underestimated the complexity of the diagnostic market and neglected differences between tests and therapy.

2. The paper reached the somewhat troubling conclusion that "the differentiation between HSV-1 and HSV-2 by [monoclonals] to glycoprotein gA and gB may well depend on the cells in which the viruses are grown."

3. See also the overview of this work in Pereira (1982).

4. The Rawls group also explored, as Pereira had done, the use of anti-HSV monoclonal antibodies as a tool for passive immunization (i.e., in vaccine research). See Balachandran, Bacchetti, and Rawls (1982a) and Dix, Pereira, and Bohringer (1981).

5. The same observer, however, also stressed the superiority of viral isolation over immunofluorescence-antibody techniques and supported Pereira's claim that intratypic variation made the use of monoclonal antibody cocktails necessary. Pereira's suggestion that "pooled monoclonal antibodies for typing HSV-1 and HSV-2 in the clinical laboratory may be necessary" was also taken up by Hsiung et al. (1984:73).

5

Between Nature and Culture: Constructing Novelty, Patenting Inventions

> An *innovation* is something new, newly proposed, or newly created; *The product line for the spring contains several innovations.* Innovative can apply either to what is created—*His proposal was very innovative*—or to the creator—*She's an unusually innovative designer.* Since an *innovation* is of itself something new, a new *innovation* is tautological and substandard.   Wilson (1993:147–148)

> Are hybridomas inventions? In a word, yes.   Raub (1981)

In 1980, the NIH issued guidelines "indicating that hybridomas and their products should be considered as inventions" (Zack and Scharff 1982:15).[1] William Raub's earlier quotation summarizes the NIH position. In his presentation on NIH policies on hybridomas, Raub went on to explain that, while in theory almost all hybridomas produced under any Public Health Service grant should be reported as inventions, in practice "such comprehensive reporting seem[ed] neither necessary nor desirable"; only a small number of hybridomas "of obvious commercial interest" were likely to be reported. Raub also noted that hybridomas presented special problems for NIH grant and contract policies, as no identical hybridomas were likely to be produced, therefore raising, in addition to issues of patenting, the question of the preservation and distribution of these unique specimens.

The NIH position was echoed during the "Science Meets Law" conference, held in October 1981 at Cold Spring Harbor (Plant et al. 1982; Carey 1983). The conference format provided for presentations by distinguished researchers on the scientific issues (mainly genetic engineering and monoclonal antibodies), and presentations on legal issues by patent experts. Each session was followed by an open forum in which the two camps engaged in general discussion. This neat separation between legal and scientific issues was not respected in the presentations. Moreover, as far as hybridoma technology was concerned, the speakers and discussants explored the question of how (not whether) and under what circumstances hybridomas, as well as their products and applications, could be patented.

About 10 years later, the palpable uncertainty of the 1981 Cold Spring Harbor conference that had, from the outset, surrounded patents in the hybridoma field because, among other things, of Milstein's alleged failure to patent hybridoma technology (see later discussion), had to a large extent evaporated, as instanced in the exponential growth of patents in the hybridoma field briefly discussed in Chapter 3 (see Figures 3.4 and 3.5). Perhaps more significant, however, is the fact that two of the main areas of application of hybridoma technology were by then characterized by the presence of strong patents. In the immunoassay field, Hybritech, a biotech startup that had recently been acquired by Eli Lilly, had successfully defended a key patent against another biotech startup—Monoclonal Antibodies Inc.—and had subsequently obtained a very favorable out-of-court settlement after suing one of the giants in the field, Abbott Laboratories. These developments were paralleled in the area of lymphocyte surface antigens that grew out of hybridoma technology and that fostered diagnostic and therapeutic innovations in major medical domains, such as transplantation, lymphomas, and leukemias. Here Ortho Pharmaceutical Corporation (Johnson & Johnson) had reached an out-of-court settlement first with Becton-Dickinson and, subsequently, with Coulter Corporation on the so-called OKT antibody series and the use of these antibodies in flow-cytometric equipment (see later discussion and Chapter 3).

This is not to say that obtaining a patent in the hybridoma technology area was unproblematic. Hybritech's patent, for example, had followed a tortuous path. At first rejected by the Patent Examiner, it was issued after the introduction of modifications that became the target of a subsequent dispute with Monoclonal Antibodies Inc. The patent was then invalidated by a first judgment in that dispute and reinstated by a Federal Court of Appeals. Perhaps more significantly, Cetus's (another biotech startup) repeated attempts since 1981 to patent monoclonal antibodies against human fibroblast interferon were given a deathblow in January 1992 by the U.S. Patent and Trademark Office (PTO) Board of Patent Appeals, prompting two patent attorneys to ask whether the end of monoclonal patents was in sight (McGough and Burke 1992). From our perspective, however, the point is not whether a particular patent was sustained or rejected, nor whether an entire class of claims will eventually fall under an unpatentability clause, but the very fact that monoclonal antibodies entered the patent arena.

Thus, as we shall see, Cetus's failure, far from tolling the death knell of patenting in this area, has prompted discussion of the circumstances under which a *prima facie* case of unpatentability can be overcome. Indeed, hundreds of patents involving monoclonal antibodies have been issued since the 1992 PTO decision in the Cetus case.

Thus, following their redefinition as tools, hybridomas were translated into inventions. But what does that mean? A good way of characterizing our claim is to differentiate it from other claims that resort to a similar terminology. Historians and philosophers of science, for instance, have long drawn distinctions between invention and discovery. Hacking (1983:162) has noted that inventions are distinct from either theories or experiments. Invention has a practical character and is capable of leading on its own to new technologies and new theoretical analysis. Rheinberger (1993b), in turn, has put the invention/discovery distinction to a different use by claiming that "[s]cience is not about discovering things, it is about inventing things."[2] His is an attempt to replace the conventional wisdom whereby scientists recognize (discover) things out there with the by now also fairly conventional trope of scientists (de)constructing facts.

Our purpose is different from both Hacking's and Rheinberger's. The analysis of hybridomas' redescription as, and thus transformation into, a new kind of object does not imply that any of the categories used to account for hybridoma technology, and its products are more or less true of it. Rather, we argue that hybridomas became inventions (in, say, 1980) once they began to be treated as such in laboratory and legal practice.[3] In other words, our remark is ethnographic, not philosophical. Our claim should not be read as a matter of (re)labeling, if by that term we mean the mere attribution of a (new) tag to the same object. The attribution of a new name is, in itself, an event and as such transcends the object. As Ivins Jr. (1969:180) has noted, "at any given moment the accepted report of an event is of greater importance that the event, for what we think about and act upon is the symbolic report and not the concrete event itself." In other words, objects emerge as events and an event cannot be dissociated from its (re)descriptions; insofar as they are new, hybridomas and monoclonal antibodies count as events.

In the case of hybridomas and monoclonal antibodies, their redescription as inventions was correlative with the development of a new set of practices that redefined the entire domain. These practices redefined, in turn, their object(s). Some transformations, such as the creation of new forms of interaction between industrial, clinical, and academic institutions, are obvious and/or have been largely commented upon (see Chapter 4). Others were more subtle. For instance, some commentators have noted that in certain domains patents became an important component of the literature that had to be regularly scanned by scientists and clinicians. This is evidenced by a survey of patents (the written expression of inventions) and scientific publications (the textual translation of discoveries) concerning clinically relevant monoclonal antibodies over a $2^{1}/_{2}$-year period that showed that the former amounted to about half of the latter (Koch and Bennedsen 1989/1990:389).[4]

Still, one could maintain that, by and large, patents and publications—inventions and discoveries—belong to distinct social worlds, that invention is the "contemporary counterpart [of discovery] in the domain of practical life" (Luttenberger 1992). From this point of view, the redescription of hybridomas as inventions has to be equated with their diffusion into the commercial field, where a different kind of scientist (industrial researchers) and a different kind of professional (lawyers) perform distinct technical and textual operations. This argument is routinely made by both scientists and social scientists. Consider, for instance, Milstein's (1993:11) claim that "lawyers and scientists do not speak the same language or use the same criteria," or Greg Myers's (1995) sophisticated textual analysis of the distinctiveness of the scientific and commercial arenas.[5]

However, we find this description inadequate on at least four counts. First, as previously noted, we are confronted with the simultaneous transformation of the various settings in which hybridoma technology is implemented, a transformation that could be (anachronistically) traced back to the last sentence of Köhler and Milstein 1975 *Nature* paper ("[Hybridomas] could be valuable for medical and industrial use"). Second, there is the obvious intermingling, rather than sheer opposition, of science and law in this process. Third, the creation and shifting of boundaries between the relevant social arenas (e.g., the field of commercial immunoassays as opposed to the basic study of antigen-antibody interactions) are the result of the ongoing process of redescription of hybridomas as inventions, as evidenced, for instance, in patent litigations.[6] Last but not least, as previously indicated, what was modified were not only practices concerning hybridomas—or, in other words, the context in which they evolved—but, we argue, the entities themselves.

While the trend whereby scientific research finds itself increasingly the object of legal dispute has been analyzed in terms of the possible impact of commercial practices on fundamental research (Panem 1984; Weiner 1986; Markle and Robin 1985),[7] patent litigations will provide here a window through which to observe the transformation of monoclonal antibodies into inventions. It is our claim that science and law were interactively involved in that process; in other words, instead of contrasting these two sets of practices as parallel or even denouncing them as outright opposites, we shall look at how legal and scientific discourses opened up a new field of action. Interestingly enough, one of the results of this redescription was to destabilize established routines, so that, for instance, science, which usually bears the marks of objectivity and certainty, came to be seen as uncertain and subject to interpretation when viewed in relation to the issue of invention.

Under present U.S. patent law, a number of conditions must be satisfied in order for a process or substance to be taken under the description of a patentable object (Cooper 1982; Greenlee 1982; Wegner 1982; Plant 1986). Four are central to the cases we discuss: a) non-obviousness, that is, the invention must not be obvious "for a person of ordinary skill in the art, guided by all the patents and printed publications to which he might look for guidance" (Cooper 1982:119; Wegner 1982:153–158); b) novelty, that is, the applicant must be the first inventor or, in legal terms, no "prior art" (prior invention of the same device or process) must be shown to exist; c) enablement, that is, the patent must disclose how to make and use the invention, again for "a person of ordinary skill in the art"; and d) distinct claiming, that is, the different claims described in a patent must have well-marked boundaries. Of particular interest to us is the presumption of non-obviousness that an applicant has to overcome in order to obtain a patent. In order to demonstrate novelty and non-obviousness, the (prospective) patent holder must demonstrate non-identity *and* discontinuity. The validity of a patent can be denied by showing continuity *or* identity, a process clearly reminiscent of the arguments discussed in Chapter 1.

Indeed, patent disputes over hybridoma technology provide excellent examples of the production of conflicting accounts of the dynamics of scientific research. During patent litigation, the research process itself is under scrutiny. This is so because one of the central questions of patent litigation is the determination of originality. In order to determine originality, it is necessary to investigate the process of scientific discovery (Brannigan 1981) to establish whether or not the proposed object of discovery is indeed novel and non-obvious. While the presence of discovery is a condition of possibility for the establishment of invention, the latter cannot be reduced to the former. In Chapter 1 we saw how the fact/technique distinction was constitutive of discovery accounts. In invention accounts, this dichotomy becomes a distinction between nature and (technical) culture. Do the advantages of a given discovery naturally flow from the entities that constitute the discovery or is human agency the decisive factor?

To understand why this translation is crucial, a possible misconception has to be corrected. Given the scientific and technical nature of the objects involved in patent disputes, one might suspect that contentions over novelty, non-obviousness, and criteria of identity would relate to (i.e., both resort to and concern) scientific and technical facts. It is less the facts of science, however, that are at issue in a patent dispute than the process of their production. In particular, the establishment of the singularity or novelty of a scientific/technical object presupposes the articulation of a discourse on the dynamics of scientific discovery and development.

Although representations of scientific activities (e.g., discovery accounts and disciplinary histories) can also be objectified and accepted as a canon, it is clear that there can be no undisputed representation of scientific activity *in the same way* that there is an undisputed representation of a scientific result such as, say, the double-helix structure of DNA (Woolgar 1976; Latour and Woolgar 1986; Latour 1987). This lack of agreement is, to a large extent, based on the fact that the objects of scientific discourse offer no internal evidence of their emergence. To put it another way, the facts of scientific discovery can be constructed as social, psychological, and historical facts and, as such, are open to the same interpretative strategies used in the corresponding social science disciplines or in their popular versions. The recourse to social, historical, psychological, and other criteria of identity is a recurrent strategy amongst, for instance, expert scientific witnesses in their attempt to establish the existence of, and hence priority over, a given entity.

Representations of continuity are predicated upon arguments about identity. Questions of identity engender not only arguments about what counts as the same but, also, about what belongs in the same category (van der Belt 1988; van der Belt and Rip 1987). Issues of identity give access to prior, taken-for-granted theories about the sociotechnical division of work. These theories, in turn, reshape the objects they entail. For instance, the content of categories such as fundamental research and industry, can be explored by showing how during a patent trial expert witnesses construct different distributions of the research and development continuum, relating technical statements and devices to social (sub)groups that then become criteria of identity for both human and nonhuman actors. Thus, several processes are simultaneously at work. One is the redescription of hybridomas and their products as techno-legal objects resulting from the intermingling of science and law. Another is the establishment of a novel identity predicated upon discontinuity. Yet another is the mobilization of a nature/culture or social/technical frame. The last two processes are interdependent. The first is dependent upon them.

The main body of the chapter will be devoted to a detailed analysis of the transcripts of scientific expert witnesses in the course of the already-mentioned Hybritech-Monoclonal Antibodies Inc. court proceedings. First, however, the main themes and categories relevant to the transformation of hybridomas into inventions will be introduced by analyzing several disputes that never made it to court because legal proceedings were not initiated (at least at the time of this writing), because an out-of-court settlement was reached, or because the patent, in spite of a protracted struggle, was never issued in the first place. This initial discussion will provide a background to the analysis that follows.

Milstein Versus Wistar

As pointed out in the previous section, one of the interesting characteristics of the 1981 "Science Meets Law" conference held at Cold Spring Harbor was that the separation between scientific and legal issues was not respected by the speakers. In other words, lawyers repeatedly asked scientists about the possible scientific basis of this or that legal distinction, while scientists integrated legal categories into their presentations. For instance, in their overview of monoclonal antibody technology, the scientists Donald J. Zack and Matthew D. Scharff (1982) speculated on the legal consequences of the biochemical and biophysical properties of the new kind of antibodies. Their discussion was informed in part by events that had already shaken the field, namely, two U.S. patents, granted to Philadelphia's Wistar Institute, covering hybridoma technology as applied to viral and tumor antigens, but also by a sense of what the next obvious domains of dispute would be given present patent law *and* state-of-the-art research.

In Chapter 1 we discussed the Koprowski affair, that is, the dispute between Milstein and the team lead by Hilary Koprowski at the Wistar Institute in Philadelphia concerning their respective role and contribution to hybridoma technology. That dispute broke out when in 1977 and 1978 the Wistar scientists filed two very broad patents covering a "[p]rocess for providing viral antibodies by fusing a viral antibody producing cell and a myeloma cell to provide a fused cell hybrid culture and collecting viral antibodies," and a "[m]ethod of producing tumor antibodies" (Koprowski, Gerhard, and Croce 1977b; Koprowski and Croce 1978). The patents were based on work executed using myelomas obtained from Milstein's laboratory, although apparently no agreement of any sort had been signed between Milstein and Koprowski when the cells were first transferred from Cambridge to Philadelphia (Koprowski and Croce 1980). Milstein, it will be recalled, had not filed a patent.[8] The two U.S. patents, issued in 1979 and in 1980, were severely criticized by Milstein and other scientists, who felt that the patents' subject matter was little more than the basic technique described in the 1975 *Nature* paper or, at best, an obvious application of it.[9]

The question of "obviousness in light of Milstein and Köhler's previous work" resurfaced in subsequent patent disputes and Patent and Trademark Office decisions. The interesting point, for now, is to note that in contrast to what many would see as the fundamental issue, that is, whether or not the Philadelphia researchers had appropriated what was in fact Köhler and Milstein's accomplishment, Zack and Scharff's remarks on the Wistar case at the 1981 Cold Spring Harbor conference focused on a more practical issue. Because the Wistar patent mentioned the use of a particular myeloma cell line, could somebody, simply by using another myeloma mutant, work around the patent? In other words, the question was redefined pragmatically as one of articulating concrete scientific practices and resources (for instance, the availability and use of different cell lines) with legal notions circumscribing the boundaries of innovation. Moreover, this process implied a discussion of which elements should be deemed constitutive of hybridoma technology in ways similar to those discussed in Chapter 1 (e.g., the Koprowski and Schwaber cases). Obviously, the process of ascribing the status of invention to hybridoma technology had reached an advanced stage: Scientific and legal resources were being used jointly to work out the details of that particular transformation. This strategy became even more apparent in relation to a second issue that led to an open patent dispute.

Ortho Versus Becton-Dickinson

Browsing through the proceedings of the 1981 Cold Spring Harbor conference, one finds questions such as the following, addressed by a Harvard molecular biologist, Mark Ptashne, to Matthew Scharff: "Can't you, for legal purposes, define a class of monoclonal antibodies or antibodies that will recognize, within a certain affinity range, a given antigen? Differences within that class become trivial. That is a legal question, but isn't that the obvious thing?" In addition, there is the following question, addressed by Johnson & Johnson's counsel, Geoffrey Dellenbaugh, to Scharff: "You said that you doubted that it would be possible to make—or if you wanted to get around it, you could make different monoclonal antibodies to the same antigen. How would you distinguish those from each other?" (Plant et al. 1982:26, 24).

In their presentation, Zack and Scharff had indeed noted that "the chances of any two investigators making a hybridoma which is producing exactly the same antibody molecule is very small." In other words, two monoclonal antibodies would differ by one or more of several variables, namely, electrophoretic mobility, specificity, biological activity, affinity for antigen, and amino acid sequence. Thus, "if novelty is the crucial criteria [sic] and it is to be defined by chemical structure," most monoclonal antibodies could be considered novel. Ptashne and Dellenbaugh framed the same question differently and raised the question of *equivalence* by asking whether a patent issued for a monoclonal antibody directed against a specific antigen would cover all monoclonal antibodies that could be raised against the same antigen in the future. *Functional equivalence* expressed in terms of a given reactivity range, rather than structural chemical considerations, would define the identity of a given monoclonal antibody or set of monoclonal antibodies (see also Greenlee 1982:131 and Wegner 1982:157).

Dellenbaugh no doubt had in mind a set of patents for specific monoclonal antibodies and hybrid cell lines producing them that were filed in 1979 and 1980, and issued in 1981 to his company.[10] Ortho's monoclonals, known as the OKT series, were directed against different types of T cells and were involved in the construction of new classes of immunological entities of widespread laboratory and clinical significance, known as lymphocyte subsets.[11] In September 1984 Ortho filed a patent infringement suit against Becton-Dickinson.[12] The latter had been selling diagnostic (research) kits containing monoclonal antibodies directed against the "same"[13] type of T cell as the OKT monoclonal antibodies. Becton-Dickinson's monoclonal antibodies had been developed independently from Ortho's by researchers at Stanford University, the Sloan-Kettering Cancer Research Institute, and the University of Alabama.

Becton-Dickinson responded by filing antitrust counterclaims asserting "fraud in procurement" and/or "pushing patents ... that ... are ... invalid or not infringed" (*BioEngineering News* 1985a). The Ortho suit raised the following issue. While lawyers and scientists agreed that a conventional pharmaceutical compound could be accurately described by giving its chemical structure, there was disagreement about whether this was possible with an antibody, given its size, complexity, mode of production, and mode of action. The established solution to this problem that concerned biological material in general was to deposit the hybridomas producing the antibody in a recognized culture collection.[14] While this would take care of the description issue, however, it did not address the question of novelty, which involved the discrimination of the patented antibody from other (similar) antibodies.

A "mere" technical solution to this issue[15] was of course not available, because the problem was not the lack of identity criteria but the choice between those criteria. To choose meant to settle upon an identity that was simultaneously specific enough not to dissolve the claim and broad enough to cover "equivalent" antibodies that had been or could be produced by competitors. How then was an antibody identity to be established? When should one antibody be perceived as the same as or equivalent to another when considering patent infringement?

Ortho's approach, obviously, was to identify monoclonal antibodies according to functional criteria. Ortho's attorney later argued the case against Becton-Dickinson by citing the early antibiotics industry, an analogy that has been invoked by other writers (Dellenbaugh, personal communication, January 1986; Woodruff and Miller 1981). There, substances isolated from living organisms and shown to produce a chemically unknown substance that killed microorganisms had been patented by describing their characteristics (that is, their reactivity with a panel of microorganisms, their infrared spectrum, etc.). A given antibiotic could be construed, however, *in principle* (i.e., even if its structure was for the moment unknown), as a chemically well-defined substance. With monoclonal antibodies, according to Zack and Scharff's argument, the chances were infinitely small that someone—even using the same myelomas and fusion technique—would end up with structurally identical antibodies. Furthermore, it was not clear that monoclonal antibodies could be considered functionally equivalent if, in reacting against the same antigen, they reacted with different sites on the antigen or exhibited a different binding strength to the antigen.

The Ortho–Becton-Dickinson case was settled out of court, thus leaving these issues unresolved and, more importantly for the present purpose, depriving us of what would most certainly have been a fascinating continuation of the exchanges between lawyers and scientists that took place in 1981 at Cold Spring Harbor.[16] One important conclusion can nonetheless be drawn for the Ortho–Becton-Dickinson case. In that dispute the debate focused on the issue of equivalence, as opposed to, for instance, the question of whether the production of the OKT series would have been an obvious application of the Milstein and Köhler technique to just another antigen. In other words, one could have argued that, because hybridoma technology had become a well-known technique, the idea of applying it to all sorts of microorganisms and cells required no further inventive step. Indeed, at the 1981 Cold Spring Harbor meeting, the following exchange took place between James Watson and a German patent expert:

> *Watson:* I am confused by *obviousness*. By your definition, I somehow believe that if we made a monoclonal antibody against insulin, you would say that that is not obvious, and therefore we could get a patent on it. But I would think that is the most obvious thing in the world. It requires no new knowledge. Virtually anyone can do it. . . .
> *Vossius:* Posing the problem may be obvious, but then finding the solution may not be obvious.
> *Watson:* What is obvious? I mean, a rather stupid technician working for 6 months . . . (Plant et al. 1982:188).[17]

As will become evident through comparison with the cases discussed in the next section, the decisive element in the Ortho–Becton-Dickinson case was that the OKT antibodies were deemed to have revealed the existence of previously unknown antigens (see also Nenning and Bourcevet 1990:855; McGough and Burke 1990) and thus to be instrumental in the development of a new field of inquiry. They derived their undisputed innovative character from their antigenic target or, more broadly, from their association with lymphocyte subset research. From this point of view, what seems to matter is not hybridoma technology or monoclonal antibodies per se but, rather, the experimental system. Here monoclonal antibodies are part of a larger collection that includes not only the antibody but also the antigen and other items that account for the biomedical relevance of that antigen.[18]

Ex Parte Old and *Ex Parte Erlich*: Yes, No, Maybe

In 1981 Cetus applied for a patent on monoclonal antibodies against a species of human interferon. The application was rejected by the Patent Examiner and the decision upheld in 1986 by the PTO Board of Patent Appeals and Interferences (*Ex parte Erlich*; McGough and Burke 1992). The examiner had argued that the alleged invention described in the patent was obvious both because the method used to produce monoclonal antibodies was a "step by step" application of the process developed by Köhler and Milstein and because the antigen to which this process was applied—human fibroblast interferon—was a "known antigen of unquestioned research interest as antiviral or antitumor agent." In other words, according to the Patent Examiner, Cetus had taken a well-known technique and applied it straightforwardly to a well-known target in order to obtain predictable results.

Nonetheless, in appealing this decision, Cetus had grounds for optimism; other patents had been issued for specific monoclonals, and, more particularly, a 1985 decision of the PTO Board of Appeals had reversed a judgment rejecting a patent on monoclonal antibodies directed against malignant human renal cells (*Ex parte Old*). *Ex parte Old* was, at first sight, strikingly similar to the Cetus case. The Examiner in Chief, in a dissenting opinion, had indeed argued that

> The application of admittedly known standard techniques to admittedly known renal cancer cell lines to produce expected hybridomas which produce expected monoclonal antibodies to recognize antigens or epitopes, while laudatory, does not give rise to a patentable invention. . . . Although one may not anticipate with specificity just which antigens will be recognized, it is clear to one of ordinary skill in the art from the relevant teachings that antigenic material will be recognized.
>
> (Ibid.:200).

But the majority of the board had rejected this reasoning on the basis of the unpredictability argument:

> Although the technique underlying hybridoma technology is well recognized, nevertheless, the results obtained by its use clearly are unpredictable. Hybridoma technology is an empirical art in which the routineer is unable to foresee what particular antibodies will be produced and which specific surface antigens will be recognized by them. Only by actually carrying out the requisite steps can the nature of the monoclonal antibodies be determined and ascertained; no "expected" results can thus be said to be present. Hence, it may be "obvious to try" the Kohler [sic]-Milstein technique as applied to malignant cells, but such is not the standard under which obviousness under [patent law] must be established. (Ibid.).

The 1985 decision shifted the burden of novelty from human agency to the unpredictable workings of nature and thus seemed to open the way for the patentability of every monoclonal one could produce (an argument referred to, in legalese, as the "inventive uniqueness of each type of monoclonal antibody"). In what could be perceived as a reversal of the decision, however, the PTO Board of Appeals in the Cetus case upheld the rejection on grounds of obviousness. The board specifically addressed the unpredictability issue, arguing that while the production of anti-interferon monoclonal antibodies might have involved "tedious and laborious" screening steps, the "level of skill in this art had developed sufficiently since the publication in 1975 of the work of Kohler [sic] and Milstein that one having all the applied references before him at the time the invention was made would have proceeded to produce monoclonal antibodies specific for human fibroblast interferon *with a reasonable expectation of success*" (*Ex parte Erlich*:1016, our emphasis). "Reasonable expectation of success" was used to counter the unpredictability argument, because "obviousness under [patent law] does not require absolute predictability" (ibid.). Arguing further that "each case is determined on its own merit," the board stated that both its previous 1985 decision and the fact that several patents had been granted for monoclonals were irrelevant for the present case.

Cetus refiled its application in 1987 and, following another rejection by the Patent Examiner, once again submitted its case to the PTO Board of Appeals. This time, Cetus had an additional reason to be optimistic. In 1986 a Federal Court of Appeals had upheld the validity of Hybritech's patent on the use of monoclonal antibodies in a sandwich immunoassay, allegedly recognizing the "empirical nature" of hybridoma technology (see the following for a detailed discussion of the Hybritech patent). The 1992 Board of Appeals decision was once again negative, however, for basically the same reasons advanced in the 1986 decision. The "each-case-must-be-determined-on-its-own-merit" argument was again used to dismiss the relevance of the 1985 decision concerning antibodies against malignant human renal cells and the continued issuance of patents directed to hybridomas and monoclonal antibodies. The Hybritech decision was also found to be of no relevance because it did not concern monoclonal antibodies per se, all the more so given that even when monoclonal antibodies were mentioned, the court recognized that their production was "admittedly old after Kohler [sic] and Milstein showed how to produce them."

More importantly for our present purpose is the fact that Cetus's argument, according to which the production of monoclonal antibodies to a given antigen at the time of the invention was empirical in nature and thus unpredictable, was found faulty. The board decided that because the antigenicity of human fibroblast interferon and its potential therapeutic value were well known, as was "classical hybridoma technology," there was a "reasonable expectation of success" that made the entire enterprise obvious by providing "ample motivation." In explaining its decision, the Board of Appeals relied on a list of publications that included the 1977 Galfré et al. *Nature* paper co-authored by Milstein and several 1977 and 1978 articles by the Koprowski team (see Chapter 1). In addition, the board cited a 1988 Court of Appeals decision concerning anti-HBsAg monoclonal antibodies (*In re Wands*).[19] The appeal concerned a patent rejected on the grounds that the application of its teachings required "undue experimentation." After four unsuccessful fusions, the applicant had succeeded in producing 143 high-binding hybridomas. Only nine of the successful hybridomas had been submitted to further testing, and four had proven to fall within the claims of the patent. In rejecting the patent, the examiners had argued that this showed the unpredictability and unreliability of the applicant's method: Only four (2.8%) of 143 hybridomas could be described as a certified success.

The Court of Appeals disagreed. It began by raising the success rate to 44.4% (four hybridomas out of nine, there being grounds to believe that several untested hybridomas would also have fallen within the claims) and went on to declare that "an 'experiment' is not simply the screening of a single hybridoma, but is rather the entire attempt to make a monoclonal antibody against a particular antigen" (ibid.:1407). In other words, hybridoma technology was a well-known technique at the time of the application; its routine use against a given antigen led to the production of several hybridomas, not all of which could be expected to be positive; the screening of hybridomas to determine which one produced the desired antibody was part of hybridoma technology; thus, no "undue experimentation" was required nor could the results be called "unpredictable." Ironically, predictability (or, more precisely, lack of unpredictability) was used in the HBsAg case to argue for the validity of the patent and for the opposite purpose in the Cetus case. After these repeated rejections, Cetus abandoned its patent application.

Several comments are here in order. First of all, the patent cases make a clear case for symmetry. As we have seen, social scientists (e.g., Weiner 1986) as well as scientists (Milstein 1993; Ekins 1989) looked at the patenting trend with suspicion, pointing to the gap between, or even to the mutually exclusive character of, science and law. While not denying that differences can be established, we would argue that the PTO Board of Appeals opinion in the Cetus case could have been underwritten by several of those same scientists who are critical of the way the patent system is administered. Not only was the case for obviousness based on the same research and review articles scientists cited,[20] but the examiners also used the rhetoric that can be found in the review articles examined in Chapter 3.

For instance, they spoke of the "veritable explosion of research applying [Köhler and Milstein's] method to obtain monoclonal antibodies specific to a wide variety and number of antigens," that followed the publication of the 1975 *Nature* paper (*Ex parte Erlich*:1013). On the other hand, the 1985 decision that supported the "inventive uniqueness" of every monoclonal antibody could be cited as a *prima facie* example of the opposite trend, whereby purely semantic distinctions of no scientific import were used by lawyers to impose decisions that ran against scientific common sense on scientifically illiterate judges or patent examiners.

In this respect, apparently contradictory decisions taken by the PTO Board of Appeals in the matter of inventive uniqueness of monoclonal antibodies mirror the division expressed in scientific circles. Not only are scientific witnesses of recognized stature available to both sides of the dispute, but several scientists obviously regard the inventive uniqueness of monoclonal antibodies as a sound principle. In other words, legal decisions reflect scientific attitudes towards the properties and characteristics of monoclonal antibodies. Moreover, the two PTO decisions are not necessarily contradictory, not only from a legal point of view,[21] but also from what we could call a native epistemic viewpoint.

If, as we have argued, what counts in the scientists' eyes are not monoclonal antibodies or hybridomas as such but, rather, the experimental system of which they are part, then a strong case can be made for a different treatment of, say, monoclonal antibodies directed against a chemically well-defined molecule, such as interferon, and monoclonal antibodies recognizing elusive tumor markers. The refusal of the legal system to operate a social synthesis, to provide, in other words, an overview of what should count as obvious at a given time, can thus be linked to a similar lack of transcendence in scientific practice, as evidenced, for instance, by the lack of epistemic unity among different specialties, research fronts, and so on.

The Cetus case also illustrates the role of the nature/culture distinction, as exemplified by the use of the unpredictability argument in the translation of monoclonal antibodies into inventions. The fact that this theme can be used to argue for or against the granting of a patent need not trouble us here. It is the presence of the theme, rather than its use, that is of interest in the present case. In the next section, we shall have ample opportunity to discuss it.

Finally, the answer to the practical question of whether, in the light of the cases discussed so far, monoclonal antibodies per se are patentable, is multiple: yes, no, maybe. A resounding yes follows from the 1985 "inventive uniqueness" decision. A qualified no follows from the Cetus case. A cautious maybe follows not only from the fact that monoclonal antibodies continue to be patented, but also from the fact that monoclonal antibodies resulting from some "improvement" to the basic technique or monoclonal antibodies that target previously unknown antigens overcome the limits set by the Cetus decision (Nenning and Bourcevet 1990:855; McGough and Burke 1992:1083). This range of answers is indicative of the ongoing redefinition of monoclonal antibodies as inventions, a process we now analyze in detail by using the transcripts of the Hybritech-Monoclonal Antibodies Inc. dispute.

Hybritech Versus Monoclonal Antibodies Inc.

In the Wistar case, hybridoma technology as a technique was at stake. In the Ortho–Becton-Dickinson and Cetus cases, the relevant issue was the monoclonal antibodies per se. In all these cases the hybridoma field was directly concerned. At first sight, and as noted by the PTO Board in the 1992 Cetus decision, this was not the case in the Hybritech-Monoclonal Antibodies Inc. dispute, because the immediate object of litigation was an immunoassay technique that predated the development of hybridomas.

Because the use of monoclonal antibodies was instrumental in the technique as patented by Hybritech, however, not to speak of the fact that the litigants were two young biotech companies created for the express purpose of commercially exploiting hybridoma technology, the Hybritech-Monoclonal Antibodies Inc. dispute was largely seen as relevant to the hybridoma field. Indeed, it was the first test case out of which some of the uncertainties surrounding patents in that field were to be resolved. In the words of a biomedical scientist (Ekins 1989:258): "[T]he reality of the present situation is that, by successfully patenting the use of antibodies produced by Milstein and Köhler's technique, commercial companies have succeeded in implicitly patenting the invention itself." It should be added that the trial transcripts of the Hybritech–Monoclonal Antibodies Inc. dispute do indeed contain long passages devoted to the definition of the characteristics, properties, and status of monoclonal antibodies.

Although the first sales arising from the hybridoma technique involved monoclonal antibodies alone, the second and far more significant phase of commercialization came from the inclusion of monoclonal antibodies in diagnostic kits. Hybritech was one of the first companies created to exploit this market.[22] In 1980 Hybritech filed a patent describing a method of using monoclonal antibodies in a diagnostic kit. The patent, issued in 1983, was supposed to protect all present and future kits marketed by Hybritech under the trademark TANDEM, which in 1981 had become the first monoclonal product to receive clearance from the Food and Drug Administration (FDA). It described the use of a technique known as a "sandwich immunoassay"[23] in which two antibodies were used to detect the presence of a given antigen in body fluids. While the sandwich technique had been earlier developed and marketed with antibodies produced by traditional methods, Hybritech's patent provided for the use of monoclonal antibodies.

The fun began in March 1984, when Hybritech sued Monoclonal Antibodies Inc., alleging that the latter's pregnancy tests infringed the Hybritech patent. In August 1985, the U.S. District Court in San Francisco declared Hybritech's patent invalid on five independent grounds, including that "the patent teaches nothing new in art" and that the "art alleged to be taught was obvious and logical to anyone skilled in the field."[24] After this initial judgment, Hybritech—now in a difficult financial position—was taken over by the multinational firm Eli Lilly, who decided to appeal.

In the appeal hearing of September 1986, the judgment was reversed.[25] On a final appeal in November 1986 the reversal was upheld. Hybritech's position was endorsed by the refusal of the U.S. Supreme Court in April 1987 to hear any further appeal on the validity of the patent (107 S. Ct. 1606; *Biotechnology News* 1987a,b). Hybritech lost no time in filing suit against Abbott (apparently the first company to commercialize the sandwich assay, albeit without monoclonal antibodies).[26] Abbott and Hybritech subsequently settled out of court (Ezzel 1989).

Several university-based and industrial scientists acted as expert witnesses during the Hybritech–Monoclonal Antibodies Inc. trial. Their testimony is recorded verbatim in the trial transcripts. In addition to the transcripts, we have examined the judges' opinions in this case.[27] What follows brings to the fore the transformation of monoclonal antibodies into techno-legal objects. It does so through a detailed exploration of the themes and categories invoked by scientists and lawyers during the proceedings. Our analysis begins with a discussion of the establishment of identity in the somewhat esoteric topic of immunoassay systems. While immunoassay systems are not necessarily related to hybridoma technology (although, as we shall see, whether or not this was the case, and to what extent, became a controversial issue), this topic sets the stage for the subsequent analysis of exchanges directly concerned with monoclonal antibodies.

Establishing Identities: Is IRMA a RIA?

Among the central issues raised during the trial was the question of the identity or difference between two types of immunoassays, so-called (competitive) radioimmunoassays (RIA) and immunoradiometric assays (IRMA). Monoclonal Antibodies Inc.'s lawyers, in order to establish the existence of "prior art" and thus to invalidate Hybritech's patent because of lack of novelty, claimed that two immunologists from Stanford University, Dr. Herzenberg (a figure familiar to readers of Chapter 3) and his student Dr. Vernon Oi, had carried out sandwich assays using monoclonal antibodies before Hybritech. The latter replied by claiming that Herzenberg and Oi's experiments involved competitive RIA, and not IRMA, and that only IRMA qualified as sandwich assays.

To understand the issues involved, some technical background is necessary. It should be pointed out, however, that during the trial several different versions of what constitutes a sandwich assay were presented. What follows should be conceived of as an arbitrary point of entry into the debate and not an attempt to establish *a priori* definitions of the contested entities around which the trial was constructed.

Generally speaking, an immunoassay is a method of using antibodies to detect antigens, that is, substances of clinical interest, such as bacteria, viruses, and hormones (see Chapter 4). Once produced, the antibody is mixed with a patient's specimen. If the antigen is present, it forms a complex with the antibody. A variety of methods (including fluorescent, radioactive, or enzymatic labels) are used to determine whether or not the reaction has taken place and therefore whether or not the antigen is present in the patient specimen (and thus, for example, whether or not a woman is pregnant).

In recent years, there has been increasing use of solid phase immunoassays. Here, an antibody (or an antigen) is attached to a solid surface, such as the side of a plastic test tube or a small plastic bead. At this point there are several ways of making an immunoassay. We offer two. In the first case, the solid phase is coated with an antibody. A radioactively labeled antigen similar to the antigen suspected to be present in the patient specimen is mixed with the specimen and the mixture is added to the solid phase. If no antigen is present in the patient specimen, then only radioactively labeled antigen will bind with the antibody; if, however, the patient specimen contains the antigen, both kinds of antigen compete for the antibody and the measured amount of radioactive antigen-antibody complex is less. This is called a *competitive RIA*.

In the second case, the solid phase is coated with a first antibody. The specimen is added to the solid phase and, if antigen is present, it will bind to the solid phase through the antibody. A second, radioactively labeled antibody is then added, which binds to the antigen bound to the first antibody, creating a sandwich where the bread is the antibody and the filling the antigen. This is called an *IRMA*. Further distinctions can be drawn between forward IRMA (as described earlier); reverse IRMA, where labeled antibody and specimen are first mixed and then poured into the test tube; and simultaneous IRMA, where all ingredients are mixed simultaneously. Figure 5.1, used as an illustration in both the District Court and the Court of Appeal opinion, represents the sandwich assay.

Further complications ensue when the antibody is used as an antigen. One can,

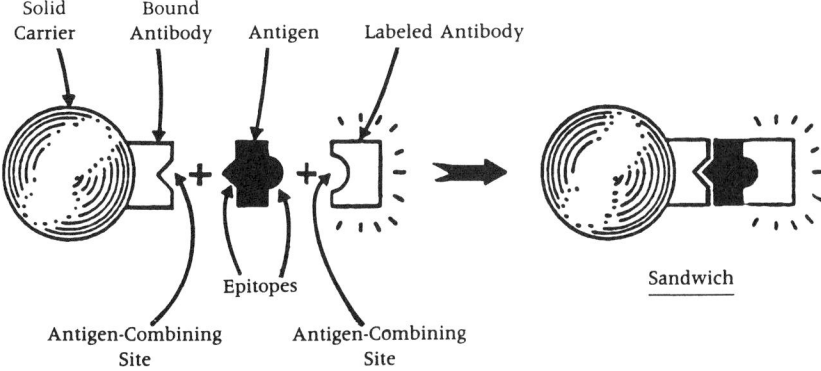

Figure 5.1. Schematic representation of a sandwich assay. (Source: 623 F. Supp. 1344, D.C. Cal. 1985, and 802 F.2d 1367, Fed. Cir. 1986.)

for example, attach an antigen to the solid phase, allow it to react with a first antibody, and then detect the complex using a second, labeled antibody that reacts with the first antibody now construed as an antigen. While a number of distinctions can be made, whether or not they are deemed significant, or even held to exist, is a matter of debate. For instance, in the present litigation it was maintained by Hybritech that IRMA and RIA were distinct kinds of immunoassay, whereas Monoclonal Antibodies Inc. reduced the difference to insignificance.

This distinction and the ambiguities surrounding it are not a lawyers' invention. Both the distinction and its problems of application are extent in scientific practice. For example, according to a recent textbook (Ekins 1981:6), one should distinguish between two types of immunoassays: Type I (i.e., IRMA) "is based on the use of an *excess* (usually large) of antibody over analyte [antigen]," Type II (i.e., RIA) "rel[ies] on the use of an amount of antibody *less than* the amount of analyte in the system." Accordingly, Type I relies upon labelling of the antibody and is thus also called a *labelled antibody* assay; Type II relies upon labelling the analyte and is called a *labelled analyte* or *labelled antigen* assay (Ekins 1981:11). The text goes on to affirm the existence of a major difference between the two assays despite procedural similarities:

> These two forms of assay inevitably share many methodological features: nevertheless the fundamental difference in the concepts on which they rely manifest itself, *inter alia*, in the manner in which assays of each type should be "designed", and in their relative sensitivity and specificity characteristics. This difference arises essentially from the differing impact of the Law of Mass Action on systems of each type.
> (Ekins 1981:7).[28]

Having stressed the difference, however, the author is forced to acknowledge the lack of consensus in practice: "Unfortunately, the clarity and logical advantages of such a nomenclature have not prevailed, and terms such as "RIA," for example, are often applied indiscriminately to techniques falling into both Type I and Type II categories" (Ekins 1981:11).

In the Hybritech-Monoclonal Antibodies Inc. litigation, arguments raised against the distinction between RIA and IRMA were offered by Dr. Herzenberg, who acted as a Monoclonal Antibodies Inc. witness:

> I don't make a big distinction in my mind, between an assay where one adds reactant "A" before "B" or "B" before "A." I call them all radioimmunoassay—IRMA's, sandwich assays. All the names people have tried to give product identification to what they are doing—for instance, soap. All soaps are practically the same—deterginents [sic]. Enormous amounts of money are spent advertising the differences between one brand and another. They are all basically the same. (11.1333).[29] ... Just reverse the order of the reactants without making much of a fuss about it. (11.1373–1374).

Dr. Herzenberg not only denied the utility of drawing the distinction; he also accounted for its origin by equating it with attempts to turn existing immunoassay techniques into private or personal property: "I don't think—I don't appreciate the—these artificial distinctions which are made between one kind of radioimmunoassay and another in terms of saying this one is mine and that one is—you know, is yours" (11.1336).

Those interested in such an undertaking were described by Dr. Herzenberg as "the people in the specific sub, sub-field, which they have self-designated as commercial radioimmunoassays." The project of this peculiar technosocial world is " . . . to distinguish between one kind of sandwich and another. They call the IRMA type sandwich antibody, antigen, antibody as the sandwich. Anything else they call two step radioimmunoassay" (11.1376–1377).

By designating commercial radioimmunoassays as the name of a "specific sub, sub-field," Dr. Herzenberg not only managed to reduce a number of supposedly universal technical distinctions to the opinion of particular social groups, he also proposed a representation of the R&D continuum that combined technical and social entities. The world of commercial radioimmunoassays, in this view, was an intermediary between the worlds of pure science and corporations. Another intermediary unit, clinical chemists, was evoked by Ms. Blakemore, another Monoclonal Antibodies Inc. witness.

From the vantage point of pure science—which claims universality—the distinction between IRMA and RIA was merely the expression of a will to distinguish. When asked to give an acontextual definition of a sandwich assay, Dr. Herzenberg responded by contextualizing the definition of definition:

> Q. What is your definition of a sandwich assay?
> A. Do you mean how I would define a sandwich assay to someone who just wanted to know how you would carry out an assay involving two antibodies and an antigen? Or do you want me to use the definitions—as I say, that has become current among the people who want to distinguish from one kind of radioimmunoassay from another and, you know, have made a sub-categorization of sandwich. Which one would you like? (11.1376–1377).

From the preceding we see that the witness for the defendant was able to trivialize the distinction between IRMA and RIA by pushing those who invoked the distinction to the margins of science. The court setting, however, allowed for the same procedure to be turned against Dr. Herzenberg. As can be seen from the following exchange, Hybritech's lawyer was able to redefine the relevant domain of expertise so as to exclude Dr. Herzenberg:

> *Q.* Doctor, isn't it true that you consider yourself to be a leader in the field of immunology?

A. I hate to think I am so immodest, but I think people told me I am. Yes, I think I am a good immunologist.
Q. But you are not an expert in the field of developing commercially useful immunoassays; is that correct?
A. Well, there are some commercially very useful immunoassays which I have had a lot to do developing. There are others I haven't.
Q. You are not a leader in the field of immunoassays; isn't that right?
A. Of the kind of immunoassays that I believe you would consider in that particular field, I am not . . . (11.1405–1406).

Underlying this discussion is the interpretation of the category of non-obviousness. It is apparent from the opinions of the District Court and of the Federal Court of Appeal that non-obviousness is not to be measured in absolute terms but in relation to a given sociohistorical situation. To the question, non-obvious for whom?, the law answers "for any person of ordinary skill in the art." The latter stipulation is, of course, open to interpretation (Greenlee 1982:128). In this case, *person* was translated into social world; for instance, the social world of pure science or the social world of developers of commercial immunoassays. The District Court found that Hybritech's alleged invention was obvious "to those in the scientific and commercial world." The Court of Appeal found that the reasoning in this instance called on distinctions advanced by experts from yet other social worlds, including representatives of what the presiding judge termed the *real world*, that is, market forces and end-users. Accordingly, commercial success, which for the District Court was merely the icing of the cake, ranked for the Court of Appeal among the deciding criteria of non-obviousness.

The vision of Monoclonal Antibodies Inc.'s witness as a theoretical, if not esoteric, immunologist, and not a *bona fide* member of the community of commercial radioimmunoassay developers, was further reinforced by Hybritech's senior scientist's analysis of Oi and Herzenberg's work. In addition to claiming repeatedly that Oi and Herzenberg had performed a competitive RIA rather than an IRMA, Dr. David offered a gloss of their work that shifted it far beyond the realm of clinical or commercial reality:

Q. Do you read page 1012 [of a paper by Drs. Herzenberg and Oi] here as describing a sandwich assay with monoclonal antibodies?
A. I don't read it as describing a sandwich immunometric assay.
Q. What do you read it was? What kind of an *assay* is it?
A. It is an *experiment* in which they were developing an understanding of the *nature* of the antigen rather than the *existence* or *quantity* of the antigen.
Q. They say that the second column here describes a sandwich assay with monoclonal antibodies.
A. I think the difference of opinion lies in the interpretation of the word "assay." In their case, they are *observing the nature of an antigen*. They call that an assay. In

Between Nature and Culture 187

our case we are *determining the presence of an antigen*. And we call this an assay. It is a different type—it is a completely different kind of assay. (14.1862; our emphasis).

Upholding the distinction between nature and presence was an opposition between academic and commercial science, as evoked by the opposition between *experiment* and *assay* as well as the opposition between *observing* and *determining*. Science and *industry* appeared, in other words, not as *a priori* entities on which sociologists might ground their explanation but as the result of contingent constructs or rhetorical resources within an agonistic field (Latour and Woolgar 1986:237). Again, the lawyer's counterstrategy was to deny the context and to cling to universal definitions,[30] such as those contained in a dictionary:

Q. [To Dr. David] Do you also say that it is not an assay what Oi-Herzenberg did?
A. I say my definition of an assay and the definition on the context of the assay as described in the patent is [sic] a different definition.
Q. What does your definition of an assay come from?
A. An assay, like many other words, can have multiple meanings. . . . An assay, *as we use it in the context of the TANDEM assay*, is an assay to determine presence or concentration of something, not the nature of something.
Q. Do you define assay in the patent?
A. I think it is implicit in the context of the patent. . .
Q. [The lawyer hands to the witness Webster's dictionary] Read definitions two and three [of the word assay], please?
A. No. 2 is "examination and determination as to characteristics, as weigh, measure, or quality." Number 3 is "analysis as of an ore or drug to determine the presence, absence, or quantity of one or more components."
Q. Under that dictionary definition, doesn't Oi-Herzenberg fit the term "assay," sir, either one of those?
A. I would say it fits examination and determination as to characteristics. . . . For the record, I would say, to complete the answer to the last subject, the assay as it is used in the patent fits no. 3 in Webster's definition. (14.1908–1911; our emphasis).

In response to Monoclonal Antibodies Inc.'s attempt to establish an identity between RIA and sandwich assays, Hybritech's witnesses (in the following quote, Mr. Greene) managed to dissolve the logical identity into a historical discontinuity:

Q. By the way, RIA does include sandwich assays, does it not?
A. I don't think of it as including sandwich assay, no.
Q. Don't many immunologists use that term for a sandwich assay?
A. I think some people do use the term RIA to cover both labelled antigen and labelled antibody. *We developed, over a period of time, the practice that they were distinctive enough procedures that we should use these two different terms*. And I

suspect many immunologists today would make the distinction.... I didn't really understand the significance of the difference, I don't think very clearly, until I really started getting involved in depth at Hybritech. (1.73–75; our emphasis).

Dr. Gary David, one of the co-inventors on the Hybritech patent and the company's senior scientist, made similar comments when confronted by Monoclonal Antibodies Inc.'s lawyer with an excerpt from the minutes of a Hybritech meeting where the term *RIA kit* was used to designate what the Hybritech people claimed were early discussions of their future TANDEM concept. This time it was Monoclonal Antibodies Inc.'s lawyer's turn to stress the difference between competitive RIA and IRMA, with the witness claiming that "... many individuals in that time frame used the term incorrectly. And I may well have been and was in fact one of those individuals. I did not distinguish between RIA and IRMA." (5.406).

A second strategy adopted by Monoclonal Antibodies Inc. was to deny the novelty of Hybritech's patent by abandoning the identity of IRMA and RIA, and focusing instead on the assay system as a whole in order to establish a continuity between polyclonal and monoclonal kits. For example, Ms. Blakemore, an industrial scientist acting as a Monoclonal Antibodies Inc. expert witness, stated that the use of monoclonal or polyclonal antibodies within the same assay system did not make any real difference because the real inventive step was the system. Blackmore's position is reminiscent of the contrast drawn in Chapter 4 between RI's Dr. Smith and Bio-Bucks's Dr. K. with respect to the role and centrality of monoclonal antibodies in the production of a diagnostic kit.

To sum up, Monoclonal Antibodies Inc.'s lawyer followed two routes in an attempt to establish prior art: a) because RIA = IRMA and a RIA with monoclonal antibodies had already been produced by Drs. Herzenberg and Oi, Hybritech's patent was invalid; b) because the invention of IRMA (as opposed to RIA) was what really mattered and because IRMA had already been developed, albeit with polyclonal antibodies, the patent was, again, invalid.

Hybritech's lawyer's reply to route a) was to attempt to have Dr. Herzenberg acknowledge the existence of meaningful differences between the two types of assay. To do so he brought forward a set of technical statements, which, inevitably, lent themselves to historical and social interpretation. For instance, he asked whether, *as of 1977*, competitive RIA could be run in one step whereas IRMA had to be run in two steps, and whether, *as of 1977*, there were any *commercial* IRMAs on the market that were designed to run in one step. While agreeing with the existence of some of these differences, Dr. Herzenberg still claimed: "It is exactly the same. Since antibody and antigen are complementary molecules, to me it is not a *philosophical, logical* difference." (11.1379–1380, our emphasis).

The questions posed by Hybritech's lawyer formed the basis for distinguishing the two types of assay. They advanced the notion, subsequently ratified by the Court of Appeal, that lack of prior art, and thus "novelty," were to be judged from a historical perspective, without indulging in anachronism. Dr. Herzenberg here opposed them by clinging to supposedly universal criteria, allowing him to construe IRMA as the same as RIA.[31] This involved decomposing the diagnostic kit into its constitutive elements (namely, antibodies), which could be represented as "natural objects" and thus as ahistorical entities. This move was resisted by the Court of Appeal, which stated that the invention referred to the diagnostic kit as a package, not to its individual components. Hybritech's reply to route b) was necessarily a response to the accusation of substitution.

Mere Substitution or Inventive Step?

According to Monoclonal Antibodies Inc.'s lawyers, Hybritech's "innovation" was mere substitution. It was claimed that Hybritech had simply taken a sandwich assay kit developed by an industry leader, Abbott, and substituted their monoclonal antibodies for Abbott's polyclonal antibodies. Had this proven an accurate description of Hybritech's research program, the Hybritech patent might have been dismissed on the grounds of "obviousness" or lack of an inventive step.

While Hybritech did not deny using their monoclonal antibodies in conjunction with Abbott's assay system, they did deny that this constituted substitution or that it was an obvious maneuver. It was first of all argued that by using their monoclonal antibodies in Abbott's kit, they weren't really using Abbott's kit because the latter was by nature a polyclonal kit. In other words, the moment the polyclonals were removed from Abbott's kit, the latter ceased to exist. As Dr. David explained:

> *Q.* What you did is you substituted your monoclonal for their polyclonal and ran their test, isn't that what you did?
> *A.* I don't think so. Their test was polyclonal. (6.555).

Saying that using the kit without the polyclonals meant that the kit per se had not been used, however, led back to the problem of substitution. As Monoclonal Antibodies Inc.'s lawyer, pursuing the previous line of questioning pointed out:

> *Q.* . . . Let's put it in this way: You ran the test with their antibody, their polyclonal, and then you ran it again using your monoclonal instead, isn't that true?
> *A.* We ran the kit according to their instructions with our antibodies, yes.

> Q. So the first time you ever did this you substituted a monoclonal for the polyclonal; isn't that right? (6.555).

But, again, Hybritech's witness remained unmoved:

> A. I don't think it was a direct substitution. (6.555).

The difference between a direct substitution and what Hybritech claimed to have done (i.e., an "indirect substitution," or one that appeared obvious only in retrospect) was expressed as a problem of intention. First, it was announced in terms of the psychological difference between knowing that one was making a substitution and thinking that one was making an improvement or inventive step. Thus, in response to the question:

> Q. So your main concern at that time was to figure out a configuration where your monoclonals could be substituted for the polyclonals in immunoassays that were then on the market, among other things; correct? (1.76–77),

Mr. Greene replied:

> A. Well, I—I don't think we were at the time looking at it directly as substitution. We were trying to figure out how to use monoclonal antibodies to dramatically improve on the performance of immunodiagnostic procedures. (1.76–77).

In other words, to appreciate what Hybritech had done, it was necessary to understand their intentions.

An additional, related argument directed against the charge of obviousness consisted in stressing the "inherent uncertainty" involved in dealing with "natural systems," a claim that can be related to the unpredictability argument discussed in the Cetus case. While the advantages of substitutions in artificial, closed systems can be relatively easily foreseen, one could not know in advance what variables were relevant to the behavior of a natural system. This, according to Dr. David, made Hybritech's research program novel:

> A. I still feel that it was not obvious [to use monoclonal antibodies]. And I think it comes down to the fact that we have a very complex system here. We, in the beginning, did not know what kind of tradeoffs there would be in using monoclonal antibodies in a sandwich assay. It was quite possible that by—we didn't feel that it was a simple substitution. We felt that if we were to select monoclonal antibodies, we didn't know what we would be running into in terms of assays, sensitivity, or reliability. We didn't know what factors were critical. (14.1883).[32]

Uncertainty, by virtue of being presented in naturalistic terms, and not, say, as the result of rhetorical construction (Campbell 1985), thus became a resource in the debate.

The differences stressed in these first two lines of argumentation were grounded in the perception (social and scientific) of the degree of difficulty of undertaking such an operation. According to Dr. David, an immunoassay contained two technical levels of understanding: a macro level (or procedural level) and a molecular level. Different classes of people working at these levels formed different ideas about what is obvious and therefore different intentions. To those working at the macro level, "essentially lay immunologists," the idea of substitution may have appeared obvious. To the second class of individuals, "who have a much clearer picture of this because of their orientation," the substitution appeared neither obvious nor easy. Furthermore, because non-obviousness is in these matters the criterion prescribed by law, Dr. David introduced a subtle distinction between obvious and reasonable:

> *A.* I don't think it was obvious that it would work.
> *Q.* I see. It wasn't obvious that it was [sic: would] work, but it was obvious to go ahead and do it?
> *A.* I think it was reasonable, logical to try to do it. (14.1885).

The inventiveness of Hybritech's "substitution" was further corroborated by a fourth line of argumentation, by another Hybritech witness, Dr. Alfred Nisonoff, a well-known immunologist from Brandeis University and the author of a standard immunological textbook. Given his similar scientific status, Dr. Nisonoff's testimony was used to counter Dr. Herzenberg's testimony. According to Dr. Nisonoff, the substitution of monoclonal antibodies for polyclonal antibodies was novel when viewed from a historical perspective. When Hybritech began its research in 1979, Nisonoff explained, it was generally believed that monoclonal antibodies were too weak a substance (i.e., had too low an affinity)[33] to have much commercial use. Nisonoff went on to substantiate this historical claim on the basis of perceptions fostered by his own social circle. Under cross-examination he stated:

> *Q.* Now with regards to these low affinity monoclonal antibodies that you talked about, you believe that there were some immunologists in 1979 that thought monoclonal antibodies had low affinities; is that what you testified to?
> *A.* Yes.
> *Q.* Who were those immunologists?
> *A.* In my talking to people at meetings, there was a general impression around that monoclonal antibodies tended to have low affinity.[34] (12.1525).

Nisonoff's statement can be termed a *characterization* (Pomerantz 1987), that is, a vague statement ("people at meetings," "a general impression around") influenced by the judgment of the person who is uttering it. The counterevidence introduced by Monoclonal Antibodies Inc.'s lawyers was of the opposite kind, insofar as it consisted of quotes from several papers written by individual scientists at a particular time, predicting the application of monoclonal antibodies to the field of immunoassays. While the District Court accepted Monoclonal Antibodies Inc.'s evidence as an indication of obviousness, the Court of Appeal disagreed by resorting to a distinction between "obvious" and "obvious to try."[35] This was not a totally unexpected argument because, as previously discussed, the PTO Board of Appeals had also resorted to it in validating a patent on monoclonal antibodies directed against malignant human renal cells. The board had qualified as "a well established axiom" the statement according to which "'obvious to try' is not the same as 'obviousness.'" So well established, in fact, that ad hoc semantic constructions such as "obvious to try with a reasonable good chance for success" were deemed unable to undermine it (*Ex parte Old*:200).

These points can be reduced to two schemata of interpretation corresponding to what Erving Goffman (1986:21) called the two *primary frameworks* used by individuals in Western society to organize their experience: natural frameworks and social frameworks. In the present case, the social framework made use of diachronic and synchronic categories. The debate took a historical turn, for example, when it was argued (as Dr. David and Dr. Nisonoff did) that other scientists back in the late 1970s thought that monoclonal antibodies were poor reagents for a sandwich assay and that it was thus not self-evident to use them in such an assay. The argument was also expressed in synchronic terms through a distinction between "lay immunologists," who, while using antibodies and antigens and carrying out immunoassays, nonetheless did not "have a very clear picture of what happens at the molecular level," and those immunologists "who would have a much clearer picture of this because of their orientation, their experience" (4.316–320).

In the preceding statements, Dr. David connected technical statements to social distinctions, as did Dr. Herzenberg, who linked the IRMA/RIA distinction to the existence of the subworld of commercial radioimmunoassays. In other words, by resorting to a social framework the distinction between the social and the technical was increasingly blurred, the social presenting itself as constitutive of the technical and vice-versa.[36] In response to Dr. David's classification, Monoclonal Antibodies Inc.'s lawyer claimed that immunologists could not be divided into two groups but were more likely to be distributed along a normal distribution curve (6.489). He thus tacitly acknowledged that technical statements were coextensive with social distinctions.

Using a natural framework Dr. David argued that the reason Hybritech's assay system was not to be conceived of as a "mere substitution" of polyclonal antibodies with monoclonal antibodies was that it "worked" in a different way. The reasons why it worked in a different way were twofold: a) Monoclonal antibodies used in the assay had been selected for high affinity; b) in order to avoid so-called steric hindrance (i.e., interference between the two antibodies when binding to the antigen), they had also been selected so as to react with remote binding sites (so-called epitopes) on the antigen (6.507). It should be noted that both reasons referred to representations of what was happening at the molecular level, as opposed to, for instance, representations of the procedures used to construct and/or to perform the assay (what one actually does at the lab bench as opposed to what is supposedly going on in the realm of the invisible).

In what follows, we show that different representations of molecular reality were advanced and that the dispute surrounding them mobilized once again historical and social arguments. We shall see that the natural framework of interpretation, when challenged, shifted to a social framework (Gilbert and Mulkay 1984:63). We shall further see that the debate concerning the legitimacy (for the purpose at hand) of drawing a distinction between procedural and molecular representations was framed in terms of what could be properly attached to technical manipulations and skills, and what could be ascribed to the intervention of uncontrollable natural events or, to use the ancient Greeks' dichotomy, in terms of the opposition between *techné* and *physis* (Schadewaldt 1979).

Contested Realities: Molecular and Procedural Representations

Let us begin with the conflicting representations of the status of events at the molecular or invisible level. Again, some technical background is necessary in order to follow the debate.

Antibodies attach themselves to antigens by binding to specific locations: these sites are called *antigenic determinants* or *epitopes*. There is, however, a certain terminological ambiguity, grounded in metonymy, because one can speak of antibodies reacting with antigens, antigenic substances, antigenic determinants, or epitopes. This ambiguity was exploited during the trial. For instance, considerable attention was devoted to the question of whether an epitope was to be considered identical to an antigenic determinant or to an antigen. One of the reasons why this question was important was that it was tied to a previous argument about prior art.

As the reader will recall, Monoclonal Antibodies Inc. claimed that Drs. Herzenberg and Oi had performed monoclonal sandwich assays prior to Hybritech. Hybritech's Dr. David responded to this challenge by arguing that Drs. Herzenberg and Oi's work, whose acknowledged goal was to determine the number of binding sites present on each of the two arms of a Y-shaped antibody by treating an antibody as antigen, dealt with observing the nature of an antigen (the number of epitopes) and not with determining its presence. By equating epitopes to antigenic substances, one could have undermined the nature/presence distinction. This gave rise to a number of exchanges, of which the following excerpts are representative:

> *Q.* [To Dr. David] Isn't an epitope an antigenic substance?
> *A.* An epitope is not an antigenic substance. An antigenic substance includes a number of epitopes. An epitope is not equated with an antigenic substance. (14.1908–1909)
>
> *Q.* [To Dr. Oi] And you weren't determining the presence or absence of the antigen, were you?
> *A.* Absolutely. These antigens, remember, are epitopes. (3.125).[37]

The controversy over the semantic field of terms such as *antigenic substance* and *epitope* was linked to the more general question of what constituted an "appropriate" representation of molecular events. Let us recall that, according to present immunological wisdom, antibodies are produced by specific cells, with each cell (and its clones, i.e., genetically identical cells) producing one particular kind of antibody specific to a particular antigenic determinant. As polyclonal antibodies are a mix of (monospecific) antibodies, they can bind to different antigenic determinants on the same antigen as well as to other antigens.

Monoclonal antibodies are monospecific antibodies produced by the clones of a single cell; they attach themselves to a single location on a given antigen. Such is, in general terms, the class of particulars inhabiting the molecular realm. Representations of the functions of these particulars led to different representations of the difference between monoclonal and polyclonal immunoassays. As one Hybritech witness pointed out:

> *Q.* Mr. Greene, would you represent a sandwich assay, using polyclonal antibodies in the same way that you would represent a sandwich assay using monoclonal antibodies?
> *A.* No, I would not draw[38] them in the same fashion, if that's what you mean.
> *Q.* Okay. And are there differences in your view?
> *A.* Yes, there's differences in—in the picture that you would look at on a molecular level (2.48–49).[39]

This picture was fleshed out in greater detail by another Hybritech witness, Dr. David:

> *A.* In the [monoclonal] case, we have an antibody bound to an antigen, which in turn is bound to a second labeled antibody. Each of these again is bound by a very

precise, specific epitope on the surface of the molecule. In the polyclonal situation, you can have a number of things happen. [The witness gave several examples of the "number of things" which can happen] Now, in the monoclonal situation you have one antibody, labeled antibody, bound to the solid support through a bridge created by one antigen. In the case of polyclonal antibody you can have that and you can have various configurations of that, or, more likely, you can have two, three, four, more antibodies with labels on them bound to the solid support. (4.307–313).

This molecular picture was, however, contested. Despite the apparent specificity of Dr. David's representation, alternative descriptions of what was happening at this level were advanced by the expert witnesses. The central issue was whether or not the binding of a monoclonal antibody to an antigenic site should be considered the same kind of event as the binding of a polyclonal antibody to an antigenic site. The status of Hybritech's sandwich assay (novelty or obvious development) depended on the acceptance of one of the contending representations of the molecular realm. Once again, this apparently purely technical issue was explored through a social framework.

The differences between polyclonal and monoclonal systems alluded to by Hybritech were first of all historical. According to Mr. Greene, evolution in the language used to describe binding events had resulted in a sort of incommensurability between monoclonal and polyclonal assays. Prior to the advent of monoclonal antibodies, it was argued, binding sites on the antigen were referred to as *antigenic determinants*. Following the introduction of hybridoma technology, the term *epitope*, proposed many years earlier by the renowned immunologist Niels K. Jerne, had spread rapidly and had become the dominant description of molecular events.[40] The renewed understanding of molecular processes provided by monoclonal antibodies had the retroactive effect of making previous descriptions of the polyclonal assay system obsolete. Before monoclonal antibodies,

> A. [By Mr. Greene] Well, typically, the sandwich assay ... historically—and this derives really from times before monoclonals were either invented or well understood—was represented in very simple fashion as—as being antibody, antigen, antibody.... Nobody really paid attention on the molecular level. (2.49–52).

Now,

> ... And, in fact, the sandwich you form, it is now known—now that monoclonals are available to really study this phenomenon—that the sandwich formation that occurs in a polyclonal system is really a very complex thing.... And so during the washing process of a polyclonal it's unpredictable what you're going to end up with as a result of this heterogeneity. (Ibid.).

Moreover, in addition to creating new complexity, monoclonal antibodies had the advantage of solving previously unknown problems:

> Now the beauty, of course, of the monoclonal system is that . . . you're now precisely controlling the binding locations. You have designed this so that the steric hindrances that—proteins don't like to get together; they have charges that keep them apart. And you can design this in an optimal configuration (Ibid.).

From Mr. Greene's and Dr. David's point of view, the newly found complexity of polyclonal systems had the effect of redescribing Hybritech's understanding of what it had done in the course of research:

> A. [By Mr. Greene] Well, I think what was—what was not understood was the advantage of being able to precisely define the binding sites and the sandwich geometry that was feasible with the homogeneous antibodies, and got around some of these problems that—that occur with polyclonal systems. In fact, if you look at textbooks back in 1975, '76, I think you will find just the very simple description, without all this complexity that actually occurs. . . . My impressions from the time were that people working with antiserum at that point did not think in terms of specific binding sites to any great degree. (2.53–54).

The historical discontinuity claimed by Hybritech could be experienced not only through reference to an invisible molecular realm. Procedural, witnessable advantages, grounded in the molecular machinery, were also trotted out. Standards for novelty could correlatively be reduced to matters of perception evolving over time. In the following exchange, Hybritech's witness explained that the company's customers did not at first see any significant difference between polyclonal and monoclonal kits. As the customers came to appreciate the product, they legitimated Hybritech's patented perception:

> Q. [To Mr. Greene] . . . Basically, your invention was to take the existing sandwich assays, which were using polyclonal antibodies, and now instead to use monoclonal antibodies instead of the polyclonals. Correct?
> A. I—I have trouble saying "yes," simply because in fact that was the original perception that—that some of our customers had; and on that basis they weren't interested in our product. And so we had to explain to them that we were using these antibodies in a very different fashion. That the problems that they had associated up until that point with IRMA's had been overcome by our new design, and that the result would be much better than—that they were ordinarily used to seeing.
> Q. You were using them in a different fashion. Weren't the kits almost exactly the same, in terms of where the antibodies were in the tubes, and so forth?
> A. Well, there were parts of the kit that looked very similar to the conventional products on the market, yes. But the procedure is—is significantly enough different that the laboratories liked it. . . . (1.82–83).

Hybritech's arguments referred to ways to legitimize perceptions by attributing them to a) what the customers thought, b) what the researchers thought, c) what the researchers thought they were thinking at the time (self-reference or attribution), and d) what other researchers thought or thought they were thinking. What, however, according to Hybritech's witnesses, should be conceived of as a variously grounded incommensurability, providing new foundations for the actual working of sandwich assays, became in the account of another witness, Ms. Blakemore, a simple and inconsequential matter of terminology:

> A. I think there is—has been a lot of discussion about the use of monoclonal antibodies which recognize different epitopes and which do not block each other.... Now, I think in—when we were developing [sandwich] assays with polyclonal antibodies, we used to call these binding sites or antigenic sites. I think in the language of monoclonal antibodies these sites are called epitopes. (8.918–919).

Pursuing this line of argument, the witness stated that the properties of antibodies were independent of the way the antibody was produced. For instance, an antibody remained an antibody whether it had been harvested from the serum of a rabbit (and could thus be considered of polyclonal origin) or whether it had been obtained through cell fusion methods and had thus been dubbed monoclonal. From this point of view, the possible advantages of using monoclonal antibodies, and thus the characteristics of an immunoassay, naturally flow from the antibodies' intrinsic or general properties, such as their affinity, and not from the skills deployed in obtaining them: from *physis*, not from *techné* (see, for instance, 8.954, 8.958, 9.973). By establishing an identity of substance between monoclonal and polyclonal antibodies, the witness reinforced the representation of Hybritech's assay system as a mere substitution. Conversely, to deny the validity of the term *substitution*, was to deny the identity. The well-known philosophical dictum "no entity without identity" (Strawson 1976) had to be inverted: no identity without entity.

Debate over what should be attributed to *physis* and what to *techné* was also at the center of a connected line of reasoning. One way of contesting Hybritech's patent claim was to argue that the patent did not teach either how to produce high-affinity antibodies or how to produce and select monoclonal antibodies reacting with remote epitopes, the two salient properties of the assay system. This is the enablement condition prescribed by patent law. Monoclonal Antibodies Inc.'s strategy here was not to claim that Hybritech's patent concealed essential technical details in the way trade secrets do; it was claimed that the enablement clause could not be respected because there was nothing new to teach.

Of course, the enablement clause, like the non-obviousness clause, was open to interpretation. It was claimed, and accepted by the District Court, that the patent did not contain sufficiently detailed descriptions teaching how to make the sandwich assay other than by trial and error; the patent could also be seen to fail the related test of the distinct claim clause by being indefinite, because, for instance, and to quote the District Court, there is "no standard set of experimental conditions which are used to estimate affinities." A competing interpretation, ratified by the Court of Appeal, was to state that the enablement clause referred to "persons of ordinary skill in the art." Given the fact, to quote the Court of Appeal, that the process required "sophisticated, competent people to perform the screening and that the screening process is labor-intensive and time consuming," then it was possible to speak of "screening methods used to identify the necessary characteristics, including affinity, of the monoclonal antibodies used in the invention." Furthermore, the language needed to be only as precise "as subject matter permits" (see also *In re Wands*).

Just as Hybritech's lawyer had represented Drs. Herzenberg and Oi's work as "theoretical," Monoclonal Antibodies Inc.'s lawyer was able to represent Hybritech's research as crass empiricism. Hybritech's scientists, it was claimed, had simply made a selection of monoclonal antibodies that worked:

> *Q.* [To Dr. David] Isn't it true that in 1979 Doctor Amshey had done the very same thing and that is select antibodies for remote or separate sites on an antigen?
> *A.* I sure don't see an indication that he has done it.
> *Q.* He suggested it, didn't he?
> *A.* I don't see any indication that they—the term *remoteness*—any indication of how far apart these determinants are.
> *Q.* Obviously far enough apart to work, aren't they?
> *A.* They are presumably far enough apart to fit two antibodies on.
> *Q.* Isn't that all you mean when you say that you select them so that they will be remote?
> *A.* As I went through in considerable detail more than once, no.
> *Q.* Isn't that total nonsense, Doctor David? You don't know where those antigen binding sites are on those molecules. You just screen them until they work, isn't that true? ...
> *A.* We screen them until they are sufficiently far apart that they don't interfere with each other.
> *Q.* You don't know how far apart, do you?
> *A.* In actual units, no.
> *Q.* In any units?
> *A.* We know we can bind one to the antigen without the effect of binding the other.
> *Q.* So what you are doing is running the screen until you got two antibodies that work in the assay, isn't that really what you are doing?
> *A.* That work best in the assay.
> *Q.* Work best in the assay. So you pick your two antibodies, and all you know is that they both bind to the antigen and don't interfere with one another. That is all you know. You don't know how far apart they are, isn't that true?
> *A.* I didn't say you had to know how far apart they were. I said you had to select them such that they were sufficiently far apart.
> *Q.* You had to select them so they are sufficiently far apart so they would work, isn't that true?
> *A.* So that they work optimally.

> *Q.* You don't know if they are an opposite sides of the antigen or the same side, or anything of that nature, when you select them, do you?
> *A.* That's correct. (14.1914–1916).

Monoclonal Antibodies Inc.'s lawyer's view was evidently shared by Monoclonal Antibodies Inc.'s expert witness, Ms. Blakemore:

> *A.* . . . As I said at the start of my testimony, a requirement of sandwich assays that is well known from the time sandwich assays were first reported in the literature was that the analyte, or the thing that you were trying to measure, has got to be able to be bound simultaneously by two antibodies—by at least two antibodies—one on a solid face [sic: phase] and one that is labeled. Now, I think it goes without saying that if these—if one of these antibodies blocks the binding of the other one so that a sandwich cannot form, that these pairs of antibodies can't be used. (8.950–951).

Monoclonal Antibodies Inc.'s argument against Hybritech at the molecular level was thus threefold. First, if a kit worked that meant that the antibodies were far enough apart on the antigen so as not to interfere with each other. Distance here was merely functional, it could not be measured. Secondly, the means of producing such antibodies could only be trial and error. Selecting the ones that "worked" meant you had no means of selection other than trial and error. And finally, the properties of affinity associated with the monoclonal antibodies selected were not the result of any special procedure. Their affinity was inextricably bound up with the fact that they did work. The affinity was not selected for. It was an *a posteriori* calculation that allowed Hybritech to construct a criterion of identity for their monoclonal antibodies and thus claim them, and therefore the assay system, as theirs.

In relation to this latter issue, Herzenberg argued that the claim to have obtained antibodies of a specific affinity was fundamentally erroneous. According to Herzenberg, "You can't really measure affinity—and this is an important factor—you can't measure affinity if it is properly defined, when the antibody, even the monoclonal antibody, has the opportunity of binding at two sites on the antigen molecule."[41] Herzenberg, it will be recalled, had been called to testify because he had allegedly developed, prior to Hybritech, a monoclonal assay similar to that patented by the plaintiff. Hybritech lawyers, however, maintained that Herzenberg's assay did not count as prior art, as he had failed to calculate the affinity of the antibodies used in his assay. To this he replied: "I think we did the same kind of measurements as were done in the patent application. You have to have a certain affinity and avidity, as I explained earlier to the court, to be able to get the assay to work. So we just determined whether the assay would work or not, and that would be an implicit measurement of affinity and avidity" (11.1403).[42]

To sum up, just because Hybritech constructed a criterion of identity for the entity, did they discover or produce a new entity? From a philosophical point of view, there is no easy answer to this question (e.g., Hamlyn 1984:56). Our purpose, however, has not been to offer yet another philosophical solution to this vexing issue. Rather, we have adopted an ethnographic viewpoint in order to describe how practical solutions were provided for the purpose at hand. In particular, we have seen how novelty was made cognitively and morally accountable through recourse to the distinction between *physis* and *techné*, this distinction being circumscribed by the legal categories of enablement and distinct claim.

Interestingly enough for us and our readers, the two camps in the dispute also touched upon an issue that we raised in Chapter 3, namely, whether the spread of hybridoma technology was to be conceived of as a passive diffusion process, that is, whether the meaning and subsequent use of an innovation are from the outset contained within the innovation, or whether the process should be analyzed as an active process of translation, wherein subsequent users of the innovation create at the same time new uses for the innovation and the market for its use and, by virtue of these actions, modify the status (social, economic, ontological, etc.) of the object (Callon 1989). A way of restating Monoclonal Antibodies Inc.'s and Hybritech's positions on the issue of molecular and procedural representations is to ask whether, once monoclonal antibodies became a practical option following Köhler and Milstein's 1975 *Nature* article, their meaning and future uses were obvious to the point of naturally flowing from the antibodies themselves. This was Monoclonal Antibodies Inc.'s claim.

Hybritech maintained that their use of monoclonal antibodies was novel and far from evident. Here we are thus confronted not only with a philosophical or a historical argument, but also with opposing models of the spread of innovation. Those models were instrumental in deciding whether or not monoclonal antibodies and their applications could indeed be translated into inventions.

Conclusions

Various authors, including ourselves (Mackenzie, Keating and Cambrosio 1990), have claimed that scientific opinion in the court has very different consequences from such opinion in its original context: divorced from that context they take on a kind of flexibility that can be extremely useful for a patent attorney. In the patent arena, scientific arguments are divorced from the tacit understandings that regulate their use in the scientific arena and can thus be (mis)used to appropriate scientific discoveries. A similar opinion was made public by those scientists who expressed "a sense of outrage" at what they considered the manufacturer's hijacking of Köhler and Milstein's discovery through the use of "misleading and specious" arguments (Ekins, personal communication, January 26, 1994; Ekins 1989:256). Our argument, in this chapter, is different. Without passing judgment on the speciousness of this or that claim (after all, distinguished scientists acted as witnesses on both sides of this and other disputes), and without resorting to *a priori*, mythical characterizations of science and law as different domains of normative practice, we have followed the translation of monoclonal antibodies and their applications into (patentable) inventions. The dynamics of this movement is independent of the validity of the arguments used in any particular case.

Patents and patent trials are ostensibly predicated upon the establishment of priority, as expressed through the notions of novelty and non-obviousness. In turn, the establishment of priority entails the identification of an entity as singular or novel to the extent that it is distinguished from like or similar entities that are either its predecessor or contemporary. The problem of ownership of a contested object is continuous with its establishment as an autonomous entity. The accomplishment of the latter task involves, as we have seen, the construction of identity criteria for the object in question. Technical arguments, in the course of this process, are juxtaposed and interfaced with social, historical, economic, or philosophical arguments. The social becomes coextensive with and constitutive of the technical as much as the latter participates in the redefinition of the former.

The Hybritech-Monoclonal Antibodies Inc. dispute clearly shows how much of the debate over the identity of technical objects is expressed in terms of a classification of the techno-social units (institutions and experimental systems) performing the work and in terms of temporal discontinuities, both of which color the intentions of the actors. For example, whether or not IRMA was the same as RIA depended on where and when you did your work, and not on what it was you did. In other words, what one did could not be accounted for independently of a context, which, in fact, became the content. The different contexts, in other words, gave rise to differing interpretations of the degree to which human manipulation of natural entities may reorganize these entities to the extent that they acquire a new identity.

To Monoclonal Antibodies Inc., for example, much of Hybritech's intervention into the molecular representation of monoclonal antibodies was without issue and did nothing to change the monoclonals' identity. Obviously, for Hybritech their intervention was the constitutive act of a new mode of existence of monoclonal antibodies. The predictability of monoclonal antibodies against human interferon, malignant renal cells, or lymphocyte subsets was alternatively grounded in the natural, invisible configuration of the antigenic landscape or in the artificial intervention of highly skilled scientists. Not only, thus, were these operations predicated upon the use of dichotomous interpretative frameworks (social framework vs. natural framework, *physis* vs. *techné*), but, in the end, those two frameworks became increasingly blurred: monoclonal antibodies were at once natural substances *and* artificial tools, able to carry out human intentions at the microscopic level.[43]

The antagonistic debate over the existence or lack thereof of the new entity not only revolved around the constitutive period and the setting of the alleged invention, it also evoked the invention's subsequent transformations within peculiar technosocial worlds. The subsequent transformations, in turn, redefined the original properties of the invention. For instance, while lawyers from both sides tried to assess the general attitude of the scientific community concerning potential uses and properties of monoclonal antibodies in diagnostic assays at the time of the alleged invention, the existence of the new entity was also predicated upon its subsequent commercial fate. At the same time, different levels and modalities of representation of the invention's inner workings were proposed according to the techno-social worlds considered relevant for assessing the invention's destiny, thus once again collapsing the distinction between the social and the natural.

It should by now be clear that the analysis of the argumentation and rhetoric of scientists and lawyers during the patent trial is more than a discussion of literary devices if by the latter we mean a set of discursive tools that only affect representations of antibodies as opposed to the antibodies themselves. The problems raised during the proceedings and the solutions proposed by expert witnesses were grounded in a seamless web of technical, philosophical, economic, and social distinctions. These distinctions collapsed descriptions of the invention with representations of the techno-social networks, which provided the conditions of existence of the latter. Monoclonal antibodies and the practices involving their use would no longer be the same.

NOTES

1. The text cites the following reference: *NIH Guide for Grants and Contracts (supplement, special announcement). NIH policy relating to reporting and distribution of hybridomas produced under grants and contracts* (May 1, 1980).

2. Rheinberger adds that "invention has always been and will continue to be an ongoing process of deconstruction," thus introducing his notion of "unintended inventions."

3. We are aware of the existence of national differences in this domain, but these are immaterial to our general argument. It is ironic to note, in this respect, that during the disappearance of the German Democratic Republic (GDR), an East German scientific journal published a two-part article (Nenning and Bourcevet 1990) originating from the Karl-Marx University in Leipzig. The first part discussed possibilities for patenting monoclonals in the GDR; the second part, wherein East Germany was already referred to as "the former GDR," discussed the international patent situation in the monoclonal area.

4. The survey they quote is reported in Dordick (1988). For a historical discussion of the importance of patents in the emergence of large technical systems, see Hughes (1989:138–159). It should

Between Nature and Culture 203

also be added that in the postbiotechnology era, the list of items used in curriculum vitae for tenure or promotion in academic biomedicine includes patents.

5. See, however, Webster and Packer's (1994) analysis of the emergent culture of patenting within academic science, focusing on how university-based scientists reconstruct their research so that it can lead to patents and how they exploit patents to secure continuity in their research.

6. From this point of view, "social arenas" or "social worlds," often used by writers in the symbolic-interactionist tradition, are better described as "worlds of action." On the former, see, for example, Clarke (1990); on the latter, see Dodier (1993).

7. See also Milstein's (1993) comment: "It remains a fact that the specter of patents is not only introducing new tensions in the scientific community, but also having serious undesirable effects on basic developments that largely rely on curiosity-driven research." For a forceful critique of the ballistic metaphor of impact, see Akrich (1989).

8. The fact that Milstein did not patent hybridoma technology has been ascribed to various reasons and motives, ranging from a scientific ethos not yet corrupted by commercial pressures to an abysmal blunder on the part of British patent authorities, which evoked the bitter memories of the penicillin affair, another British discovery that was commercially exploited by American companies. An example of the latter argument can be found in Wade (1980). The author claims that prior to the publication of the 1975 *Nature* article, Milstein had contacted a British government official, suggesting that the technique be patented, only to be told that it was not possible. Milstein subsequently asked recipients of myeloma cell lines to state, in writing, that they would not pursue commercial applications, believing that this would "reserve his position" by maintaining the technique in the public domain. Proponents of the scientific ethos explanation do not necessarily contest the former account but qualify it by pointing to Milstein's lack of aggressiveness in pursuing the patent option and to his eagerness to make his results public. Of course, both these accounts entertain the presupposition that hybridoma technology, as we understand it today, was an instantaneous product of the 1975 experiment. As shown in Chapters 1 and 3, this presupposition is also disputed. After the initial failure to patent hybridoma technology, Milstein patented rat myeloma cell lines developed in his laboratory; see Milstein and Wright (1980).

9. In an obvious reference to this episode, Milstein (1993) noted, "What is an obvious extension of previously established facts (as far as scientific judgment is concerned) can also be construed as novel (in legalistic terms), and thus merit patenting." This critique was also shared by the British Patent Office, which rejected a similar application submitted by the Wistar Institute, arguing that the process Wistar was trying to patent did not go beyond prior art and that it was an "obvious" application of Milstein's technique. The office decision cited an editorial in the biomedical periodical *Lancet*, which had suggested, as early as 1977, the use of monoclonals against viral antigens; see Dickson (1983). It should be added that whereas in the United States a patent can be filed up to one year after the original claims have been made public, in the United Kingdom, by publishing results one immediately relinquishes the right to patent.

The eligibility of Wistar's patent applications was also challenged in Japan, again on the basis of "prior art"; see Clark (1986) and Budiansky (1984). Many American companies seem to share this point of view, because work potentially covered by the Wistar patents is being pursued by many firms without licenses. One may guess that this general attitude is based on the assumption that the Wistar patents would not withstand a legal test in the patent court as well as on the assumption that the Wistar institute would not engage in costly legal disputes.

10. For a list of these patents, see Fox (1984). This development is closely linked to the use of the flow cytometer (a cell-sorting device) for which patents were also issued. On flow cytometry, see Keating and Cambrosio (1994).

11. The opening of a new research front as well as a new clinical market has been often related to the development of the OKT series and of the monoclonal antibodies produced by other laboratories against similar targets. On the constitution of lymphocyte subsets, see Cambrosio and Keating (1992), Scott (1985), and Klausner (1985). Ortho's OKT monoclonals were produced in a joint effort by Ortho's scientists (namely, Patrick Kung) with researchers from Harvard Medical School's Sidney (now Dana) Farber Cancer Research Institute (namely, Stuart Schlossman and Ellis Reinherz).

Results of this work were published as early as 1979 in highly visible journals such as *Science* and the *Proceedings of the National Academy of Sciences;* see Reinherz et al. (1979a,b) and Kung et al. (1979). Patents began to be filed and the cell lines (hybridomas) deposited at the ATCC the same year. Products containing these monoclonals began to be sold in 1980, soon after the patent applications were filed in 1979 and 1980.

12. *U.S. District Court of Delaware, Ortho Diagnostic Systems v. Becton-Dickinson Inc.* Civil Action #8-1-519, 21 September 1984. The Ortho–Becton-Dickinson litigation had been preceded by an episode in which Ortho's attorney caused an outcry by sending letters to about two dozen scientists (from both commercial companies and fundamental research institutions, including the NIH and universities) who had requested samples from the ATCC, warning that use of the samples "may constitute infringement of one or more of Ortho's patents, *regardless of whether the thus produced antibody is subsequently used or sold*" (our emphasis).

Instead of buying monoclonals from Ortho, scientists were suspected of obtaining samples of hybridomas for experimental use at a nominal cost from the ATCC and producing the monoclonals they needed (or inventing around by producing functionally equivalent hybridomas). NIH patent attorneys replied that the NIH did not consider the experimental use of samples to be an infringement because experimental use of an invention had not traditionally been regarded as such. In this case, however, the research market constituted, at least at the beginning, an important share of the OKT monoclonals market. Thus OKT monoclonals taken from ATCC hybridomas and used as reagents in the research process could, the Ortho attorney argued, cause "clear economic harm to Ortho," in which case the "rationale . . . excepting experimental use from infringement should not apply." On this episode see Fox (1984).

13. The identity of various reagents and T cells was not given *a priori* but was the result of a complex construction process, as indicated in Chapter 3. Moreover, it can be argued that the different subclasses of T cells did not preexist the monoclonal antibodies that recognized them but, rather, were constituted through the latter. On this topic see Cambrosio and Keating (1992).

14. Patents in general are required to provide a detailed description of the invention enabling "anyone skilled in the art" (though what "skilled in the art" amounts to can in itself be a complex issue) to reproduce the invention (although, of course, one is not supposed to use this information without a license). In the case of many biological inventions, it is generally accepted as impossible (as yet) to offer any kind of description or recipe that, of itself, would allow "anyone skilled in the art" to reproduce such an invention. As a result, at a meeting convened by the World Intellectual Property Organization (WIPO) in 1974, an international agreement was established requiring that specimens of biological material submitted for patenting (e.g., hybridomas) be deposited in specialized repositories (such as the American Type Culture Collection) and made available to anyone on request. The agreement, known as the Budapest Treaty, was ratified in 1980 (Marcus 1981; Wegner 1982:159–173).

This agreement led to a strange reversal of the original situation. Unlike more traditional inventions in which the description contained in the patent does not necessarily allow an immediate reproduction of the invention, in the case of hybridomas the transfer of the cell line is a *de facto* complete transmission of the invention. One complication arising from this fact was the inability of institutions to opt for the know-how option if their patent application was unsuccessful. As it was required that the cell be deposited on application (and accessible to all for research purposes), if the patent application was rejected, the cell line was in the public domain and unprotected. A decision by the U.S. Board of Patent Appeals and Interferences, however, first left the exact meaning of the deposit requirement open to negotiation—see Elman (1985); *BioEngineering News* (1985c,1986a)—and then allowed the deposition to be delayed until it is established that the application has "allowable subject matter"—see *Biotechnology News* (1987a,b). Further complications have arisen from the lack of a clear distinction between research and commercial applications.

15. "The test for novelty will surely present a challenge to the biologist and chemist who must define the new cell, be it microbial or hybridoma, to distinguish it from other cells previously existing. But basic science tells us that the new cell is different, different in the combination of its DNA components, with resulting differences in function or structure, or both. Where differences exist, they certainly should be definable and their novelty probable." (Woodruff and Miller 1981:1080).

16. The settlement was strongly in favor of Ortho. Becton-Dickinson paid Johnson & Johnson $5

million for damages and royalties in return for nonexclusive licenses for the patents, excluding therapeutic uses. In announcing the settlement, Ortho's spokesperson noted that the company planned "to defend the patents vigorously against others who are infringing"; see *BioEngineering News* (1986b). And so it did, by suing Coulter and reaching, in that case too, an out-of-court settlement.

17. With regards to the role of technicians in science, see Shapin (1989).

18. See Rheinberger (1993a:470); "Instruments by themselves are not the moving forces of the scientific goings-on: it is their embedment into experimental systems that count."

19. HBsAg is the acronym of Hepatitis B Surface Antigen. On anti-hepatitis monoclonal antibodies and Wands's team at the Massachusetts General Hospital, see Chapter 4.

20. The 1986 PTO decision even mentioned in a footnote the above-quoted Watson-Vossius Exchange at the 1981 Cold Spring Harbor meeting but dismissed it as not necessarily indicative of the "skill in the art" at the time of the invention; however, a 1981 review article was cited as acceptable evidence.

21. This was stressed in the PTO opinion.

22. On Hybritech's beginnings, see Prescott (1983) and Schneider (1985).

23. An *immunoassay* is an analytical device composed of various chemical and biological reagents, and uses the antibody-antigen reaction as a method for detecting or measuring the amount of the antigen; an *immunoassay (diagnostic) kit* is a prepackaged combination of the same with instructions. It uses antibodies as the active ingredient to detect or measure substances in patient specimens. For a definition of a *sandwich assay,* as well as further details on immunoassays, see the later discussion.

24. U.S. District Court, Northern District, California. *Hybritech v. Monoclonal Antibodies Inc.* #C-81-0930. August 28, 1985. *Hybritech Incorporated v. Monoclonal Antibodies, Inc.* 623 F. Supp. 1344–1357; 227 USPQ, 215–223 (N. D. Cal. 1985). For a detailed commentary on the judgment, see *Biotechnology Law Report* (1985).

25. U.S. Court of Appeals for the Federal Circuit. *Hybritech v. Monoclonal Antibodies Inc.* Appeal #86-531, September 19, 1986. *Hybritech Incorporated v. Monoclonal Antibodies, Inc.,* 802 F.2d 1367–1385, 231 USPQ 81 (Fed. Cir. 1986).

26. *Hybritech Incorporated v. Abbott Laboratories,* 4 USPQ2d 1001 (C. D. Cal. 1987); *Hybritech Incorporated v. Abbott Laboratories* 849 F. 2d 1446, 7 USPQ 2d 1191 (Fed. Cir. 1988); see *McGraw-Hill's Biotechnology Newswatch* (1986); Ezzell (1986, 1987).

27. U.S. Case law establishes a basic distinction between fact and opinion. The examination and cross-examination of witnesses is seen as a fact-finding activity, whereas the evaluation of the evidence gathered by this activity on the basis of legal categories is up to the court. This division of labor is less clear cut than previously thought; see Pomerantz (1987). The judges' opinions remain the place to look for the most explicit discussion of legal categories. In the present case, we have at our disposal two opposing opinions: one from the District Court and one from the Court of Appeals (623 F.Supp 1344 D.C.Cal. 1985; 802 F.2d 1367 Fed. Cir. 1986).

28. This point is noteworthy because it refers to a fundamental opposition (often implicit or, as in this case, explicit) between, on the one hand, procedural steps (what one actually does and can witness with his or her own senses) and, on the other hand, representations of what supposedly goes on at a molecular (invisible) level. This opposition surfaced several times during the Hybritech–Monoclonal Antibodies Inc. trial (see below). In this case the opposition is between procedural steps and kinetics as an abstract (mathematical) underlying reality; in other cases, the opposition is between procedural steps and iconic models of molecular events (antibodies represented as little "Ys," antigens as geometrical shapes with little "bumps," etc.); on this issue, see Knorr-Cetina and Amann (1990) and Cambrosio, Jacobi, and Keating (1993).

29. The first number refers to the volume of the trial transcripts (United States District Court, Northern District of California, *Hybritech Incorporated vs. Monoclonal Antibodies Inc.,* C 84-0930 SC), the second number to the page(s); in this case, volume 11, page 1333.

30. As pointed out in Asad (1986:153): "Sense or nonsense, like truth or falsehood, applies to [socially situated] *statements* and not to abstract concepts." The tension between situated statements and abstract concepts ran through the patent trial. Lawyers constantly tried to elicit "universal" statements from expert witnesses, while the latter replied by contextualizing their statements. From the

point of view of a sociologist of science, the scientists' strategy of contextualization must appear somewhat paradoxical, because the statement that scientific practice is locally situated is generally seen as a (contested) outcome of recent work in this discipline, more precisely, as an outcome of so-called laboratory studies.

Following the pioneering work of Latour and Woolgar (1986), several sociologists of science have undertaken fieldwork within laboratories. The latter, so the story goes, by using an ethnographic approach, were able to debunk the myth of universal science. In a patent trial such as this one, debates over identities are first and foremost debates over the context for which the identity is to be considered as valid.

31. Dr. Herzenberg's answer contained a second element, namely, the idea, acknowledged by all immunological textbooks, that antibodies could be used as antigens and thus elicit an antibody response. Here structure was opposed to function: Antibodies, while they have a specific physicochemical structure, can function as antigens. Oi and Herzenberg's experiments, and therefore scientific practice, involved precisely the use of antibodies as antigens. The structure/function opposition was also exploited as a rhetorical device to undermine the distinctions drawn by Hybritech.

32. Conversely, Dr. David argued that he could not know what was going on in Abbott's polyclonal assay:

Q. [To Dr. David] What else did you do that was different from what Abbott did?
A. I don't know, because I don't know the precise [assay] conditions . . . of a couple of their antibodies, for example. (14.1924–1925).

33. The question of affinity (the strength of binding between antigen and antibody, to use a simplistic definition), while it played a central role during the trial and continued to play such a role in the more recent Hybritech-Abbott litigation, is highly complex. In order not to overburden the reader with technical details, we shall not deal with this here; see, however, Keating, Cambrosio, and Mackenzie (1992).

34. Several witnesses were asked to assess the general attitude of the scientific community back in the seventies, that is, at the time of Hybritech's alleged invention. By answering this question, witnesses were simultaneously defining who or what should count as "the scientific community."

35. Neither did predictions qualify as prior art, insofar as they failed the test of reduction to practice.

36. The recent sociological approach known as *sociology of translation* insists on the methodological principle that the technical/social distinction cannot be used as an analytical resource because it is the result of the dynamic one seeks to study. See, for example, Callon and Law (1989) and Latour (1987).

37. At the end of a long exchange, the witness seemed to be somewhat exasperated by what could be described as terminological pointillism, as shown by the following remark:

Q. Isn't *antigen* the proper term for that [a predetermined amount of protein]?
A. You can call almost anything you want antigen, so, yes. (3.130).

38. Witnesses were actually asked to draw on a paper board or to use a flannel board to (re)present the molecular events they were describing. Besides this direct use of iconography, witnesses' discourse concerning the molecular realm very often referred to visual elements. The iconographic dimension greatly contributed to smoothing the constant shift from actual lab bench operations to the operations supposedly taking place at the molecular level. See, on visual language in science, Lynch and Woolgar (1990), as well as, more particularly, on visual language in immunology, Cambrosio, Jacobi, and Keating (1993).

39. A way of undermining similar statements was, of course, to contest the technical competence of the witness:

Q. [To Mr. Greene] And it is your feeling that the sandwich simultaneous assay worked better with the monoclonals?
A. Yes.
Q. Why is that?

A. Because for one thing there is not the kind of interference on a molecular level that occurs when you mix the labeled antibody with the antigen at the same time as you're putting it into proximity with a solid-phase antibody.

Q. Well, I'm not talking about a *theoretical answer* now, sir. You're not really competent to give a theoretical scientific answer, are you? I'm just trying to establish *from a user's standpoint* why you think the assay would work better . . . (1.87, our emphasis).

The lawyer's argument introduced a shift, linked to technical competence, from one representational level (the molecular one) to another (the procedural one). Oteri, Weinberg, and Pinales (1973) have shown, in the case of the cross-examination of chemists in drugs cases, how expert discourse can be undermined through the interrogation of competence.

40. The meaning of the term *epitope,* however, is still contested in immunological circles. For instance, a group of French immunologists (e.g., Cazenave and Coutinho 1993:47) insist on defining it on purely operational grounds, denying that an epitope is an intrinsic property of an antigen and arguing that it is defined by the antibodies recognizing it. Every antigen, according to this point of view, has as many epitopes as there are different kinds of specific antibodies capable of recognizing them.

41. In Herzenberg's view, the Hybritech researchers had measured avidity "which is the strength of binding with two binding sites" (11.1362). Interestingly enough, in a 1988 Court of Appeals decision in another case, one reads the following passage: "The examiner, the board, and [the applicant] all point out that, technically, the strength of antibody-[antigen] binding is measured as *avidity,* which takes into account multiple determinants on the [antigen] molecule, rather than affinity. Nevertheless, despite this correction, all parties then continued to use the term 'affinity'. We will use the terminology of the parties" (*In re Wands*:1405 footnote 26, emphasis in the original).

42. Hybritech's expert witness the following day, Brandeis University immunologist Alfred Nisonoff, pointed out: "It is generally understood and accepted that one can determine affinities with bivalent antibodies, report them as affinities without knowing positively that bivalent attachment doesn't occur, and I can document that." This was, however, quickly qualified by the statement that the patenting scientists had measured "functional affinity . . . if you wanted to be a purist." (Ibid., Vol. 12, pp. 1494, 1496). *Functional affinity* (as opposed to *intrinsic affinity*) is the term used by some immunologists to denote what others call avidity.

43. This argument is developed by Rheinberger (1993a,b) in relation to genetic engineering.

Epilogue

A question raised in the introduction to this book—and one that was, in part, prompted by colleagues who attended presentations of this book's material and by one of the book's reviewers—concerns the context within which the monoclonal antibody revolution took place. Explicitly or implicitly, to speak of a context is to reduce whatever is being contextualized to the elements that make up the context. Within a narrative it introduces a teleology, as the context is held to explain the contextualized event, to make it intelligible. No doubt, extraterrestrial anthropologists will one day spend some time examining the strange hold that final causes have on the human race, and so we shall add nothing further here.[1] Some remarks concerning hybridoma technology are, however, warranted.

In September 1993, the Wellcome Trust's History of Twentieth Century Medicine Group, in association with the Institute of Contemporary British History, held a "Witness Seminar" on monoclonal antibodies, during which key players in the development of hybridoma technology were invited to reflect upon their accomplishments (Tansey and Catterall 1994; Catterall and Tansey 1995). Introducing the meeting, Dr. Robert Bud, Head of Life and Environmental Sciences at the London's Science Museum, "examined the context of the monoclonal antibody story." This he did by evoking the rapid development, especially in the United States, of commercial biotechnology, a movement characterized by the meeting of venture capital and science in the creation of hundreds of "biotech startup companies," as well as by a rising concern about the potential dangers of the new techniques that culminated in the drafting of guidelines and other controversial forms of regulation of fundamental and commercial biotechnology (Tansey and Catterall 1994:323).

The blossoming of hybridoma technology could thus be explained by the fact that it became, along with recombinant DNA and, a distant third, new fermentation technologies, one of the three legs of what the U.S. Office of Technology Assessment (1984) popularized under the name of *new biotechnology*.[2] Biotechnology itself, of course, would seem in need of some further contextualization in terms, for instance, of the evolving structure of the chemical and pharmaceutical industries, the rise of the diagnostic industry, the transformation of health care, and so on.

It is not our intention to deny that commercial biotechnology constitutes one of the contexts that actors have used to make sense of monoclonal antibodies. One could, however, have chosen to engage in a quite different kind of contextualization by concentrating, for instance, on the paradigm of present-day immunology—clonal selection theory—which is echoed in the very term mono*clonal* antibodies. As is well known, immunology was dominated for several decades, "the 50-odd years between about 1910 and 1960" (Silverstein 1989:329), by immunochemistry and, correlatively, by instructionist theories of antibody formation.[3] According to the latter, antibodies existed prior to immunization not as specific molecules, but as unfolded, nonspecific proteins. Introduction of an antigen into an organism provided a surface or template about which the proteins could wrap themselves and thus acquire the properties associated with specificity.

In the 1950s, the clonal selection theory associated with Niels Jerne and Frank Macfarlane Burnet advanced the idea that the antigen did not act as a template about which formless proteins wrapped themselves into the shape of antibodies, but as a mechanism of selection. Antibodies with different specificities preexisted in the body and were produced by cells, one cell producing only one kind of antibody. The introduction of an antigen stimulated the reproduction of antibody-producing cells of a corresponding specificity. By shifting the immunological focus from chemistry to biology, or, more precisely, to genetics, clonal selection theory could thus be credited with providing the immunogenetic context within which Köhler and Milstein worked. In other words, by adopting clonal selection theory as the relevant context, monoclonal antibodies become an articulation of the clonal selection paradigm.[4] As in the case of biotechnology, immunobiology and the clonal selection theory can, in turn, be contextualized by placing them within the transformation of the life sciences after World War II, characterized by the rise of molecular biology,[5] the reconfiguration of biomedical research and clinical practices, with which immunology entertains a close relationship (for instance, transplantation), and so on.

If, for some tastes, the biotechnology story sounds too externalist (the technical accomplishments get lost in a sea of social and economic factors), and if the clonal selection story sounds too conceptual (how could free-floating ideas manage to constrain laboratory life?), one could delegate the job of providing a context for hybridoma technology to material practices. This context would consist of the various techniques available to and mobilized by Köhler and Milstein: cell culture techniques and related equipment and reagents, cell lines, and other artificial organic material, including inbred strains of mice, and so on.[6] Because these techniques and materials have a history, and because Köhler and Milstein worked in a specific historical juncture, technique and materials could serve as an explanatory context for hybridoma technology.

These various contexts are often differentiated by their level of generality, as expressed in spatial terms: commercial biotechnology thus appears as a "broader social context" than the "narrower technical circumstances" provided by equipment and tools. Some scholars would argue that all these levels are indeed relevant and should be simultaneously taken into account (Fujimura 1987). In practice, however, some kind of context, deemed to be of more immediate relevance or to possess a greater explanatory power, is given precedence over the others. In certain cases, enforcement of explanatory hierarchies can be aggressive. The reviewer of a historical anthology of landmark articles in immunology, for instance, attacked the editor's presentation of Köhler and Milstein's 1975 *Nature* paper by arguing that she had "completely ignored the context within which Milstein's research had taken place" (Corbellini 1993:521).[7] The editor had actually provided a context, namely, genetic engineering and the risks associated with biotechnology, but this context was dismissed as irrelevant and contrasted with the "relevant" immunogenetic context, namely, Milstein's more than a decade-long involvement in the search for proof that somatic mutations lay at the root of antibody diversity.

In spite of the heat produced by such debates, the question of which of the various candidate contexts should count as "the right one" is ultimately idle. In a sense all these contexts are relevant, and in another sense none of them are, for they all imply that the meaning of a scientific innovation is given in advance, that, in the end, there are no surprises. The object we have described—hybridoma technology as an expanding network of relations—has no clearly defined limits. Indeed, to place monoclonals within a pregiven context would have been to adopt a narrow approach unable to capture the multiple, intersecting modes of existence (Simondon 1989) of monoclonals as (bio)technical objects: everyday tools of laboratory practice, therapeutic molecules (Borrebaeck and Larrock 1990), a starting point for new attempts at improving on nature (Winter and Milstein 1991; Bain, Hoekstra, and Lerner 1992),[8] tools in the development of new instrumentation, and intellectual property.

The sociotechnical network whose ramifications we have attempted to trace calls upon any number of theories, both large and small, ad hoc and paradigmatic, to underwrite the daily routines that establish connections between practices, players, reagents, and institutions. It is precisely because of this heterogeneity that fixed limits—epistemological or social—that would define an *a priori*, clear-cut context are at best an illusion and at worst a distortion. It seems to us that events that are pulled together under the description of discovery, invention, or innovation offer practitioners the opportunity of creating a new context for their work. In other words, the intention of discovery is ultimately decontextualization, and that is the process we have described.

NOTES

1. But see, for a more terrestrial treatment of the same question, Latour (1988).
2. For further information on the rise of biotechnology, see, for example, Yoxen (1983), Kenney (1986), Wright (1986), Krimsky (1991), and Bud (1993).
3. What follows is an extremely simplified summary of a more complex history. For more details, see Silverstein (1989), Moulin (1991), and Keating, Cambrosio, and Mackenzie (1992).
4. Goding (1983:5–6) explicitly links the development of hybridoma technology to clonal selection theory.
5. Conversely, the molecular biological revolution has been partly identified with the development of tools such as monoclonal antibodies. As noted by Silverstein (1989:348), "The availability of such pure reagents [monoclonal antibodies] has provided one of the most powerful tools of the current revolution in molecular biology and has opened up new avenues of investigation in many basic and clinical sciences."
6. The history and sociology of biomedical techniques, equipment, and research materials, including laboratory animals, have received much recent attention. See, for instance, Borell (1987), Brown and Henderson (1983), Clarke (1987), Clarke and Fujimura (1992), Kay (1988), Kohler (1991), Löwy and Gaudillière (1994), and Oudshoorn (1990).
7. The book under attack is Bibel (1988).
8. Interestingly enough, some of these new approaches involve a "return to immunochemistry"; see Getzoff et al. (1988:1).

References

Abrams, Paul G., Jeffrey L. Rossio, H.C. Stevenson, and K.A. Foon. 1986. "Optimal Strategies for Developing Human-Human Monoclonal Antibodies." *Methods in Enzymology* 121:107–119.

Akrich, Madeleine. 1989. "La construction d'un système socio-technique. Esquisse pour une anthropologie des techniques." *Anthropologie et Sociétés* 13(2):31–54.

Anderson, Warwick. 1992. "The Reasoning of the Strongest: The Polemics of Skills and Science in Medical Diagnosis." *Social Studies of Science* 22:653–684.

Anscombe, G.E.M. 1957. *Intention*. Oxford: Basil Blackwell.

Armstrong, David. 1977. "Clinical Sense and Clinical Science," *Social Science and Medicine* 11:599–601.

Art To Science In Tissue Culture. 1983. "Cell Fusion with P.E.G.: Is It Reproducible?" 2:1–2.

Asad, Talal. 1986. "The Concept of Cultural Translation in British Social Anthropology." In *Writing Culture*, eds. James Clifford and George E. Marcus, pp. 141–164. Berkeley, CA: University of California Press.

ATCC. 1985. American Type Culture Collection. *Catalogue of Cell Lines and Hybridomas*. Fifth Edition. Rockville, MD: American Type Culture Collection.

Bachelard, Gaston. 1953. *Le Matérialisme Rationnel*. Paris: Presses Universitaires de France.

Bain, J.D., D.M. Hoekstra, and Richard A. Lerner. 1992. "Semisynthetic Combinatorial Antibody Libraries: A Chemical Solution to the Diversity Problem." *Proceedings of the National Academy of Sciences of the United States of America* 89:4457–4461.

Balachandran, N., D. Harnish, R.A. Killington, Silvia Bacchetti, and William Rawls. 1981. "Monoclonal Antibodies to Two Glycoproteins of Herpes Simplex Virus Type 2." *Journal of Virology* 39:438–446.

Balachandran, N., Silvia Bacchetti, and William E. Rawls. 1982a. "Protection Against Lethal Challenge of BALB/c Mice by Passive Transfer of Monoclonal Antibodies to Five Glycoproteins of Herpes Simplex Virus Type 2." *Infection and Immunity* 37:1132–1137.

Balachandran, N., D. Harnish, William E. Rawls, and Silvia Bacchetti. 1982b. "Glycoproteins of Herpes Simplex Virus Type 2 as Defined by Monoclonal Antibodies." *Journal of Virology* 44:344–355.

Balachandran, N., Barbara Frame, Max Chernesky, Edmund Kraiselburd, Yamil Kouri, Doris Garcia, Carol Laveky, and William E. Rawls. 1982c. "Identification and Typing of Herpes Simplex Viruses with Monoclonal Antibodies." *Journal of Clinical Microbiology* 16:205–208.

Barski, Georges, Serge Sorieul, and Francine Cornefert. 1960. "Production dans des cultures in vitro de deux souches cellulaires en association de cellules de caractère «hybride»." *Comptes Rendus de l'Académie des Sciences* 251:1825–1827.
Bartal, A.H. and Y. Hirshaut. 1987. "Preface." In *Methods of Hybridoma Formation*, eds. A.H. Bartal and Y. Hirshaut, pp. v–vi. Clifton, NJ: Humana Press.
Bazin, Hervé. 1986. "Hybridomes et anticorps monoclonaux." *Biofutur* 44:15–17.
Bibard, Laurent. 1991a. "Histoire d'une innovation: le cas d'un médicament." *Revue économique* 42:273–300.
Bibard, Laurent. 1991b. *La place et le rôle des sciences dans les innovations techniques. Quelques cas en biotechnologie*. Thèse de Doctorat. Paris: École des Hautes Études en Sciences Sociales.
Bibel, Debra J., ed. 1988. *Milestones in Immunology: A Historical Exploration*. Madison, WI: Science Tech.
BioEngineering News. 1985a. "Deposit Case before CAFC." 6(19):1.
BioEngineering News. 1985b. "More from ATCC Conference: Access to Culture May Cause Row." 6(20):1.
BioEngineering News. 1986a. "Battle Continues in Ortho v. Becton-Dickinson Patent Case." 7(3):1–2.
BioEngineering News. 1986b. "Becton, Ortho in Historic $5 Million Monoclonal and Cytometry Settlement." 7(39):1.
BioEngineering News. 1986c. "Americans Sex Ignorant?" 7(40):2.
Bio/Technology. 1983. "Electrofusion: A Faster, More Efficient Technique for Hybridoma Production." 1:390–391.
Biotechnology Law Report. "Monoclonal Antibodies Inc. Wins Patent Infringement Lawsuit Brought by Hybritech, Inc." 1985. 4:302–305.
Biotechnology News. 1987a. "Supreme Court Upholds Hybritech Patent." 7(10):1.
Biotechnology News. 1987b. "Rules Eased on Organism Deposits for U.S. patents." 7(11):4.
Boltanski, Luc. 1990. *L'amour et la justice comme compétences*. Paris: Métailié.
Borrebaeck, Carl A.K. and James W. Larrock, eds. 1990. *Therapeutic Monoclonal Antibodies*. New York: Stockton Press.
Borell, Merriley. 1987. "Instruments and an Independent Physiology: The Harvard Physiology Laboratory, 1871–1906." In *Physiology in the American Context, 1850–1950*, ed. Gerald L. Geison, pp. 293–321. Bethesda, MD: American Physiological Society.
Bozeman, Marc H. 1982. "The Regulation of Hybridoma Products." In *The Impact of Hybridoma Technology on the Medical Device and Diagnostic Product Industry. Proceedings of the Educational Seminar. HIMA Report No. 82–1*, ed. Timothy J. Henry, pp. 63–82. Washington D.C.: Health Industry Manufacturers Association.
Brannigan, Augustine. 1981. *The Social Basis of Scientific Discoveries*. Cambridge, England: Cambridge University Press.
Brock, William H. 1981a. "Purity." In *Dictionary of the History of Science*, eds. W.F. Bynum, E.J. Browne, and Roy Porter, p. 352. Princeton, NJ: Princeton University Press.
Brock, William H. 1981b. "Reagent." In *Dictionary of the History of Science*, eds. W.F. Bynum, E.J. Browne, and Roy Porter, pp. 361–362. Princeton, NJ: Princeton University Press.
Brock, William H. 1992. *The Fontana History of Chemistry*. London: Fontana.

Brown, Russel J. and H.M. Henderson. 1983. "The Mass Production and Distribution of HeLa Cells at the Tuskeegee Institute, 1953–1955." *Journal of the History of Medicine and Allied Health Sciences* 38:415–431.

Brownlee, G.G., T.M. Harrison, M.B. Matthews, and César Milstein. 1972. "Translation of Messenger RNA for Immunoglobulin Light Chains in a Cell-free System from Krebs II Ascites." *FEBS Letters* 23:244–248.

Brownlee, G.G., E.M. Cartwright, Nicholas J. Cowan, J.M. Jarvis, and César Milstein. 1973. "Purification and Sequence of Messenger RNA for Immunoglobulin Light Chains." *Nature New Biology* 244:236–240.

Bud, Robert. 1993. *The Uses of Life: A History of Biotechnology*. Cambridge, England: Cambridge University Press.

Budiansky, Stephen. 1984. "Disclosure Threat to Japanese Rights." *Nature* 307:97.

Bulletin of the World Health Organization. 1981. "The Role of Genetic and Molecular Characterization of Viruses in Relation to Influenza Surveillance and Epidemiology: A WHO Memorandum." 56:875–879.

Burrin, Jacky and David Newman. 1991. "Production and Assessment of Antibodies." In *Principles and Practice of Immunoassay*, eds. Christopher P. Price and David J. Newman, pp. 19–52. Basingstoke, England: Macmillan.

Business Week. 1979. "Venturing into Medical Technology." (16 April):107–112.

Bussard, Alain E. 1966. "Antibody Formation in Nonimmune Mouse Peritoneal Cells after Incubation in Gum Containing Antigen." *Science* 153:887–888.

Bussard, Alain E. 1984a. "How Pure are Monoclonal Antibodies?" In *Monoclonal Antibodies: Standardization of their Characterization and Use. Developments in Biological Standardization*, Vol. 57, eds. M. Barme and W. Hennessen, pp. 13–15. Basel: Karger.

Bussard, Alain E. 1984b. "The Universe of Immunoclones. How to Keep Track of Them?" In *Monoclonal Antibodies: Standardization of their Characterization and Use. Developments in Biological Standardization*, Vol. 57, eds. M. Barme and W. Hennessen, pp. 5–7. Basel: Karger.

Bussard, Alain E. and Jacqueline Pages. 1978. "Establishment of a Permanent Hybridoma Producing a Mouse Autoantibody." In *Origin and Natural History of Cell Lines. Proceedings of a Conference held at the Accademia Nazionale dei Lincei, Rome, Italy, October 28–29, 1977*, eds. Claudio Barigozzi, pp. 167–179. New York: Alan R. Liss.

Bussard, Alain, Micah I. Krichevsky, and Lois D. Blaine. 1985. "An International Hybridoma Data Bank: Aims, Structure and Function." In *Monoclonal Antibodies Against Bacteria*, Vol. 1, eds. Alberto J.L. Macario and Everly Conway de Macario, pp. 187–311. Orlando: Academic Press.

Buttin, Gérard and Pierre-André Cazenave. 1980. "L'hybridation des cellules lymphocytaires." *Bulletin de l'Institut Pasteur* 78:7–47.

Buttin, Gérard, G. Le Guern, L.K. Phalente, E.C.C. Kin, L. Medrano, and Pierre-André Cazenave. 1978. "Production of Hybrid Lines Secreting Monoclonal Anti-Idiotypic Antibodies by Cell Fusion on Membrane Filters." In *Lymphocyte Hybridomas. Current Topics in Microbiology and Immunology, 81*, eds. Fritz Melchers, Michael Potter, and Noel L. Warner, pp. 27–36. Berlin: Springer Verlag.

Callon, Michel, ed. 1989. *La science et ses réseaux*. Paris: La Découverte.

Callon, Michel. 1994. "Is Science a Public Good?" *Science, Technology, & Human Values* 19:395–424.

Callon, Michel and Bruno Latour. 1986. "Les paradoxes de la modernité. Comment concevoir les innovations?" *Prospective et Santé* (Winter):13–25.

Callon, Michel and John Law. 1989. "On the Construction of Sociotechnical Networks: Content and Context Revisited." *Knowledge and Society: Studies in the Sociology of Science Past and Present* 8:57–86.

Calvino, Italo. 1985. *Mr Palomar*. London: Secker & Warburg.

Cambrosio, Alberto and Peter Keating. 1992. "A Matter of FACS: Constituting Novel Entities in Immunology." *Medical Anthropology Quarterly* 6:362–384.

Cambrosio, Alberto, Camille Limoges, and Eric Hoffman. 1992. "Expertise as a Network: A Case Study of the Controversies over the Environmental Release of Genetically Engineered Organisms." In *The Culture and Power of Knowledge. Inquiries into Contemporary Societies*, eds. Nico Stehr and Richard V. Ericson, pp. 341–361. Berlin: De Gruyter.

Cambrosio, Alberto, Daniel Jacobi, and Peter Keating. 1993. "Ehrlich's 'Beautiful Pictures' and the Controversial Beginnings of Immunological Imagery." *Isis* 84:662–699.

Campbell, Ailsa M. 1984. *Monoclonal Antibody Technology. The Production and Characterization of Rodent and Human Hybridomas*. Amsterdam: Elsevier.

Campbell, Ailsa. 1994. "Review of *Methods of Immunological Analysis: Volume 1, Fundamentals; Volume 2: Samples and Reagents*." *Immunology Today* 15:92–93.

Campbell, Brian L. 1985. "Uncertainty as Symbolic Action in Disputes Among Experts." *Social Studies of Science* 15:429–453.

Carey, Norman. 1983. "Science Meets Law (Review of *Patenting of Life Forms*)." *Nature* 302:458–459.

Catterall, P.P. and E.M. Tansey. 1995. "Technology Transfer in Britain: The Case of Monoclonal Antibodies." *Contemporary Record*, forthcoming.

Cazenave, Pierre-André and António Coutinho. 1993. "Immunité et vaccination." *Pour la science* 193:42–50.

Clark, Thomas J.M. 1986. "L'impact économique des anticorps monoclonaux." *Biofutur* 44:121–133.

Clarke, Adele E. 1987. "Research Materials and Reproductive Science in the United States, 1910–1940." In *Physiology in the American Context, 1850–1950*, ed. Gerald L. Geison, pp. 323–350. Bethesda, MD: American Physiology Society.

Clarke, Adele E. 1990. "A Social Worlds Research Adventure. The Case of Reproductive Science." In *Theories of Science in Society*, eds. Susan E. Cozzens and Thomas F. Gieryn, pp. 15–42. Bloomington, IN: Indiana University Press.

Clarke, Adele E. and Joan H. Fujimura, eds. 1992. *The Right Tools for the Job: At Work in Twentieth-Century Life Sciences*. Princeton, NJ: Princeton University Press.

Clifford, James. 1990. "Notes on (Field)notes." In *Fieldnotes. The Makings of Anthropology*, ed. Roger Sanjek, pp. 47–70. Ithaca, NY: Cornell University Press.

Cipolla, Carlo M. 1965. *Guns, Sails and Empires: Technological Innovation and the Early Phase of European Expansion, 1400–1700*. New York: Minerva Press.

Coffino, P., Barbara Knowles, S.G. Nathenson, and Matthew D. Scharff. 1971. "Suppression of Immunoglobulin Synthesis by Cellular Hybridization." *Nature New Biology* 231:87–90.

Cohn, Melvin. 1967. "Natural History of the Myeloma." *Cold Spring Harbor Symposia on Quantitative Biology* 32:211–221.

Cohn, Melvin. 1981. NCI Contract Proposal.

Collins, Harry M. 1985. *Changing Order. Replication and Induction in Scientific Practice*. London: Sage.
Collins, Harry M. 1987. "Expert-Systems and the Science of Knowledge." In *The Social Construction of Technological Systems. New Directions in the Sociology and History of Technology*, eds. Wiebe E. Bijker, Thomas P. Hughes, and Trevor Pinch, pp. 329–348. Cambridge, MA: MIT Press.
Collins, Harry M. 1990. *Artificial Experts. Social Knowledge and Intelligent Machines*. Cambridge, MA: MIT Press.
Collins, Harry M. 1992. "Hubert L. Dreyfus, Forms of Life, and a Simple Test for Machine Intelligence." *Social Studies of Science* 22:726–739.
Collins, Harry M., R.H. Green, and R.C. Draper. 1985. "Where's the Expertise?: Expert Systems as a Medium of Knowledge Transfer." In *Expert Systems 85*, ed. Martin Merry, pp. 323–334. Cambridge, England: Cambridge University Press.
Collins, H.M., G.H. de Vries, and W.E. Bijker. 1990. "The Grammar of Skills." Unpublished manuscript.
Conway de Macario, Everly, and Alberto J.L. Macario. 1985. "Monoclonal Antibodies for Bacterial Identification and Taxonomy: 1985 and Beyond." *Clinics in Laboratory Medicine* 5:531–544.
Cooper, Iver P. 1982. *Biotechnology and the Law*. New York: Clark Boardman Company.
Corbellini, Gilberto. 1993. "La scoperta della storia dell'immunologia." *Physis* 30:517–526.
Cotton, R.G.H. and César Milstein. 1973. "Fusion of Two Immunoglobulin-Producing Myeloma Cells." *Nature* 244:42–43.
Coutinho, Antonio. 1993. "A VRM Network that Refers to the Somatic Self: Medical Prospects and Difficulties." Paper presented at the Conference "Conceptual Issues in Immunology: Experimental and Clinical Foundations." Boston University, May 5–6.
David, Gary S., W. Present, J. Martinis, Robert Wang, Richard Bartholomew, W. Desmond, and E. Dale Sevier. 1981a. "Monoclonal Antibodies in the Detection of Hepatitis Infections." *Medical Laboratory Sciences* 38:341–348.
David, Gary S., Robert Wang, Richard Bartholomew, E. Dale Sevier, Thomas H. Adams, and Howard E. Greene. 1981b. "The Hybridoma. An Immunochemical Laser." *Clinical Chemistry* 27:1580–1585.
Day, Eugene, D. 1990. *Advanced Immunochemistry*, 2nd Edition. New York: Wiley-Liss.
de Pinho, R.A., L.B. Feldman, and Matthew D. Scharff. 1986. "Tailor-Made Monoclonal Antibodies." *Annals of Internal Medicine* 104:225–233.
de Weck, A.L. 1987. "Foreword." In *Monoclonal Antibody Production Techniques and Applications*, ed. Lawrence B. Schook. New York: Dekker.
Descombes, Vincent. 1977. *L'inconscient malgré lui*. Paris: Éditions de Minuit.
Diamond, Betty A. and Matthew D. Scharff. 1982. "Monoclonal Antibodies." *JAMA* 248:3165–3169.
Dickson, David. 1983. "Wistar Denied Monoclonal Antibody Patent in U.K." *Science* 222:1309.
Diamond, Betty A., Dale E. Yelton, and Matthew D. Scharff. 1981. "Monoclonal Antibodies. A New Technology for Producing Serologic Reagents." *The New England Journal of Medicine* 304:1344–1349.
Dix, Richard D., Leonore Pereira, and Richard Bohringer. 1981. "Use of Monoclonal Antibody Directed Against Herpes Simplex Virus Glycoproteins to Protect Mice

Against Acute Virus-Induced Neurological Disease." *Infection and Immunity* 34:192–199.

Dodier, Nicolas. 1993. *L'expertise médicale*. Paris: Métailié.

Dorkick, J.S. 1988. "Patents and Literature." *Applied Biochemistry and Biotechnology* 19:271–296.

Dreyfus, Hubert L. 1992. "Response to Collins, *Artificial Experts*." *Social Studies of Science* 22:717–725.

Dubiski, S. 1987. "Foreword." In *The Rabbit in Contemporary Immunological Research*, ed. S. Dubiski, pp. ix–xi. Burnt Mill, England: Longman.

Dutton, Gail. 1993. "FDA Rewrites Pts-To-Consider for Monoclonals and Cell Lines." *Genetic Engineering News* 13(8):1 and 29.

Edwards, Ray. 1985. *Immunoassay. An Introduction*. London: William Heinemann Medical Books.

Eisenberg, Roselyn J., Deborah Long, Leonore Pereira, Berge Hampar, Martin Zweig, and Gary Cohn. 1982. "Effect of Monoclonal Antibodies on Limited Proteolysis of Native Glycoprotein gD of Herpes Simplex Virus Type 1." *Journal of Virology* 41:478–488.

Ekins, Roger. 1981. "Merits and Disadvantages of Different Labels and Methods for Immunoassay." In *Immunoassays for the 80s*, eds. A. Voller, A. Bartlett and D. Bidwell, pp. 5–16. Baltimore, MD: University Park Press.

Ekins, Roger. 1989. "A Shadow over Immunoassay." *Nature* 340:256–258.

Elman, Gerry. 1985. "Lundak Decision Overturns Time Requirement for Depositing Biotech Sample." *Genetic Engineering News* 5(10):11.

Ephrussi, Boris. 1970. *Hybridization of Somatic Cells*. Princeton, NJ: Princeton University Press.

Eshhar, Zelig. 1985. "Monoclonal Antibody Strategy and Techniques." In *Hybridoma Technology in the Biosciences and Medicine*, ed. Timothy A. Springer, pp. 3–41. New York: Plenum Press.

Ex parte Erlich. 3 USPQ2d, 1011–1018.

Ex parte Old. 229 USPQ, 197–200.

Ezzel, Carol. 1986. "Hybritech Versus Abbott." *Nature* 324:506.

Ezzel, Carol. 1987. "Hybritech Wins Court Injunction over Sandwich Assays." *Nature* 327:5.

Ezzel, Carol. 1989. "Abbott and Hybritech Settle Dispute." *Nature* 340:418.

Farr, A.D. 1981. "Hepatitis: A Laboratory Growth Industry." *Medical Laboratory Sciences* 38:301–302.

Fauci, Anthony S., H. Clifford Lane, and David J. Volkman. 1983. "Activation and Regulation of Human Immune Responses: Implications in Normal and Disease States." *Annals of Internal Medicine* 99:61–75.

Fazekas De St. Groth, Stephen. 1985. "Monoclonal Antibody Production: Principles and Practice." In *Handbook of Monoclonal Antibodies. Applications in Biology and Medicine*, eds. Soldano Ferrone and Manfred P. Dierich, pp. 1–10. Park Ridge, NJ: Noyes Publications.

Fazekas De St. Groth, Stephen and Doris Scheidegger. 1980. "Production of Monoclonal Antibodies: Strategy and Tactics." *Journal of Immunological Methods* 35:1–21.

Ferguson, Eugene S. 1985. "La fondation des machines modernes: des dessins." *Culture Technique* 14:183–207.

Ferguson, Eugene S. 1992. *Engineering and the Mind's Eye*. Cambridge, MA: MIT Press.

Fisher, Lawrence M. 1991. "Biologists Re-Engineer Antibodies." *The New York Times* (5 March):C1 and C3.
Fjermedal, Grant. 1984. *Magic Bullets*. New York: Macmillan.
Fleck, Ludwik. 1979. *Genesis and Development of a Scientific Fact*. Chicago: The University of Chicago Press.
Foster, H.L. and M.W. Balk. 1982. "Histocompatibility and Isoenzyme Differences in Commercially Supplied 'BALB/c' Mice: A Reply." *Science* 217:381.
Fox, Jeffrey L. 1984. "Encroaching on Research Freedom." *Science* 224:584–586.
French, Deborah, Ellyn Fischberg, Susan Buhl, and Matthew Scharff. 1986. "The Production of More Useful Monoclonal Antibodies." *Immunology Today* 7:344–346.
Fujimura, Joan H. 1987. "Constructing 'Do-Able' Problems in Cancer Research: Articulating Alignment." *Social Studies of Science* 17:257–293.
Fujimura, Joan H. 1988. "The Molecular Biological Cancer Research Bandwagon: Where Social Worlds Meet." *Social Problems* 35:261–283.
Fujimura, Joan H. 1992. "Crafting Science: Standardized Packages, Boundary Objects, and 'Translation.'" In *Science as Practice and Culture*, ed. Andrew Pickering, pp. 169–211. Chicago: University of Chicago Press.
Fujimura, Joan H. 1996. *Crafting Science, Transforming Biology*. Cambridge, MA: Harvard University Press.
Galfré, Giovanni and César Milstein. 1981. "Preparation of Monoclonal Antibodies: Strategies and Procedures." *Methods in Enzymology* 73 (Part B):3–46.
Galfré, Giovanni, S.C. Howe, César Milstein, G.W. Butler, and J.C. Howard. 1977. "Antibodies to Major Histocompatibility Antigens Produced by Hybrid Cell Lines." *Nature* 266:550–552.
Gaudillière, Jean-Paul. 1991. *Biologie moléculaire et biologistes dans les années Soixante: naissance d'une discipline*. Thèse de Doctorat en Histoire, Université Paris VII.
Gaudillière, Jean-Paul. 1993a. "NCI and the Spreading Genes. About the Production of Viruses, Mice and Cancer." Paper presented at the Sociology of the Sciences Yearbook Conference "The Practices of Human Genetics: International and Interdisciplinary Perspectives." Brandeis University, Waltham, MA, July 14–15.
Gaudillière, Jean-Paul. 1993b. "Oncogenes as Metaphors for Human Cancer." In *Medicine and Change: Historical and Sociological Studies of Medical Innovation*, ed. Ilana Löwy, pp. 213–249. Paris: John Libbey/INSERM.
Gefter, Malcolm L., David H. Margulies, and Matthew D. Scharff. 1977. "A Simple Method for Polyethylene Glycol-Promoted Hybridization of Mouse Myeloma Cells." *Somatic Cell Genetics* 3:231–236.
Genetic Engineering News. 1984. "HyClone Labs Gets Sole Commercial License to Hybrid Selection System." 4(5):19 and 34.
Genetic Engineering News. 1993. "Sales of Monoclonal Antibodies Predicted to Rise to $3.8 Billion by 1998." 13(14):3.
Getzoff, Elizabeth D., John A. Trainer, Richard A. Lerner, and Mario Geysen. 1988. "The Chemistry and Mechanism of Antibody Binding to Protein Antigens." *Advances in Immunology* 43:1–98.
Gilbert, Nigel G. and Michael Mulkay. 1984. *Opening Pandora's Box. A Sociological Analysis of Scientists' Discourse*. Cambridge, England: Cambridge University Press.
Goding, James W. 1983, 1986. *Monoclonal Antibodies: Principles and Practices*. London: Academic Press.

Goffman, Erving. 1986. *Frame Analysis. An Essay on the Organization of Experience.* Boston: Northeastern University Press.

Gold, Michael. 1986. *A Conspiracy of Cells.* Albany, NY: State University of New York Press.

Goldsby, Richard A., S. Srikumaran, and Albert J. Guidry. 1984. "Cell Culture and the Origins of Hybridoma Technology." In *Hybridoma Technology in Agricultural and Veterinary Research*, eds. Norman J. Stern and H. Ray Gamble, pp. 8–14. Totowa, NJ: Rowman & Allanheld.

Goodman, Nelson. 1978. *Ways of Worldmaking.* Indianapolis, IN: Hackett Publishing Company.

Gordon, Deborah R. 1988. "Clinical Science and Clinical Expertise: Changing Boundaries Between Art and Science in Medicine." In *Biomedicine Examined*, eds. Margaret Lock and Deborah R. Gordon, pp. 257–295. Dordrecht, The Netherlands: Kluwer.

Gosling, James P. 1990. "A Decade of Development in Immunoassay Methodology." *Clinical Chemistry* 36:1408–1427.

Government of Canada. 1981. *Biotechnology: A Development Plan for Canada. Report of the Task Force on Biotechnology.* Ottawa: Ministry of Supply and Services.

Greenlee, Lorance. 1982. "Patenting Hybridoma Technology. Plunging Farther into Uncharted Territory." In *The Impact of Hybridoma Technology on the Medical Device and Diagnostic Product Industry. Proceedings of the Educational Seminar. HIMA Report No. 82–1*, ed. Timothy J. Henry, pp. 127–132. Washington D.C.: Health Industry Manufacturers Association.

Haaijman, J.J., C. Deen, C.J.M. Kröse, J.J. Zijlstra, J. Coolen, and J. Radl. 1984. "A Jungle Full of Pitfalls." *Immunology Today* 5:56–58.

Haber, Edgar. 1977. "Introduction." In *Antibodies in Human Diagnosis and Therapy*, eds. Edgar Haber and Richard M. Krause, pp. 1–6. New York: Raven Press.

Hacking, Ian. 1983. *Representing and Intervening.* Cambridge, England: Cambridge University Press.

Hacking, Ian. 1986. "Culpable Ignorance of Interference Effects." In *Values at Risk*, ed. Douglas MacLean, pp. 136–154. Totowa, NJ: Rowman & Allanheld.

Hacking, Ian. 1992. "The Self-Vindication of the Laboratory Sciences." In *Science as Practice and Culture*, ed. Andrew Pickering, pp. 29–64. Chicago: The University of Chicago Press.

Hall, P. 1984. "The Business of Biotechnology." *Financial World* (21 March—3 April): 8–14.

Hamlyn, David W. 1984. *Metaphysics.* Cambridge, England: Cambridge University Press.

Hämmerling, Günter J., M. Reth, Hilmar Lemke, J. Hewitt, I. Melchers, and Klaus Rajewsky. 1978. "Fusion of Myelomas and T lymphomas with Immunocytes." In *Protides of the Biological Fluids. Proceedings of the Twenty-Fifth Colloquium. Brugge, 1977*, ed. H. Peeters, pp. 551–558. Oxford: Pergamon Press.

Hampar, Berge, Martin Zweig, Harvey Rabin, Conrad J. Heilman, Ralph F. Hopkins, and Russel H. Neubauer. 1980. "Test Methods Employing Monoclonal Antibodies Against *Herpes Simplex* Virus Types 1 and 2 Nucleocapsids Proteins." *United States Patent* 4,430,437, filed August 27, 1980, issued February 7, 1984.

Harlow, Ed and David Lane. 1988. *Antibodies. A Laboratory Manual.* Cold Spring Harbor, NY: Cold Spring Harbor Laboratory Press.

Harris, Alan W. and Melvin Cohn. 1970. "Physiology and Genetics of Some Lymphoid Cell Functions." In *Developmental Aspects of Antibody Formation and Structure*, Vol. 1, eds. J. Sterzl and I. Riha, pp. 275–279. Prague: Academia.

Harris, Henry. 1970. *Cell Fusion*. Cambridge, MA: Harvard University Press.

Harris, Henry and J.F. Watkins. 1965. "Hybrid Cells Derived from Mouse and Man: Artificial Heterokaryons of Mammalian Cells from Different Species." *Nature* 205:640–646.

Hasse, M. 1990. "Monoclonal Antibodies for Use in Man: Current Regulatory Situation in the Federal Republic of Germany." In *Symposium on Monoclonal Antibodies for Therapy, Prevention, and In Vivo Diagnosis of Human Disease. Utrecht, The Netherlands, 1989. Developments in Biological Standardization*, Vol. 71, pp. 213–220. Basel: Karger.

Herodotus. 1972. *The Histories*. Harmondsworth, England: Penguin Books.

Herzenberg, Leonard A. and Jeffrey A. Ledbetter. 1979. "Monoclonal Antibodies and the Fluorescence-Activated Cell Sorter: Complementary Tools in Lymphoid Cell Biology." In *The Molecular basis of Immune Cell Function*, ed. J. Gordin Kaplan, pp. 315–330. Amsterdam: Elsevier/North Holland Biomedical Press.

Herzenberg, Leonard A. and Leon Wofsy. 1977. "Cell Separation and Characterization." In *Immune System: Genetics and Regulation. ICN-UCLA Symposia on Molecular and Cellular Biology. Vol. VI, 1977*, eds. Eli Sercarz, Leonard Herzenberg, and C. Fred Fox, pp. 341–343.

Herzenberg, Leonard A., Richard G. Sweet, and Leonore A. Herzenberg. 1976. "Fluorescence-Activated Cell Sorting." *Scientific American* 243:108–117.

Hipolito, Nino. 1982. "Bureau of Medical Devices Position on Approval of Hybridoma-Derived Products." In *The Impact of Hybridoma Technology on the Medical Device and Diagnostic Product Industry. Proceedings of the Educational Seminar. HIMA Report No. 82-1*, ed. Timothy J. Henry, pp. 93–103. Washington D.C.: Health Industry Manufacturers Association.

Hirschfeld, Jan. 1980. "The Doctrine of Monospecific Antibodies." *African Journal of Clinical and Experimental Immunology* 1:23–44.

Horibata, Kengo and Alan W. Harris. 1970. "Mouse Myelomas and Lymphomas in Culture." *Experimental Cell Research* 60:61–77.

Houba, V. 1984. "The Interest of WHO in Monoclonal Antibodies." In *Monoclonal Antibodies: Standardization of their Characterization and Use. Developments in Biological Standardization*, Vol. 57, eds. M. Barme and W. Hennessen, pp. 3–4. Basel: Karger.

Howes, E.L., E.A. Clark, E. Smith, and N.A. Mitchison. 1979. "Mouse Hybrid Cell Lines Produce Antibodies to Herpes Simplex Virus Type 1." *Journal of General Virology* 44:81–87.

Hsiung, G.D., M.L. Landry, D.R. May, and C.K. Fong. 1984. "Laboratory Diagnosis of Herpes Simplex Virus Type 1 and Type 2 Infections." *Clinics in Dermatology* 2:67–82.

Hughes, Thomas Parke. 1989. *American Genesis: A Century of Invention and Technological Enthusiasm 1870–1970*. New York: Viking.

Hybridoma Techniques.1980. *EMBO, SKMB Course, Basel*. Cold Spring Harbor, NY: Cold Spring Harbor Laboratory Press.

In re Wands. 8 USPQ2d, 1400–1408.

Irvins Jr., William M.I. 1969. *Prints and Visual Communication*. New York: Da Capo Press.

Jasanoff, Sheila, Gerald E. Markle, James C. Petersen, and Trevor Pinch, eds. 1995. *Handbook of Science and Technology Studies*. Thousand Oaks, CA: Sage.

Jones, Bryn. 1983. "Division of Labour and Distribution of Tacit Knowledge in the Automation of Metal Machining." In *Design of Work in Automated Manufacturing Systems*, ed. T. Martin, pp. 19–22. New York: Pergamon Press.

Jones, Bryn and Stephen Wood. 1984. "Qualifications tacites, division du travail et nouvelles technologies." *Sociologie du Travail* 4:407–421.

Jullien, François. 1992. *La propension des choses*. Paris: Seuil.

Kahan, B., R. Auerbach, B.J. Alter, and F.H. Bach. 1982. "Histocompatibility and Isoenzyme Differences in Commercially Supplied 'BALB/c' Mice." *Science* 217:379–381.

Kahan, Jonathan S. 1986. "The Evolution of FDA Regulation of New Medical Device Technology and Product Applications." *Food Drug Cosmetic Law Journal* 41:207–214.

Kampmeier, R.H. 1993. "Herpes Simplex." In *The Cambridge World History of Human Disease*, ed. Kenneth F. Kiple, pp. 773–778. Cambridge, England: Cambridge University Press.

Kay, Lily E. 1988. "Laboratory Technology and Biological Knowledge: The Tiselius Electrophoresis Apparatus, 1930–1945." *History and Philosophy of the Life Sciences* 10:51–72.

Kearney, John F., Andreas Radburch, Nerhard Liesegang, and Klaus Rajewsky. 1979. "A New Mouse Myeloma Cell Line that has Lost Immunoglobulin Expression but Permits the Construction of Antibody-Secreting Hybrid Cell Lines." *The Journal of Immunology* 123:1548–1550.

Keating, Peter and Alberto Cambrosio. 1994. "'Ours Is an Engineering Approach': Flow Cytometry and the Constitution of Human T-Cell Subsets." *Journal of the History of Biology* 27:449–479.

Keating, Peter, Alberto Cambrosio, and Michael Mackenzie. 1992. "The Tools of the Discipline: Standards, Models and Measures in the Affinity/Avidity Controversy in Immunology." In *The Right Tools for the Job: At Work in Twentieth-Century Life Sciences*, eds. Adele E. Clarke and Joan H. Fujimura, pp. 312–354. Princeton, NJ: Princeton University Press.

Keating, Peter, Camille Limoges and Alberto Cambrosio. 1995. "The Automated Laboratory: The Generation and Replication of Work in Molecular Genetics." *Sociology of the Sciences Yearbook,* forthcoming.

Kennett, Roger H. 1981. "Hybridomas: A New Dimension in Biological Analysis." *In Vitro* 17:1036–1050.

Kennett, Roger H., K.A. Davis, A.S. Tung, and Norman R. Klinman. 1978. "Hybrid Plasmacytoma Production: Fusions with Adult Spleen Cells, Monoclonal Spleen Fragments, Neonatal Spleen Cells and Human Spleen Cells." In *Lymphocyte Hybridomas. Current Topics in Microbiology and Immunology. 81*, eds. Fritz Melchers, Michael Potter, and Noel L. Warner, pp. 77–91. Berlin: Springer Verlag.

Kenney, Martin. 1986. *Biotechnology. The Universe-Industrial Complex*. New Haven, CT: Yale University Press.

Killington, R.A., L. Newhook, N. Balachandran, William E. Rawls, and Silvia Bacchetti. 1981. "Production of Hybrid Cell Lines Secreting Antibodies to Herpes Simplex Virus Type 2." *Journal of Virological Methods* 2:223–236.

Klausner, Arthur. 1984. "Hopkins Lab Improves Hybridoma Production." *Bio/Technology* 2:743–744.

Klausner, Arthur. 1985. "Ortho Awaits Nod on Therapeutic Monoclonal." *Bio/Technology* 3:961.
Klausner, Arthur. 1987a. "'Quadromas' Yield Bispecific Antibodies." *Bio/Technology* 5:195–196.
Klausner, Arthur. 1987b. "Stage Set for 'Immunological Star Wars.'" *Bio/Technology* 5:867–868.
Klinman, Norman R. 1969. "Antibody with Homogeneous Antigen Binding Produced by Splenic Foci in Organ Culture." *Immunochemistry* 6:757–759.
Klinman, Norman R. 1975. *Clonal Analysis of the Immune Mechanism (Mice)*. Grant proposal (project number 5R01 AI08778-07, NIH-CRISP database).
Knorr-Cetina, Karin D. 1981. *The Manufacture of Knowledge. An Essay on the Constructivist and Contextual Nature of Science*. New York: Pergamon Press.
Knorr-Cetina, Karin and K. Amann. 1990. "Image Dissection in Natural Scientific Inquiry." *Science, Technology, & Human Values* 15:259–283.
Knorr-Cetina, Karin D. and Michael Mulkay, eds. 1983. *Science Observed. Perspectives on the Social Study of Science*. London: Sage.
Koch, C. and J. Bennedsen. 1989/1990. "Monoclonal Antibodies." *Current Opinion in Immunology* 2:385–391.
Köhler, Georges. 1981. "Why Hybridomas?" *Hybridoma* 1:1–4.
Köhler, Georges. 1985. *Vortrag zur Basler Ehrungsfeier am 23.1.85*. Unpublished manuscript.
Köhler, Georges and César Milstein. 1975. "Continuous Cultures of Fused Cells Secreting Antibody of Predefined Specificity." *Nature* 256:495–497.
Köhler, Georges and César Milstein. 1976. "Derivation of Specific Antibody-Producing Tissue Culture and Tumor Lines by Cell Fusion." *European Journal of Immunology* 6:511–519.
Köhler, Georges, S.C. Howe, and César Milstein. 1976. "Fusion Between Immunoglobulin-Secreting and Nonsecreting Myeloma Cell Lines." *European Journal of Immunology* 6:292–295.
Köhler, Georges, Terry Pearson, and César Milstein. 1977. "Fusion of T and B Cells." *Somatic Cell Genetics* 3:303–312.
Köhler, Georges, H. Hengartner, and César Milstein. 1978. "The Sequence of Immunoglobulin Chain Losses in Mouse (myeloma x B-cell) Hybrids." In *Protides of the Biological Fluids. Proceedings of the Twenty-Fifth Colloquium. Brugge, 1977*, ed. H. Peeters, pp. 545–549. Oxford: Pergamon Press.
Köhler, Georges, H. Hengartner, and M.J. Shulman. 1978. "Immunoglobulin Production by Lymphocyte Hybridomas." *European Journal of Immunology* 8:82–88.
Kohler, Robert, E. 1991. "Systems of Production: Drosophila, Neurospora, and Biochemical Genetics." *Historical Studies in the Physical and Biological Sciences* 22:87–130.
Kolakowsky, Stephen C. 1990. "Home Use Diagnostics: Special Considerations." In *The Medical Device Industry*, ed. Norman F. Estrin, pp. 417–433. New York: Marcel Dekker.
Koprowski, Hilary. 1969. "Centaurs of 2001." *Transactions and Studies of the College of Physicians of Philadelphia* 36:242–253.
Koprowski, Hilary and Carlo M. Croce. 1978. "Method of Producing Tumor Antibodies." U.S. Patent 4,172,124, filed April 28, 1978, issued October 23, 1979.
Koprowski, Hilary and Carlo Croce. 1980. "Hybridomas Revisited." *Science* 210:248
Koprowski, Hilary and Barbara Knowles. 1974. "Viruses, Immune Functions, and Anti-

genic Determinants in Heterokaryons and Hybrids." In *Somatic Cell Hybridization*, eds. Richard L. Davidson and Felix F. de la Cruz, pp. 71–100. New York: Raven Press.

Koprowski, Hilary, Walter Gerhard, and Carlo M. Croce. 1977a. "Production of Antibodies Against Influenza Virus by Somatic Cell Hybrids Between Mouse Myeloma and Primed Spleen Cells." *Proceedings of the National Academy of Sciences of the United States of America* 74:2985–2988

Koprowski, Hilary, Walter V. Gerhard, and Carlo M. Croce. 1977b. "Process for Providing Viral Antibodies by Fusing a Viral Antibody Producing Cell and a Myeloma Cell to Provide a Fused Cell Hybrid Culture and Collecting Viral Antibodies." U.S. Patent 4,196,265, filed June 15, 1977, issued April 1, 1980.

Koprowski, Hilary, Walter Gerhard, Tadeusz Wiktor, J. Martinis, M. Shander, and Carlo M. Croce. 1978. "Anti-viral and Anti-Tumor Antibodies Produced by Somatic Cell Hybrids." In *Lymphocyte Hybridomas. Current Topics in Microbiology and Immunology. 81*, eds. Fritz Melchers, Michael Potter, and Noel L. Warner, pp. 8–19. Berlin: Springer Verlag.

Krause, Richard M. 1970. "The Search for Antibodies with Molecular Uniformity." *Advances in Immunology* 12:1–56.

Krimsky, Sheldon. 1991. *Biotechnics and Society. The Rise of Industrial Genetics*. New York: Praeger.

Kuhn, Thomas S. 1962. *The Structure of Scientific Revolutions*. Chicago: The University of Chicago Press.

Kung, Patrick C., Gideon Goldstein, Ellis Reinherz, and Stuart F. Schlossman. 1979. "Monoclonal Antibodies Defining Distinctive Human T Cell Surface Antigens." *Science* 206:347–349.

Kusterer, Kenneth C. 1979. *Know-How on the Job. The Important Working Knowledge of "Unskilled" Workers*. Boulder, CO: Westview Press.

Lakoff, George. 1987. *Women, Fire, and Dangerous Things*. Chicago: University of Chicago Press.

Lakoff, George and Mark Johnson. 1980. *Metaphors We Live By*. Chicago: University of Chicago Press.

Latour, Bruno. 1987. *Science in Action*. Cambridge, MA: Harvard University Press.

Latour, Bruno. 1988. "The Politics of Explanation: An Alternative." In *Knowledge and Reflexivity: New Frontiers in the Sociology of Knowledge*, ed. Steve Woolgar, pp. 155–176. London: Sage.

Latour, Bruno and Steve Woolgar. 1986. *Laboratory Life. The Construction of Scientific Facts*, 2nd ed. Princeton, NJ: Princeton University Press.

Law, John. 1983. "Enrôlement et contre-enrôlement: les luttes pour la publication d'un article scientifique." *Social Science Information* 22:237–251.

Law, John and John Whittaker. 1986. "On the Malleability of People and Computers: A Focused Approach to Office Ethnography." Department of Sociology, Social Anthropology and Social Work, University of Keele, England.

Lawrence, Christopher. 1985. "Incommunicable Knowledge: Science, Technology and the Clinical Art in Britain 1850–1914." *Journal of Contemporary History* 20:503–520.

Lemke, Hilmar, Günter J. Hämmerling, and U. Hämmerling. 1979. "The Specificity Analysis with Monoclonal Antibodies of Antigens Controlled by the Major Histocompatibility Complex and by the Qa/TL Region in Mice." *Immunological Reviews* 47:175–206.

Lemke, Hilmar, Günter J. Hämmerling, Christine Höhmann, and Klaus Rajewsky. 1978. "Hybrid Cell Lines Secreting Monoclonal Antibody Specific for Major Histocompatibility Antigens of the Mouse." *Nature* 271:249–251.
Leo, John. 1982. "The New Scarlet Letter." *Time* (2 August):62–66.
Levi, Primo. 1975. *Il sistema periodico*. Torino, Italy: Einaudi.
Levy, R., J. Dilley, and L.A. Lampson. 1978. "Human Normal and Leukemia Cell Surface Antigens. Mouse Monoclonal Antibodies as Probes." In *Lymphocyte Hybridomas. Current Topics in Microbiology and Immunology. 81*, eds. Fritz Melchers, Michael Potter, and Noel L. Warner, pp. 164–169. Berlin: Springer Verlag.
Liddell, Eryl J. and A. Cryer. 1991. *A Practical Guide to Monoclonal Antibodies*. Chichester, England: John Wiley and Sons.
Littlefield, John W. 1964a. "Selection of Hybrids from Mating of Fibroblasts In Vitro and their Presumed Recombinants." *Science* 145:709–710.
Littlefield, John W. 1964b. "The Selection of Hybrid Mouse Fibroblasts." *Cold Spring Harbor Symposia on Quantitative Biology*. 29:161–166.
Littlefield, John W. 1973. "Medium for Hybrid Selection [letter]." *Science* 180:255.
Littlefield, John W. 1987. "The Early History of Mammalian Somatic Cell Fusion." In *Cell Fusion*, ed. Arthur E. Sowers, pp. 421–426. New York: Plenum Press.
Lo, Mathew M.S., Tian Yow Tsong, Mary K. Conrad, Stephen M. Strittmatter, Lynda D. Hester, and Solomon H. Snyder. 1984. "Monoclonal Antibody Production by Receptor-Mediated Electrically Induced Cell Fusion." *Nature* 310:792–794.
Löwy, Ilana and Jean-Paul Gaudillière. 1994. "Disciplining Cancer: Mice and the Practice of Genetic Purity." Paper presented at the Colloquium "Des manufactures à la facture des connaissances." Paris, 19–20 May.
Luttenberger, Franz. 1992. "Arrhenius vs. Ehrlich on Immunochemistry: Decisions about Scientific Progress in the Context of the Nobel Prize." *Theoretical Medicine* 13:137–173.
Lynch, Michael. 1982. "Technical Work and Critical Inquiry: Investigations in a Scientific Laboratory." *Social Studies of Science* 12:499–533.
Lynch, Michael. 1985. *Art and Artifact in Laboratory Science*. London: Routledge & Kegan Paul.
Lynch, Michael. 1988. "Sacrifice and the Transformation of the Animal Body into a Scientific Object: Laboratory Culture and Ritual Practice in the Neurosciences." *Social Studies of Science* 18:265–289.
Lynch, Michael and Steve Woolgar, eds. 1990. *Representation in Scientific Practice*. Cambridge, MA: MIT Press.
Macario, Alberto J.L. and Everly Conway de Macario. 1985. "Introduction: Monoclonal Antibodies Against Bacteria for Medicine, Dentistry, Veterinary Sciences, Biotechnology, and Industry—An Overview." In *Monoclonal Antibodies Against Bacteria*, Vol. 1, eds. Alberto J.L. Macario and Everly Conway de Macario, pp. xvii–xxxiii. Orlando: Academic Press.
Mackenzie, Michael, Alberto Cambrosio, and Peter Keating. 1988. "The Commercial Application of a Scientific Discovery: The Case of the Hybridoma Technique." *Research Policy* 17:155–170.
Mackenzie, Michael, Peter Keating, and Alberto Cambrosio. 1990. "Patents and Free Scientific Information in Biotechnology: Making Monoclonal Antibodies Proprietary." *Science, Technology, & Human Values* 15:65–83.
Manson, Lionel A. 1994. "Review of *Tumour Immunobiology: A Practical Approach*." *Immunology Today* 15:93–94.

March, James G. 1978. "Bounded Rationality, Ambiguity and the Engineering of Choice." *Bell Journal of Economics* 9:587–608.
March, James G. and Herbert Simon. 1958. *Organizations*. New York: Wiley.
March, James G. and Herbert A. Simon. 1970. "Decision-Making Theory." In *The Sociology of Organizations: Basic Studies*, eds. O. Grusky and G.A. Miller, pp. 93–102. New York: The Free Press.
Marcus, Irving. 1981. "International Patent Procedures." *In Vitro* 17:1086–1088.
Margulies, David H., W. Michael Kuehl, and Matthew D. Scharff. 1976. "Somatic Cell Hybridization of Mouse Myeloma Cells." *Cell* 8:405–415.
Markle, Gerald E. and Stanley S. Robin. 1985. "Biotechnology and the Social Reconstruction of Molecular Biology." *Science, Technology, & Human Values* 10:70–79.
McDade, Joseph E. 1985. "Diagnostic Applications of Monoclonal Antibodies: Infectious Disease Diagnosis." In *Monoclonal Antibodies in Clinical Diagnostic Medicine*, ed. David S. Gordon, pp. 137–155. New York: Igaku-Shoin.
McGough, Kevin J. and Daniel P. Burke. 1992. "The End of Monoclonal Patents?" *Bio/Technology* 10:1082–1083.
McGraw-Hill's Biotechnology Newswatch. 1981a. "'Instant' Monoclonal Test for Rabies Reaches Market." 1(5):7.
McGraw-Hill's-Biotechnology Newswatch. 1981b. "New Firm Puts Millions into VD Diagnostic Kits." 1(5):7.
McGraw-Hill's Biotechnology Newswatch. 1982a. "Building a Better Mouse Hybridoma." 2(4):7.
McGraw-Hill's Biotechnology Newswatch. 1982b. "Speakers at Battelle '82 Bearish on Market Future, Medical Uses of Monoclonals." 2(14):6.
McGraw-Hill's Biotechnology Newswatch. 1982c. "Mongrel Mice Caused No Major Monoclonal Losses, Hybridoma Makers Report." 2(16):5.
McGraw-Hill's Biotechnology Newswatch. 1984a. "Ames, Beckman, DuPont Compete in Theophylline Monoclonal Assay Kits." 4(1):5.
McGraw-Hill's Biotechnology Newswatch. 1984b. "FDA Gives 'Generic Okay' to Monoclonals, Biologics from Cancer Cell Lines." 4(16):6.
McGraw-Hill's Biotechnology Newswatch. 1984c. "Johns Hopkins Upgrades Hybridoma Formation for High-Affinity Monoclonals." 4(16):2–3.
McGraw-Hill's Biotechnology Newswatch. 1985a. "Allergenetics' Monoclonal Allergy Assays Square Off Against Polyclonal Tests." 5(1):7.
McGraw-Hill's Biotechnology Newswatch. 1985b. "Financial Fair-Goers Pick Med-Test Development over Monoclonal Research." 5(2):3.
McGraw-Hill's Biotechnology Newswatch. 1985c. "Monoclonals Wage Uphill Struggle for Lion's Share of Diagnostic-Test Market." 5(3):6.
McGraw-Hill's Biotechnology Newswatch. 1985d. "Syva, UCSF Disagree Over Monoclonal Chlamydia Test." 5(13):4.
McGraw-Hill's Biotechnology Newswatch. 1986. "Hybritech Sues Abbott." 6(24):3.
Medawar, Peter. 1963. "Is the Scientific Paper a Fraud?" *The Listener* (12 September):377–378.
Melchers, Fritz, Michael Potter, and Noel L. Warner. 1978. "Preface." In *Lymphocyte Hybridomas. Current Topics in Microbiology and Immunology. 81*, eds. Fritz Melchers, Michael Potter, and Noel L. Warner, pp. ix–xxiii. Berlin: Springer Verlag.
Merchant, Bruce E. 1982. "Points to Consider During Monoclonal Antibody Production."

In *The Impact of Hybridoma Technology on the Medical Device and Diagnostic Product Industry. Proceedings of the Educational Seminar. HIMA Report No. 82–1*, ed. Timothy J. Henry, pp. 83–92. Washington D.C.: Health Industry Manufacturers Association.

Milstein, César. 1980. "Monoclonal Antibodies" *Scientific American* 243:66–74.

Milstein, César. 1981. "Monoclonal Antibodies from Hybrid Myelomas (The 1980 Wellcome Lecture)." *Proceedings of the Royal Society of London* B211:393–412.

Milstein, César. 1984. "The Impact of Monoclonal Antibodies on Studies of the Differentiation of Lymphocytes." In *Leucocyte Typing. Human Leucocyte Differentiation Antigens Detected by Monoclonal Antibodies*, eds. Alain Bernard, Laurence Boumsell, Jean Dausset, César Milstein, and Stuart Schlossman, pp. 3–8. Berlin: Springer Verlag.

Milstein, César. 1986. "From Antibody Structure to Immunological Diversification of Immune Response." *Science* 231:1261–1268.

Milstein, César. 1990. *Notes for a Lecture in Miami January 1990*. Unpublished manuscript.

Milstein, César . 1993. "Patents on Scientific Discoveries are Unfair and Potentially Dangerous." *The Scientist* 7(21):11.

Milstein, César and Len Herzenberg. 1977. "T and B Cell Hybrids." In *Immune System: Genetics and Regulation. ICN-UCLA Symposia on Molecular and Cellular Biology. Vol. VI, 1977*, eds. Eli Sercarz, Leonard Herzenberg and C. Fred Fox, pp. 273–275. New York: Academic Press.

Milstein, César and Georges Köhler. 1977. "Cell fusion and the Derivation of Cell Lines Producing Specific Antibody." In *Antibodies in Human Diagnosis and Therapy*, eds. Edgar Haber and Richard M. Krause, pp. 271–284. New York: Raven Press.

Milstein, César and A.J. Munro. 1973. "Genetics of Immunoglobulins and of the Immune response." In *Defense and Recognition,* ed. R.R. Porter, pp. 199–228. London: Butterworth.

Milstein, César and J. Svasti. 1971. "Expansion and Contraction in the Evolution of Immunoglobulin Gene Pools." In *Progress in Immunology. First International Congress of Immunology*, ed. Bernard Amos, pp. 33–45. New York: Academic Press.

Milstein, César and B.W. Wright. 1980. "Rat Myeloma Cell Line which Does Not Express an Immunoglobulin Chain, YB213.0.Ag.20, Is Prepared from Cell Line Y3-Ag1.2.3 via Hybrid Myeloma Cell Line." European Patent 0,043,718, filed in the UK July 7, 1980, issued January 13, 1982.

Milstein, César, G.G. Brownlee, T.M. Harrisson, and M.B. Matthews. 1972. "A Possible Precursor of Immunoglobulin Light Chains." *Nature New Biology* 239:117–120.

Milstein, César, Kayede Adetugbo, Nicholas J. Cowan, Georges Köhler, and David S. Secher. 1978. "Expression of Antibody Genes in Tissue Culture: Structural Mutants and Hybrid Cells." In *Third Decennial Review Conference: Cell, Tissue, and Organ Culture. Gene Expression and Regulation in Cultured Cells. National Cancer Institute Monographs.*, 48, pp. 321–330. May, DHEW Publication No. [NIH] 77–1441.

Milstein, César, G.G. Brownlee, E.M. Cartwright, J.M. Jarvis, and N.J. Jarvis. 1974. "Sequence Analysis of Immunoglobulin Light Chain Messenger RNA." *Nature* 252:354–359.

Milstein, César, Kayede Adetugbo, Nicholas J. Cowan, Georges Köhler, David S. Secher, and C.D. Wilde. 1977. "Somatic Cell Genetics of Antibody-Secreting Cells: Studies of Clonal Diversification and Analysis by Cell Fusion." *Cold Spring Harbor Symposia on Quantitative Biology* 41:793–803.

Mitchell, Graham F. and Kathy M. Cruise. 1981. "Monoclonal Antiparasite Antibodies. A Shot-in-the-Arm for Immunoparasitology." In *Monoclonal Antibodies and T-Cell Hybridomas*, eds. G.J. Hämmerling, U. Hämmerling, and J.F. Kearny. Amsterdam: Elsevier.

Moulin, Anne Marie. 1990. "La métaphore du soi et le tabou de l'auto-immunité." In *Soi et Non-soi*, eds. Jean Bernard, Marcel Bessis, and Claude Debru, pp. 55–76. Paris: Seuil.

Moulin, Anne Marie. 1991. *Le dernier langage de la médecine. Histoire de l'immunologie de Pasteur au Sida*. Paris: Presses Universitaires de France.

Mulkay, Michael. 1980. "The Sociology of Science in the West." In *The Sociology of Science in East and West*, eds. Michael Mulkay and Vojin Milic. *Current Topics in Sociology* 28(3):1–84.

Myers, Greg. 1995. "From Discovery to Invention: The Writing and Rewriting of Two Patents." *Social Studies of Science* 25:57–105.

Nabholz, M., V. Miggiano, and W.F. Bodmer. 1969. "Genetic Analysis Using Human-Mouse Somatic Cell Hybrids." *Nature* 223:358–363.

Nahmias, André. 1980. "Herpes Simplex Virus Infection: Problems and Prospects as Perceived by a Peripatetic Physician." *The Yale Journal of Biology and Medicine* 53:47–54.

Nash, Martin. 1985. "On the Emergence of Commercial Products from Biotechnology." *Trends in Biotechnology* 3:219–22.

Nenning, P. and H. Bourcevet. 1990. "Zum Rechtsschutz monoklonaler Antikörper." *Die Pharmazie* 45:525–527 and 853–856.

Newmark, Peter. 1985. "The Many Merits of Monoclonals." *Nature* 316:387.

NIAID. 1981. National Institute of Allergy and Infectious Diseases. Immunology Study Group. *New Initiatives in Immunology*. Bethesda, MD: U.S. Department of Health and Human services, NIH Publication No. 81–2215, January.

NIAID. 1990. *Report of the NIAID Task Force on Immunology and Allergy*. U.S. Department of Health and Human Services, Public Health Service, National Institutes of Health, NIH Publication No. 91–2414, September.

Nigg, E.A., G. Walter, and S.J. Singer. 1982. "On the Nature of Crossreactions Observed with Antibodies Directed to Defined Epitopes." *Proceedings of the National Academy of Sciences of the United States of America* 79:5939–5943.

Nowinski, Robert C., M.R. Tam, L.C. Goldstein, L. Strong, C.-C. Kuo, L. Corey, W.E. Stamm, H.H. Handsfield, J.S. Knapp, and K.K. Holmes. 1983. "Monoclonal Antibodies for Diagnosis of Infectious Diseases in Humans." *Science* 219:637–644.

Oakeshot, M. 1951. *Political Education*. Cambridge, England: Cambridge University Press.

O'Connell, Joseph. 1993. "Metrology: The Creation of Universality by the Circulation of Particulars." *Social Studies of Science* 23:129–173.

OECD. 1988. Organisation de Coopération et de Développement Économiques, Comité de la politique scientifique et technologique. *Effets économiques à long terme de la biotechnologie*, document SPT(88)15. Paris.

Office of Technology Assessment. 1984. *Commercial Biotechnology: An International Analysis*, OTA-B-218. Springfield, VA: National Technical Information Service.

Okada, Yoshio. 1958. "The Fusion of Ehrlich's Tumor Cells Caused by HVJ Virus in Vitro." *Biken Journal* 1:103–110.

Okada, Yoshio. 1962. "Analysis of Giant Polynuclear Cell Formation Caused by HVJ Virus from Ehrlich's Ascites Tumor Cells." *Experimental Cell Research* 26:98–107.

Oteri, J.S., M.G. Weinberg, and M.S. Pinales. 1973. "Cross-Examination of Chemists in Narcotics and Marijuana Cases." *Contemporary Drug Problems* 2:225–238.

Oudshoorn, Nelly. 1990. "On the Making of Sex Hormones: Research Materials and the Production of Knowledge." *Social Studies of Science* 20:5–33.

Pages, Jaqueline M. and Alain E. Bussard. 1978. "Establishment and Characterization of a Permanent Murine Hybridoma Secreting Monoclonal Antibodies." *Cellular Immunology* 41:188–194.

Panem, Sandra. 1984. *The Interferon Crusade*. Washington, D.C.: The Brookings Institution.

Parks, David R., Leonore A. Herzenberg and Leonard A. Herzenberg. 1989. "Flow Cytometry and Fluorescence-Activated Cell Sorting." In *Fundamental Immunology*, ed. William E. Paul, pp. 781–802. New York: Raven Press.

Pasveer, Bernike. 1989. "Knowledge of Shadows: The Introduction of X-Ray Images in Medicine." *Sociology of Health & Illness* 11:360–381.

Pelissolo, Jean-Claude. 1980. *La biotechnologie, demain?* Paris: La Documentation Française.

Pereira, Leonore. 1982. "Monoclonal Antibodies to Herpes Simplex Viruses 1 and 2." In *Monoclonal Hybridoma Antibodies: Techniques and Applications*, ed. John G.R. Hurrell, pp. 120–138. Boca Raton, FL: CRC Press.

Pereira, Leonore, Tom Klassen, and J. Richard Baringer. 1980. "Type Common and Type-Specific Monoclonal Antibody to Herpes Simplex Virus Type 1." *Infection and Immunity* 29:724–732.

Pereira, Leonore, Dale Dondero, B. Norrild, and B. Roizman. 1981. "Differential Immunologic Reactivity and Processing of Glycoproteins gA and gB of Herpes Simplex Virus Type 1 and 2 made in Vero and HEp-2 cells." *Proceedings of the National Academy of Sciences of the United States of America* 78:5202–5206.

Pereira, Leonore, Dale Dondero, Danal Gallo, Veronica Devlin, and James D. Woodie. 1982. "Serological Analysis of Herpes Simplex Virus Types 1 and 2 with Monoclonal Antibodies." *Infection and Immunity* 35:363–362.

Peterson, Eric, Otwin W. Schmitt, Lynn C. Goldstein, and Robert C. Nowinski. 1983. "Typing of Clinical Herpes Simplex Virus Isolates with Mouse Monoclonal Antibodies to Herpes Simplex Virus Type 1 and 2: Comparison with Type-Specific Rabbit Antisera and Restriction Endonuclease Analysis of Viral DNA." *Journal of Clinical Microbiology* 17:92–96.

Pickering, Andrew. 1991. "Objectivity and the Mangle of Practice." *Annals of Scholarship* 8:409–425.

Pickering, Andrew, ed. 1992. *Science as Practice and Culture*. Chicago: The University of Chicago Press.

Pinch, Trevor. 1985. "Towards an Analysis of Scientific Observation: The Externality and Evidential Significance of Observation Reports in Physics." *Social Studies of Science* 15:1–36.

Pinch, Trevor. 1986. *Confronting Nature*. Dordrecht, The Netherlands: Reidel.

Pirovski, L., A. Casadevall, L. Rodriguez, L.S. Zuckier, and H.D. Scharff. 1990. "Current State of the Hybridoma Technology." *Journal of Clinical Immunology* 10(4S):5S–12S.

Plant, David W. 1986. "The Impact of Biotechnology on Patent Law." In *Biotechnology in Society. Private Initiatives and Public Oversight*, ed. Joseph G. Perpich, pp. 125–136. New York: Pergamon Press.

Plant, David W., Niels J. Reimers, and Norton D. Zinder, eds. 1982. *Patenting Life Forms. Banbury Report 10.* Cold Spring Harbor, NY: Cold Spring Harbor Laboratory Press.

Pollock, R.R., J.L. Teillaud, and Matthew D. Scharff. 1984. "Monoclonal Antibodies: A Powerful Tool for Selecting and Analyzing Mutations in Antigens and Antibodies." *Annual Review of Microbiology* 38:389–417.

Pomerantz, Anita. 1987. "Descriptions in Legal Settings." In *Talk and Social Organization*, eds. G. Button and J. Lee, pp. 226–243. Clevedon, England: Multilingual Matters.

Poncelet, P. and R. Rohcucci. 1984. "Preface." In *Flow Cytometry and Monoclonal Antibodies for Therapy Monitoring. Symposium "QUO VADIS?"—SANOFI. Montpellier, October 25–26, 1982*, pp. 1–3. Montpellier: Groupe SANOFI, Centre de recherches de Montpellier.

Pontecorvo, Guido. 1975. "Production of Mammalian Somatic Cell Hybrids by Means of Polyethylene Glycol Treatment." *Somatic Cell Genetics* 1:397–400.

Pontecorvo, Guido. 1990. "Fusing Cultured Mammalian Cells with Polyethylene Glycol." *Current Contents* (5 March):15.

Potter, Michael. 1986. "Myeloma Proteins." *Experientia* 42:967–970.

Prescott, Lawrence. 1983. "Hybritech: Portrait of a Monoclonal Specialist." *Bio/Technology* 1:156–161.

Price, Derek J. de Solla. 1961. *Science since Babylon*. New Haven, CT: Yale University Press.

Rajewsky, Klaus, G. von Hesberg, Hilmar Lemke, and Günter J. Hämmerling. 1978. "The Isolation of Thirteen Cloned Hybrid Cell Lines Secreting Mouse Strain A Derived Antibodies with Specificity for a Group A Streptococcal Carbohydrate." *Annales d'Immunologie (Institut Pasteur)*, 129C:389–400.

Raub, William F. 1981. "NIH Policies on Hybridomas." *In Vitro* 17:1089–1090.

Rawls, William E., Silvia Bacchetti, and Frank L. Graham. 1977. "Relation of Herpes Simplex Viruses to Human Malignancies." *Current Topics in Microbiology and Immunology* 77:71–95.

Ravetz, Jerome R. 1971. *Scientific Knowledge and its Social Problems*. New York: Oxford University Press.

Reinherz, Ellis L., Patrick C. Kung, Gideon Goldstein, and Stuart Schlossman. 1979a. "A Monoclonal Antibody with Selective Reactivity with Functionally Mature Human Thymocytes and All Peripheral Human T Cells." *Journal of Immunology* 123:1312–1317.

Reinherz, Ellis L., Patrick C. Kung, Gideon Goldstein, and Stuart Schlossman. 1979b. "Separation of Functional Subsets of Human T Cells By a Monoclonal Antibody." *Proceedings of the National Academy of Sciences of the United States of America* 76:4061–4065.

Rhees, Rush. 1970. "Can There be a Private Language?" In Rush Rhees, *Discussions of Wittgenstein*, pp. 55–70. London: Routledge & Kegan Paul.

Rheinberger, Hans-Jörg. 1992a. "Experiment, Difference, and Writing: I. Tracing Protein Synthesis." *Studies in History and Philosophy of Science* 23:305–331.

Rheinberger, Hans-Jörg. 1992b. "Experiment, Difference, and Writing: II. The Laboratory Production of Transfer RNA." *Studies in History and Philosophy of Science* 23:389–422.

Rheinberger, Hans-Jörg. 1993a. "Experiment and Orientation: Early Systems of In Vitro Protein Synthesis." *Journal of the History of Biology* 26:443–471.

Rheinberger, Hans-Jörg. 1993b. "Genetic Engineering and the Practice of Molecular Biology." Paper presented at the Mellon Workshop on "Genetic Engineering: Transformations in Science, Politics and Culture." Cambridge, MA, MIT, April 30 and May 1.

Rothman, Harry and D. Parkinson. 1984. "Case Study C, Monoclonal Antibodies: Historical Development and Citation Analysis." In Harry Rothman, *Analysis of Scientific Disciplines Germane to Biotechnology. Final Report*, pp. C1–C73. Biosociety Sub-programme, FAST Programme, European Community DGXII, Brussels; Technology Policy Unit, University of Aston, March.

Rouse, Joseph. 1987. *Knowledge and Power. Toward a Political Philosophy of Science*. Ithaca, NY: Cornell University Press.

Sadler, Judy. 1978. "Ideologies of 'Art' and 'Science' in Medicine. The Transition from Medical Care to the Application of Technique in the British Medical Profession." In *The Dynamics of Science and Technology*, eds. Wolfgang Krohn, Edwin T. Layton, and Peter Weingart, pp. 177–215. Dordrecht, The Netherlands: Reidel.

Salk Institute. 1977. The Salk Institute for Biological Studies. *Catalogue of Murine Immune Related Culture and Tumor Cell Lines*, Third Edition.

Salk Institute. 1979. The Salk Institute for Biological Studies. *Catalogue of Cell lines, Cancer and Immune-Related*, Fourth Edition.

Sapp, Jan. 1990. *Where the Truth Lies. Franz Moewus and the Origins of Molecular Biology*. Cambridge, England: Cambridge University Press.

Schadewaldt, Wolfgang. 1979. "The Concepts of Nature and Technique According to the Greeks." *Research in Philosophy & Technology* 2:159–171.

Scharff, Matthew D. 1981. "Cell Hybrids in Immunology." *Federation Proceedings* 38:2442–2443.

Scharff, Matthew D. 1984. "From Immunofantasy to Monoclonal Reality." In *Hybridoma Technology in Agricultural and Veterinary Research*, eds. Norman J. Stern and H. Ray Gamble, pp. 1–5. Totowa, NJ: Rowman & Allanheld.

Scharff, Matthew D. and S. Roberts. 1981. "Present Status and Future Prospects for the Hybridoma Technology." *In Vitro* 17:1072–1077.

Scharff, Matthew D., S. Roberts, and P. Thammana. 1981a. "Hybridomas as a Source of Antibodies." *Hospital Practice* 16:61–66.

Scharff, Matthew D., S. Roberts, and P. Thammana. 1981b. "Monoclonal Antibodies." *Journal of Infectious Diseases* 143:346–351.

Schmeck Jr., H.M. 1979. "Antibody Research Intensifies." *The New York Times* (23 January):C1–C2.

Schneider, Ilene. 1985. "Hybritech Balances Scientific Creativity with a Marketing Orientation." *Genetic Engineering News* 5(10):12–14.

Schon, Donald A. 1983. *The Reflective Practitioner*. New York: Basic Books.

Schwaber, Jerrold F. 1982. "Letter." *Science* 216:798.

Schwaber, Jerrold and E.P. Cohen. 1973. "Human x Mouse Somatic Cell Hybrid Clones secreting Immunoglobulins of both Parental Types." *Nature* 244:444–447.

Schwaber, Jerrold and E.P. Cohen. 1974. "Pattern of Immunoglobulin Synthesis and Assembly in a Human-Mouse Somatic Cell Hybrid Clone." *Proceedings of the National Academy of Sciences of the United States of America* 71:2203–2207.

Schwaber, Jerrold F., Marshall R. Posner, Stuart F. Schlossman, and Herbert Lazarus. 1984. "Human-Human Hybrids Secreting Pneumococcal Antibodies." *Human Immunology* 9:137–143.

Scott, M.G. 1985. "Monoclonal Antibodies. Approaching Adolescence in Diagnostic Immunoassays." *Trends in Biotechnology* 3:170–175.

Shapin, Steven. 1989. "The Invisible Technician." *American Scientist* 77:554–563.

Shay, Jerry W. 1985. "Human Hybridomas and Monoclonal Antibodies. The Biology of Cell Fusion." In *Human Hybridomas and Monoclonal Antibodies*, eds. Edgar G. Engleman, Steven K.H. Foung, James Larrick, and Andrew Rubitschek, pp. 5–20. New York: Plenum Press.

Showalter, Stephen D., Martin Zweig, and Berge Hampar. 1981. "Monoclonal Antibodies to Herpes Simplex Virus Type 1 Proteins, Including the Immediate-Early Protein ICP4." *Infection and Immunity* 34:684–692.

Silverstein, Arthur M. 1989. *A History of Immunology*. San Diego, CA: Academic Press.

Simondon, Gilbert. 1989. *Du mode d'existence des objets techniques*. Paris: Aubier.

Sinkovics, Joseph G. 1981. "Early History of Specific Antibody-producing Lymphocyte Hybridomas." *Cancer Research* 41:1246–1247.

Spinks' Report. 1980. Advisory Council for Applied Research and Development, Advisory Board for the Research Councils, and the Royal Society. *Biotechnology: Report of a Joint Working Party*. London: H.M. Stationery Office.

Spira, G., R.R. Pollock, A. Bargellesi, and Matthew D. Scharff. 1985. "Monoclonal Antibodies: A Potentially Powerful Tool in the Diagnosis and Treatment of Infectious Diseases." *European Journal of Clinical Microbiology* 4:251–256.

Springer, Timothy A., ed. 1985. *Hybridoma Technology in the Biosciences and Medicine*. New York: Plenum Press.

Staines, N.A. and A.M. Lew. 1980. "Whither Monoclonal Antibodies?" *Immunology* 40:287–93.

Star, Susan Leigh. 1983. "Simplification in Scientific Work: An Example from Neuroscience Research." *Social Studies of Science* 13:205–228.

Steplewski, Zenon and Hilary Koprowski. 1970. "Somatic Cell Fusion and Hybridization." *Methods in Cancer Research* 5:155–191.

Steplewski, Zenon, Hilary Koprowski, and Albert Leibovitz. 1976. "Polyethylene Glycol-Mediated Fusion of Human Tumor Cells with Mouse Cells." *Somatic Cell Genetics* 2:559–564.

Stokes, Terry D. 1985. "The Role of Molecular Biology in an Immunological Institute." Paper presented at the International Congress of History of Science, University of California, Berkeley.

Strawson, Peter F. 1976. "Entity and Identity." In *Contemporary British Philosophy. Personal Statements*, ed. Hywell David Lewis, pp. 193–220. London: George Allen & Unwin.

Svasti, J., and César Milstein. 1972a. "The Complete Amino Acid Sequence of a Mouse k Light Chain." *Biochemical Journal* 128:427–444.

Svasti, J., and César Milstein. 1972b. "The Disulphide Bridge of a Mouse Immunoglobulin G1 Protein." *Biochemical Journal* 126:837–850.

Swazey, Judith P. and Karen Reeds. 1978. *Today's Medicine, Tomorrow's Science. Essays on Paths of Discovery in Biomedical Sciences*. Washington, D.C.: DHEW Publication No. [NIH] 78–244.

Szybalski, Waclaw, Elizabeth Hunter Szybalska, and Giorgio Ragni. 1962. "Genetic Studies with Human Cell Lines." *National Cancer Institute Monographs*. 7:75–89.

Taggart, R. Thomas and I. Michael Samloff. 1983. "Stable Antibody-Producing Murine Hybridomas." *Science* 219:1228–1230.

Tansey, E.M. and P.P. Catterall. 1994. "Monoclonal Antibodies: A Witness Seminar in Contemporary Medical History." *Medical History* 38:322–327.

Tauber, Alfred I. 1994. *The Immune Self: Theory or Metaphor?* Cambridge, England: Cambridge University Press.

Teitelman, Robert. 1989. *Gene Dreams. Wall Street, Academia, and the Rise of Biotechnology*. New York: Basic Books.

Thévenot, Laurent. 1984. "Rules and Implements: Investment in Forms." *Social Science Information* 23:1–45.

Thompson, Keith M., David W. Hough, Peter J. Maddison, Mark D. Melamed, and Nevin Hughes-Jones. 1986. "The Efficient Production of Stable Human Monoclonal Antibody Secreting Hybridomas from EBV-Transformed Lymphocytes Using the Mouse Myeloma X63-Ag8.653 as a Fusion Partner." *Journal of Immunological Methods* 94:7–12.

Tiles, Mary. 1984. *Bachelard: Science and Objectivity*. Cambridge, England: Cambridge University Press.

Traweek, Sharon. 1984. "Nature in the Age of its Mechanical Reproduction: The Reproduction of Nature and Physicists in the High-Energy Physics Community." In *Les savoirs dans les pratiques quotidiennes. Recherches sur les représentations*, ed. Claire Belisle and Bernard Schiele, pp. 94–112. Paris: Editions du C.N.R.S.

Traweek, Sharon. 1988. *Beamtimes and Lifetimes*. Cambridge, MA: Harvard University Press.

Uhr, Jonathon W. 1984. "The 1984 Nobel Prize in Medicine." *Science* 226:1025–1028.

van den Belt, Henk. 1988. "Comment décider de l'originalité d'une invention? A.W. Hoffman et le litige du rouge d'aniline en France. 1860–1863." *Culture Technique* 18:308–317.

van den Belt, Henk and Bart Gremmen. 1990. "Specificity in the Era of Koch and Ehrlich: A Generalized Interpretation of Ludwik Fleck's 'Serological' Thought Style." *Studies in History and Philosophy of Science* 21:463–479.

van den Belt, Henk and Arie Rip. 1987. "The Nelson-Winter-Dosi Model and Synthetic Dye Chemistry." In *The Social Construction of Technological Systems*, eds. Wiebe E. Bijker, Thomas P. Hughes, and Trevor J. Pinch, pp. 135–158. Cambridge, MA: MIT Press.

Vincenti, Walter. 1984. "Technological Knowledge Without Science: The Innovation of Flush Riveting in American Airplanes, ca 1930–ca 1950." *Technology & Culture* 25:540–576.

Wade, Nicholas. 1980. "Inventor of Hybridoma Technology Failed to File for Patent." *Science* 208:693.

Wade, Nicholas. 1982. "Hybridomas: The Making of a Revolution." *Science* 215:1073–1075.

Wainwright, Milton. 1992. "The Sinkovics Hybridoma—The Discovery of the First 'Natural Hybridoma.'" *Perspectives in Biology and Medicine* 35:372–379.

Wasson, Tyler, ed. 1987. "Georges Köhler." In *Nobel Prize Winners: An H.W. Wilson Biographical Dictionary*, pp. 566–568. New York: H.W. Wilson.

Watson, James D. 1968. *The Double Helix*. New York: Atheneum.

Watson, James D. and Francis H.C. Crick. 1953. "A Structure for Deoxyribose Nucleic Acid." *Nature* 171:737–738.

Webster, Andrew and Kathryn Packer. 1994. "Patenting Culture in Science: Re-Inventing the Scientific Wheel of Credibility." Paper presented at the Conference of the European Association for the Study of Science and Technology on "Science, Technology and Change: New Theories, Realities, Institutions." Budapest, August 28–31.

Wegner, Harold C. 1982. "Hybridoma Patent Law." In *The Impact of Hybridoma Technology on the Medical Device and Diagnostic Product Industry. Proceedings of the Educational Seminar. HIMA Report No. 82–1*, ed. Timothy J. Henry, pp. 133–177. Washington D.C.: Health Industry Manufacturers Association.

Weiner, Charles. 1986. "Universities, Professors, and Patents: A Continuing Controversy." *Technology Review* 89(2):32–43.

Westerwoudt, Regine J. 1985. "Improved Fusion Methods. IV. Technical Aspects." *Journal of Immunological Methods* 77:181–196.

WHO. 1983. World Health Organization, Regional Office for Europe. *Molecular Biological and Monoclonal Antibody Techniques: Their Application to the Diagnosis, Epidemiological Study, and Control of Viral Infections of Man: Report on a WHO Meeting, Berne, 30 August–1 September 1982*. Copenhagen: World Health Organization, Regional Office for Europe; EURO Reports and Studies, vol. 88.

Wick, Mark R. 1990. "Review of *Rapid Viral Diagnosis by Immunofluorescence: An Atlas and Practical Guide*." *Immunology Today* 11:262–263.

Williams, Alan F., Giovanni Galfré and César Milstein. 1977. "Analysis of Cell Surfaces by Xenogeneic Myeloma-Hybrid Antibodies: Differentiation Antigens of Rat Lymphocytes." *Cell* 12:663–673

Wilson, Kenneth G. 1993. *The Columbia Guide to Standard American English*. New York: Columbia University Press.

Wilson, Tazewell. 1983. "Genetic Techniques Improve Hybridoma Selection." *Bio/Technology* 1:226.

Winter, Greg and César Milstein. 1991. "Man-Made Antibodies." *Nature* 349:293–299.

Woodruff, H. Boyd and Brinton M. Miller. 1981. "Patenting of Hybridomas and Genetically Engineered Microorganisms." *In Vitro* 17:1078–1080.

Woolgar, Steve. 1976. "Writing an Intellectual History of Scientific Development: The Use of Discovery Accounts." *Social Studies of Science* 6:395–422.

Wright, Susan. 1986. "Recombinant DNA Technology and Its Social Transformation." *Osiris* 2:303–360.

Yelton, Dale E. and Matthew D. Scharff. 1980. "Monoclonal Antibodies." *American Scientist* 68:510–516.

Yelton, Dale E. and Matthew D. Scharff. 1981. "Monoclonal Antibodies: A Powerful New Tool in Biology and Medicine." *Annual Review of Biochemistry* 50:657–680.

Yelton, Dale E., Betty A. Diamond, S-P. Kwan, and Matthew D. Scharff. 1978. "Fusion of Mouse Myeloma and Spleen Cells." In *Lymphocyte Hybridomas. Current Topics in Microbiology and Immunology. 81*, eds. Fritz Melchers, Michael Potter, and Noel L. Warner, pp. 1–7. Berlin: Springer Verlag.

Yelton, Dale E., David H. Margulies, Betty A. Diamond, S-P. Kwan, and Matthew D.

Schraff. 1980. "Plasmacytomas and Hybridomas: Development and Applications." In *Monoclonal Antibodies: Hybridomas: A New Dimension in Biological Analyses*, eds. Roger H. Kennet, Thomas J. McKearn, and Kathleen B. Bechtol, pp. 3–17. New York: Plenum Press.

Yewdell, J.W. and Walter Gerhard. 1981. "Antigenic Characterization of Viruses by Monoclonal Antibodies." *Annual Review of Microbiology* 35:185–206.

Young, Allan. 1992. "Making Facts and Making Time in Psychiatric Research: An Essay in the Anthropology of Scientific Knowledge." Unpublished manuscript, March.

Yoxen, Edward. 1983. *The Gene Business. Who Should Control Biotechnology?* London: Pan Books.

Zack, Donald J. and Matthew D. Scharff. 1982. "Monoclonal antibodies." In *Patenting of Life Forms. Banbury Report 10*, eds. David W. Plant, Niels J. Reimers, and Norton D. Zinder, pp. 15–23. Cold Spring Harbor, NY: Cold Spring Harbor Laboratory Press.

Zola, H. and D. Brocks. 1982. "Techniques for the Production and Characterization of Monoclonal Hybridoma Antibodies." In *Monoclonal Hybridoma Antibodies: Techniques and Applications*, ed. John G.R. Hurrell, pp. 1–57. Boca Raton, FL: CRC Press.

Zweig, Martin, Conrad J. Heilman Jr., Harvey Rabin, Ralph F. Hopkins III, Russel H. Neubauer, and Berge Hampar. 1979. "Production of Monoclonal Antibodies Against Nucleocapsid Proteins of Herpes Simplex Virus Types 1 and 2." *Journal of Virology* 32:676–678.

Zweig, Martin, Conrad J. Heilman Jr., Harvey Rabin, and Berge Hampar. 1980. "Shared Antigenic Determinants Between Two Distinct Classes of Proteins in Cells Infected with Herpes Simplex Virus." *Journal of Virology* 35:644–652.

Index

Abbott Laboratories, 109, 168, 182
Albert Einstein College of Medicine. *See also* Scharff, Matthew D.
  PEG fusogen, 42n
Allogenic immunization, 43n
Amann, K., 205n
American Type Culture Collection (ATCC), 97–98, 100
  laboratories receiving mouse myelomas from ATCC, 100, 102
Antibodies. *See also* Monoclonal antibodies; Polyclonal antibodies
  as antigens, 206n
  theories about, 210
Antigens
  antibodies as antigens, 206n
  as criteria defining monoclonal antibodies, 174–176
  differentiation antigens, 34–35, 43n
  histocompatibility antigens, 33–34
  terminological ambiguity, 193–194, 207n
Anti-influenza antibodies, 111
Antisera. *See* Polyclonal antibodies
Asad, Talal, 205n
ATCC (American Type Culture Collection), 97–98, 100
Attributional model, 5
Azaguanine, 27, 42n

Bachelard, Gaston, 104
Bacteriology, 52, 112
BALB/c mice, 11, 26
  genetic contamination, 96
Beadle, George W., 5–6
Becton-Dickinson
  distribution of monoclonal antibodies, 94, 100, 103
  FACS (fluorescence activated cell sorter), 91
  patent litigation
    Ortho vs. Becton Dickinson, 168, 174–176
Bijker, W.E., 49
Blakemore, Judith, 185, 188, 190, 197, 199
Brannigan, Augustine, 5, 171
Brock, William H., 104
Bud, Robert, 209
Bussard, Alain, 11, 12

Callon, Michel, 60, 124n, 200, 206n
Carter-Wallace, 115
CD nomenclature, 97
Cell banks, 26, 27, 43n, 99–100
Cell fusion, 40n. *See also* Fusogens; Hybridoma technology
  lymphocytes and myeloma cells failures, 24–25, 28, 29–31
Cell lines. *See also* Myeloma cell lines
  naming, 27, 42n, 78n
Centocor, 103, 108
Centre National de Transfusion Sanguine, 153
Cetus, 168–169, 176–181
Charles River Breeding Laboratories, 96
Chlamydia tests, 108
Clarke, Adele E., 203n
Clonal selection theory, 210
Cohen, E.P., 18–24
Cohn, Melvin, 24–31. *See also* Salk Institute
Cold Spring Harbor conference (1981), 167–168, 173, 174, 176
Collins, Harry M., 47, 48–49, 107
Commercialization, 41n. *See also* Diagnostic kits; Patents

Commercialization *(continued)*
 distribution of monoclonal antibodies, 94, 125n
Contextualization, 209–211
Continuity, 37–38
 Schwaber, Jerrold, and E.P. Cohen, 18–24
 Wistar Institute, 13–17
Coulter Corporation, 168
Crick, Francis, 8–9
Croce, Carl, 15, 16

Dallenbaugh, Geoffrey, 174–175
David, Gary, 186–199 passim
de Vries, G.H., 49
Descombes, Vincent, 50
Diagnostic kits, 119; 145–147, 205n
 chlamydia, 108
 hepatitis, 152–153
 herpesvirus, 137–147
 marketing to generate demand for, 114–116, 127n, 139–140
 production, 157–165
 sandwich immunoassay patents, 168, 181–200
Discoveries. *See also* Novelty; Patents
 conferring of status, 5–6
 related to fact-technique distinction, 6
Dodier, Nicolas, 203n
Draper, R.C., 49

Electrofusion, 64
Epitopes. *See* Antigens

FACS (fluorescence activated cell sorter), 91–92, 93, 125n
Fact-technique distinction, 6, 7
 hybridoma technology, 37–38
 monoclonal antibodies
  ambiguity, 7, 35–36
  related to novelty, 38
Factuality, 121–122
FDA. *See* Food and Drug Administration (FDA)
Feeder cells, 68
Ferguson, Eugene S., 49–50
First Response diagnostic kit, 114–115
Fjermedal, Grant, 38n–39n

Fleck, Ludwik, 121–122, 126n
Fluorescence activated cell sorter (FACS), 91–92, 93, 125n
Food and Drug Administration (FDA), 82, 124n
Foundational papers, 9–10, 17, 32–37
 citation analysis, 86–88
 Köhler and Milstein (1975), 9, 38n–39n, 43n
Fraud
 characterization, 5–6
Frederick Cancer Research Center, 142
Fujimura, Joan H., 62, 69, 134, 211
Fusion. *See* Cell fusion; Fusogens; Hybridoma technology
Fusogens
 chemical
  PEG (polyethylene glycol), 30, 42n–43n, 51, 64, 71
 electrofusion, 64
 viruses, 25
  Sendai virus, 25, 29, 30, 42n, 51

Generality, 81–82
 diagnostic kits, 119
 hybridoma technology, 82–85
  contingent accounts, 84–85, 91–95
  empiricist accounts, 83–84, 85–91
 research data
  citation analysis, 86–88
  immunoassays, 89–89–90
  patent analysis, 87–89
  publication data, 85–89
Genetic Systems, 135
Gerhard, Walter, 15, 111
Gilbert, Nigel G., 83, 193
Goffman, Erving, 192
Goodman, Nelson, 72
Green, R.H., 49
Greene Jr., Howard Edward, 187

Hacking, Ian, 8, 169
HAT (hypoxanthine aminopterin thymidine), 25, 26, 51, 64, 67
Hepatitis, 151–153
Herpesvirus monoclonal antibodies, 137–147

Index

Herzenberg, Leonard, 91–95, 98–99
  Hybritech vs. Monoclonal Antibodies Inc., 182, 184–199 passim
Herzenberg, Leonore, 92–95, 98–99
Horowitz Prize
  attribution to Milstein, 40n–41n
Human monoclonal antibodies, 20–21
HVJ virus. *See* Sendai virus
Hybrid cells, 25–26, 40n–41n. *See also* Cell fusion; Hybridomas
Hybridoma, 117–118, 128n
Hybridoma Cell Bank, 100
Hybridoma Data Bank, 97–98
Hybridoma technology, 37, 81. *See also* Monoclonal antibodies
  as artisanal technique, 50, 52–58, 71–72, 74–76
  art/magic/science continuum, 73–76
  diffusion, 43n, 93, 200
    availability of monoclonal antibodies, 93–95, 98–99
    United States, 92–93
  disciplinary/technical status, 60
  domains of expertise necessary, 52
  initial use, 32
  knowledge acquisition, 46, 50, 52–58, 134–135
  as magic, 69–70, 73–74
  Nobel Prize status, 6
  as object of inquiry, 3, 5, 7–8
  procedures, 50–52, 54–57, 65, 160–162. *See also* Standardization
    codification, 70–73
    improvements, 62–67, 136
    variants, 63, 67–70, 71–73
    written protocols, 58–62, 68, 73
  replication problems, 45–46, 53, 78n, 134–135, 136–137
  as a research goal, 38
Hybridomas. *See also* Monoclonal antibodies
  definition, 25
  as invention, 169–170
  precursors, 40n–41n
  unlimited supplies, 34, 74
Hybritech, 143–144, 152–153
  patents, 168

Hybritech vs. Monoclonal Antibodies Inc., 168, 181–200
Hypoxanthine aminopterin thymidine (HAT), 25, 26, 51, 64, 67

Immunoassays, 52, 125n, 182–183, 205n
  competitive IRA compared with IRMA, 182–189
  increase in use of monoclonal antibodies, 89–90, 103, 124n
  monoclonal vs. polyclonal antibodies, 89–90, 103–104, 194–196
  in pregnancy diagnostic kits, 188, 189–193
  patents, 168
  sandwich immunoassay patents, 168, 181–200
Immunology, 52, 75
  antibody theories, 210
Institut Pasteur, 153, 155
  P3-X63Ag8 myeloma cell line, 11, 12
Institute of Genetics, University of Köln
  P3-X63Ag8 myeloma cell line, 11, 12–13
Interferon, 168–169, 176–178
Invention. *See* Patents
Irvins Jr., William M.I., 169

Johnson & Johnson. *See* Ortho Pharmaceutical Corporation
Johnson, Mark, 153

Kay, Lily E., 155
Klinman, Norman, 15. *See also* Splenic fragments technique
Knorr-Cetina, Karin D., 10, 47–48, 96, 205n
Knowledge
  classification, 47–50, 76–77, 78n
  art/magic/science continuum, 73–76
  construction, 47
Knowledge transmission, 49–50
  experiential learning, 46, 52–58
  nonverbal knowledge, 50, 57–58
Knowles, Barbara, 15, 16
Köhler, Georges, 42n
  foundational papers, 9–10
  Nobel Prize, 3, 4, 31, 43n

Köhler, Georges *(continued)*
  original experiment, 28
  views on hybridoma technology, 84
Koprowski, Hilary, 11, 13–17, 39n. *See also* Wistar Institute
Krimsky, Sheldon, 133

Laboratories
  hybridoma units, 153–157
  manuals, 60–62
  receiving of mouse myelomas from ATCC, 100, 102
  receiving of rat myelomas from Milstein's laboratory, 100, 101
  scientific papers, 10
  use of P3-X63Ag8 myeloma cell line, 11, 39n, 45–46
    Institut Pasteur, 11, 12
    Institute of Genetics, University of Köln, 11, 12–13
    Wistar Institute, 11, 13–17, 39n–30n
Laboratory practice, 73. *See also* Hybridoma technology
  artisanal elements, 71–72
  levels of knowledge, 46–47
Lakoff, George, 8, 153
Lasker Foundation award, 42
Latour, Bruno, 7, 9, 47, 60, 118, 122, 124n, 172, 187, 206n
Law, John, 35, 206n
Legal issues. *See also* Patents: litigation
  integration with scientific issues, 169, 173, 179–180, 200–201
Liebert, Mary Ann, 117
Local knowledge, 47–50, 76–77
Luttenberger, Franz, 170
Lymphocytes
  classification, 97
  as fusion partners, 24, 25, 26
Lynch, Michael, 47, 48, 58, 69, 206n

March, James G., 66
Markle, Gerald E., 170
Massachusetts General Hospital, 144–145, 153
McMaster University, 144–145
M.D. Anderson Hospital, 41
Medawar, Peter, 10

Medline
  publication data re: hybridoma technology, 85–86
Mice, 11, 26, 96, 126n
Milstein, César, 42n, 56
  diffusion of hybridoma technology, 35, 84
  foundational papers, 9–10
  Nobel Prize, 3, 4, 31, 35, 43n
  non-patenting of hybridoma technology, 203n
  original experiment, 28
  views on hybridoma technology, 81, 83–84
Moewus, Franz, 5–6
Monoclonal antibodies. *See also* Diagnostic kits; Hybridomas
  availability, 99–103, 125n
    commercial distribution, 94, 125n
    initial, 93–95, 98–99
  characteristics, 104, 107, 110, 174
    compared with polyclonal antibodies, 109–110, 141
    negative factors, 106, 128n, 143–144
    purity, 104–105, 106, 127n
    reproducibility, 107–108, 127n
    specificity, 18, 84, 105–106, 107, 120, 126n–127n, 141, 143–144
    unlimited availability, 106
  commercial uses, 147
  compared with polyclonal antibodies, 105–106, 109–110
  immunoassays, 89–90, 103–104
  data bank, 97–98
  demonstration of practical properties, 35
  development, 140
  equivalence, 174–176
  as established entities, 14–15, 18–24
  human, 20–21
  naming, 97, 126n, 160–161
    formal nomenclature, 97
  novelty, criteria of, 174–176
  OKT antibody series, 168, 174–175, 176, 203n–204n
  polyclonal vs. monoclonal antibodies, 89–90, 103–104, 194–196
  in pregnancy diagnostic kits, 188, 189–193

production. *See* Hybridoma technology; Splenic fragments technique
proliferation, 97
reasons for use, 133–134
redefinition as patentable inventions, 201–202. *See also* Patents
redefinition as tools, 82–83, 85–86, 108, 112–114, 123
  initial acceptance, 110–111
  predefined uses, 142
  scientific literature, 118–123
  use in non-immunological fields, 113–114
  use in somatic cell genetics, 32
  as vehicles of standardization, 95–96, 105
Monoclonal Antibodies Inc., 168
  Hybritech vs. Monoclonal Antibodies Inc., 168, 181–200
MOPC, 21, 26–28
MRC Laboratory of Molecular Biology, 9–10. *See also* Köhler, Georges; Milstein, César
  laboratories receiving rat myelomas from MRC, 100, 101
Mulkay, Michael, 47, 83, 193
Myeloma cell lines, 26. *See also* P3-X63Ag8 myeloma cell line
  availability, 93, 135–136
  mice myelomas distributed by the ATCC, 102–103
  MOPC, 21, 26–28
  NS-1, 99
  P1, 42n
  P3, 22, 24
  rat myelomas distibuted by Milstein's laboratory, 100–101
Myeloma cells, 27, 39n
  corresponding antigens, 28
  as fusion partners, 25–26, 27
  secreting vs. nonsecreting, 44n, 64
  as source of monoclonal antibodies, 44n
Myers, Greg, 170

Nash, Martin, 76
National Cancer Institute
  Myeloma Tumor Program, 99–100
National Institute of Allergy and Infectious Diseases (NIAID), 100

Hybridoma Cell Bank, 100
  reports, 95–97, 122–123
National Institute of Health (NIH), 26
  policies on hybridomas, 167
  reports, 122
NIAID. *See* National Institute of Allergy and Infectious Diseases (NIAID)
NIH. *See* National Institute of Health (NIH)
Nisonoff, Alfred, 191–192, 193–196
Nobel Prizes
  1958, 5–6
  1984, 3, 4, 35
    attribution to Köhler and Milstein, 31
  Crick and Watson, 8–9
Non-secreting myeloma cells, 44n, 64
Novelty, 7–8. *See also* Discoveries; Fact-technique distinction; Patents
  predetermined specificity, 13–14, 18
  related to fact-technique distinction, 38
Nowinsky, Robert, 135, 140, 148–149
NS-1 cell line, 99

O'Connell, Joseph, 77, 124n
Oi, Vernon, 182, 193
OKT antibody series, 168, 174–175, 176, 203n–204n
Ortho Pharmaceutical Corporation, 100, 103
  OKT antibody series, 168, 174–175, 176, 203n–204n
  patent litigation, 168
    Ortho vs. Becton Dickinson, 168, 174–176, 204n–205n

P1 myeloma cell line, 42n
P3 myeloma cell line, 22, 24
P3-X63Ag8 myeloma cell line, 11, 78n, 79n, 99
  genetic markers, 27, 42n
  naming, 45–46
  original line, 24, 26–27
  spleen cell fusion partners, 11
  use in laboratories, 11, 39n, 45–46
    Institut Pasteur, 11, 12
    Institute of Genetics, University of Köln, 11, 12–13
    Wistar Institute, 11, 13–17, 39n–30n

Packer, Kathryn, 203n
Panem, Sandra, 170
Papers. *See* Scientific literature
Parasitology, 112
Parkinson, D., 85–86
Pasveer, Bernike, 113
Patents, 87–89, 168–170
 Cold Spring Harbor conference (1981), 167–168, 173, 174, 176
 litigation, 168–169, 170
  Ex Parte Erlich, 176–180
  Ex Parte Old, 177
  Hybritech vs. Monoclonal Antibodies Inc., 168, 181–200
  Ortho vs. Becton Dickinson, 174–176, 180–181
  Wistar Institute, 17, 173, 180–181, 203n
 lymphocyte surface antigens, 168
 Milstein, César
  non-patenting of hybridoma technology, 203n
 requirements for patentable objects, 171
  enablement, 171, 197–198, 204n
  obviousness/non-obviousness, 171, 173, 176, 177–178, 186, 190–192, 203n
PEG (polyethylene glycol), 30, 42n–43n, 64, 71
 substitution for Sendai virus, 43n, 51
Pereira, Leonore, 15–146, 142–144
Pinch, Trevor, 47
Plasmacytomas. *See* Myeloma cells
Polyclonal antibodies, 84, 125n, 126n
 monoclonal vs. polyclonal antibodies, 89–90, 103–104, 194–196
 in pregnancy diagnostic kits, 188, 189–193
Polyethylene glycol. *See* PEG (polyethylene glycol)
Pomerantz, Anita, 205n
Potter, Michael, 26–27
Pregnancy test kits
 sandwich immunoassay patents, 168, 181–200
Prizes. *See also* Nobel Prizes
 Horowitz Prize, 40n–41n
 Lasker Foundation award, 42
 preceding Nobel Prize, 43n
Protocols, 58–62

Rabies assays, 103, 108, 111
Rajewsky, Klaus, 11, 12–13, 39n, 79n
Ravetz, Jerome R., 116
Rawls, William, 144–145
Reagents. *See also* Monoclonal antibodies
 antibodies compared to chemical reagents, 104–105
 monoclonal compared to polyclonal antibodies, 28, 127n
 standardization, 92
Receptor directed system, 66
Regulation, 82, 98, 124n. *See also* Standardization
Reproducibility, 107–109
Researchers
 attitudes to hybridoma technology, 83–84, 150–151
Revolutionary metaphor, 18
Rheinberger, Hans-Jörg, 169, 202n, 205n
Rip, Arie, 172
Robin, Stanley S., 170
Rothman, Harry, 85–86
Rouse, Joseph, 124n
Royal Free Hospital, 153

Salk Institute. *See also* Cohn, Melvin
 cell bank, 99–100
 fusion experiments, 28–31
 PEG fusogen, 42n–43n
Sandwich immunoassay patents
 Hybritech vs. Monoclonal Antibodies Inc., 168, 181–200
Sapp, Jan, 5–6
Schadewaldt, Wolfgang, 193
Scharff, Matthew D., 40n
 Cold Spring Harbor conference (1981), 173, 174
Schlossman, Stuart F., 43n
Schwaber, Jerrold, 18–24
Scientific knowledge. *See* Knowledge; Knowledge transmission
Scientific literature. *See also* Foundational papers; Patents
 citation analysis
  anti-HSV monoclonals, 148

clinical standards, 116–117
disciplinary boundaries, 116–117
Hybridoma, 117–118, 128n
related to laboratory activities, 10
review articles, 40n, 118–123, 128n–129n
Secreting myeloma cells, 44n, 64
Selective mediums, 25, 64
  HAT (hypoxanthine aminopterin thymidine), 25, 26, 51, 64, 67
Sendai virus, 25, 29, 30, 42n, 51
Serology, 126n
Simon, Herbert A., 66
Simondon, Gilbert, 211
Sinkovics, Joseph G., 41n
Snyder, Solomon H., 66
Somatic cell genetics, 32
Splenic fragments technique, 13, 14, 15, 28, 40n, 43n
Standardization, 82–83, 92, 95–96, 98
  biomedical infrastructure, 96–97
  government regulation, 82, 124n
  monoclonal antibodies as vehicles of standardization, 95–96, 105
  quality control, 94
Stanford University Medical School. *See* Herzenberg, Leonard
Star, Susan Leigh, 47, 53
Steplewski, Zenon, 15, 16, 116–117
Stokes, Terry D., 155
Syva, 108

Tacit knowledge, 47–50, 76–77, 78n
Taggart technique, 64
Tambrands, 115–116
Tatum, Edward L., 5–6
Technique. *See* Fact-technique distinction
Teitelman, Robert, 39n

Textual evidence. *See* Foundational papers
Thévenot, Laurent, 82, 119, 124n

Universality. *See* Generality
University College, 141
University of Köln, Institute of Genetics. *See* Institute of Genetics, University of Köln

van den Belt, Henk, 172
Vincenti, Walter, 78n
Virology, 52

Watson, James
  Cold Spring Harbor conference (1981), 176
  double helix discovery, 8–9
Webster, Andrew, 203n
Weiner, Charles, 170
Wistar Institute
  anti-herpes monoclonal antibodies, 141
  anti-influenza antibodies, 111
  P3-X63Ag8 myeloma cell line, 11, 13–17, 39n–40n
  patent litigation, 17, 173, 180–181, 203n
  PEG fusogen, 42n
  publication difficulties, 116–117
  rabies assays, 103, 108, 111
Woolgar, Steve, 7, 47, 118, 122, 172, 187, 206n
World Health Organization, 97, 113

Xenogeneic immunization, 43n

Zack, Donald
  Cold Spring Harbor conference (1981), 173, 174

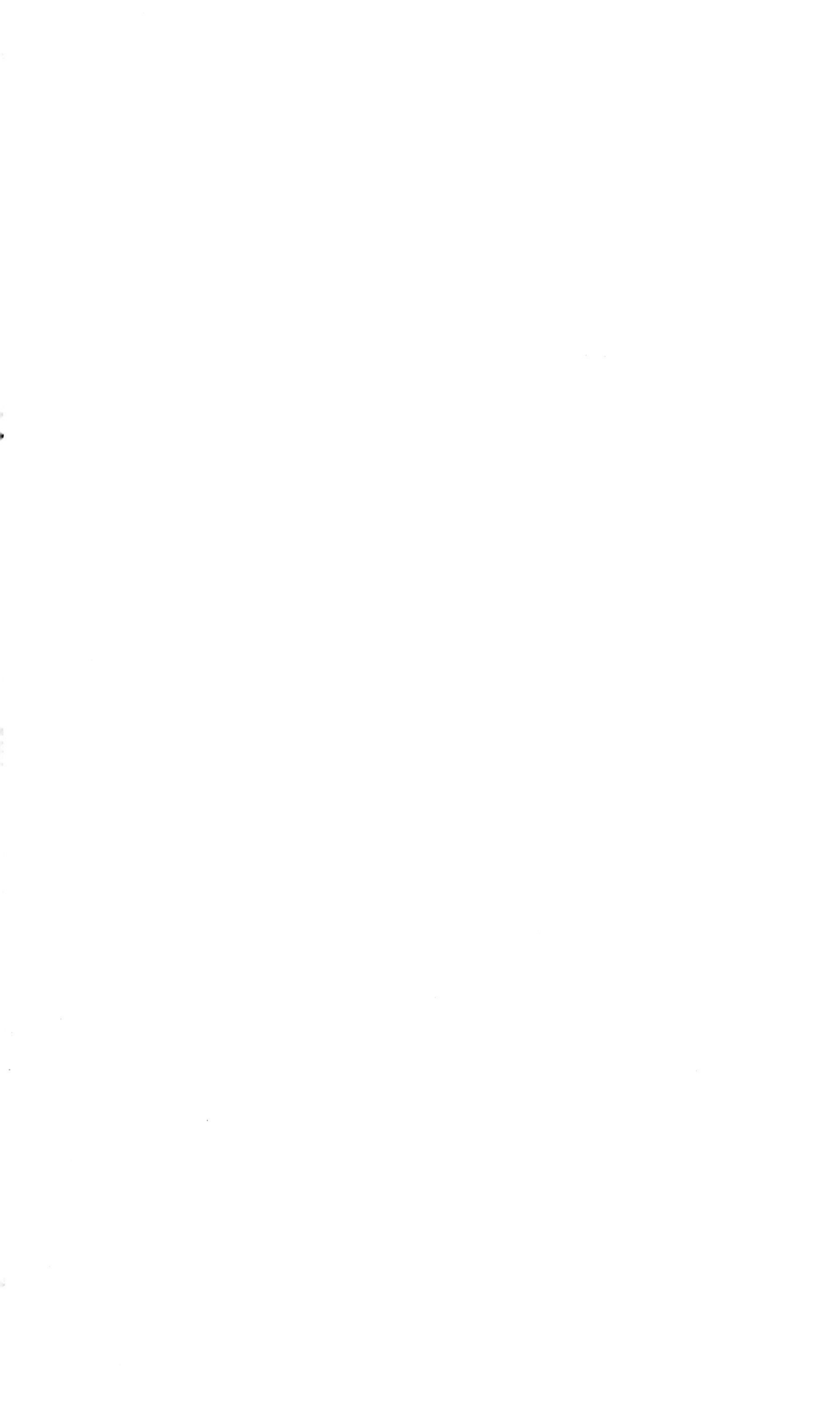